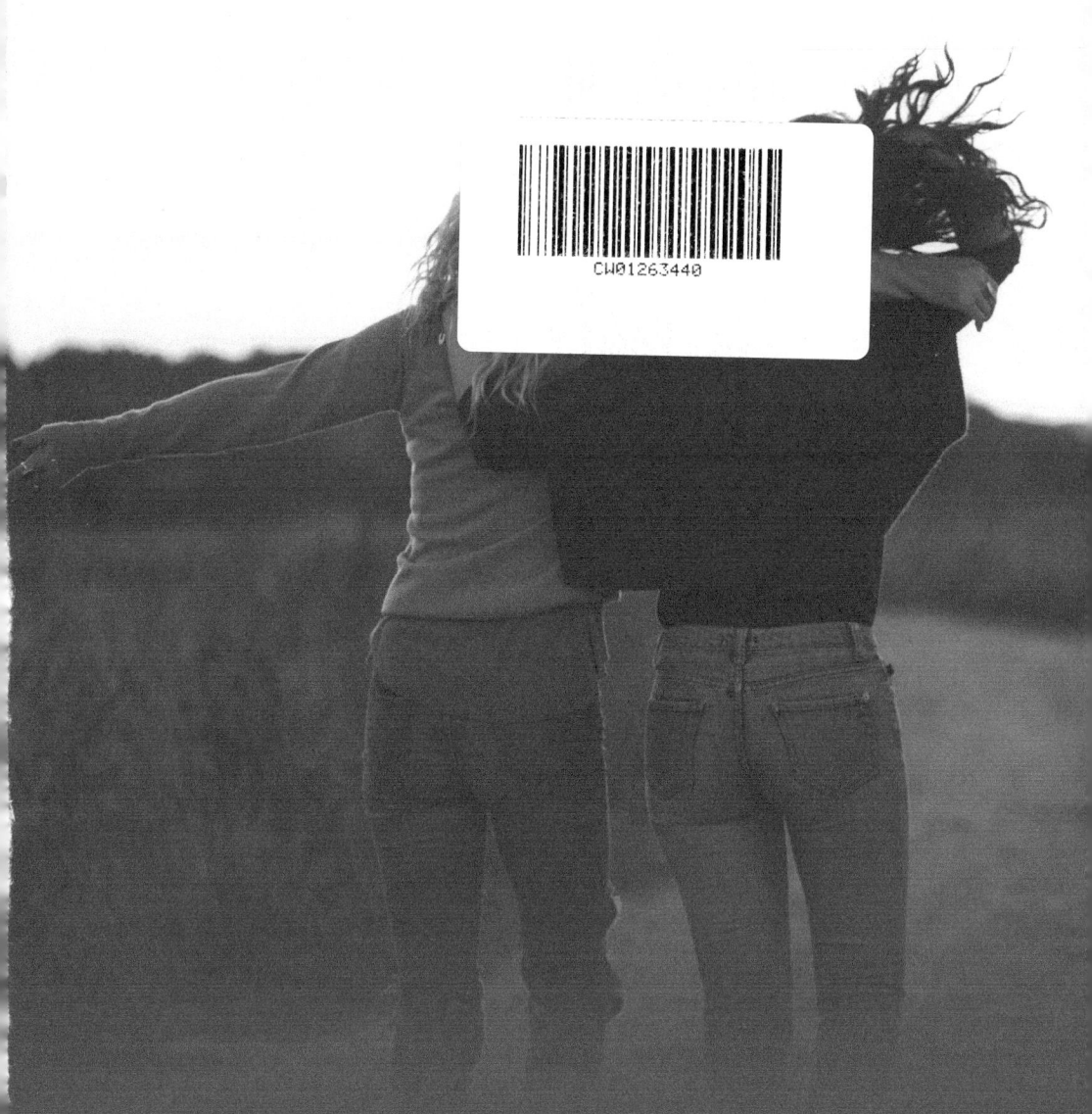

Working Relationally with Young People

A Cognitive Analytic Approach to Connecting One to One, with Families and Across Communities

Edited by Nick Barnes
and Lee Crothers

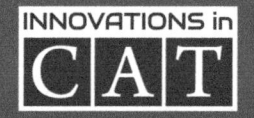

INNOVATIONS in CAT

Working Relationally with Young People

© Pavilion Publishing & Media

The authors have asserted their rights in accordance with the Copyright, Designs and Patents Act (1988) to be identified as the authors of this work.

Published by:

Pavilion Publishing and Media Ltd
Blue Sky Offices
25 Cecil Pashley Way
Shoreham by Sea
West Sussex
BN43 5FF

Tel: 01273 434 943
Email: info@pavpub.com
Web: www.pavpub.com

Published 2024

All rights reserved. No part of this publication may be reproduced, stored in a retrieval system, or transmitted in any form or by any means, electronic, mechanical, photocopying, recording or otherwise, without prior permission in writing of the publisher and the copyright owners.

A catalogue record for this book is available from the British Library.

ISBN: 978-1-803883-12-0

Pavilion Publishing and Media is a leading publisher of books, training materials and digital content in mental health, social care and allied fields. Pavilion and its imprints offer must-have knowledge and innovative learning solutions underpinned by sound research and professional values.

Editors: Nick Barnes and Lee Crothers
Cover design: Emma Dawe, Pavilion Publishing and Media Ltd
Page layout and typesetting: Phil Morash, Pavilion Publishing and Media Ltd
Printing: Halstan

INNOVATIONS in CAT

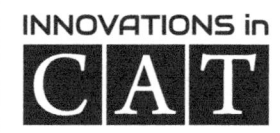

Available now in the *Innovations in CAT* series:

Reflective Practice in Forensic Settings
(Jenny Marshall and Jamie Kirkland)

Forthcoming:

Innovative Practice in Forensic Settings
(Jenny Marshall and Jamie Kirkland)

Conversations in Later Life
(Michelle Hamill, Ellen Khan and Paul Catlin)

CAT and Creativity
(Yvonne Stevens)

Praise for this book

"The rising tide of mental ill health in young people desperately needs innovation in treatment and a wider spectrum of psychosocial interventions that can engage with and strengthen their often fragile and developing sense of self and identity. The therapeutic relationship should always be a vital secure base, a space for recovery. Beyond the stability and quality of this space, relational therapies like CAT add a deeper core upon which other techniques can be selectively deployed in a personalised manner. Relational approaches are an essential pillar in effective care, and the value and benefit of other treatments are heavily dependent on the success of the trust, hope and belief that these approaches can generate."

Patrick McGorry,
Executive Director at Orygen; Professor of Youth Mental Health,
University of Melbourne

"Early on in my CAT career, I asked Tony Ryle at an ACAT conference whether anyone was using CAT with children or adolescents. He said he didn't know but he was sure it would be worth trying. This is the book I needed back then. It draws together so much expertise in, and lived experience of, CAT with young people and their carers; not to give any easy answers, but to advocate for an open, curious, collaborative attitude. This is often the most important thing we can offer young people and families but remains in short supply."

Alison Jenaway
Consultant Psychiatrist, CAT supervisor and trainer

"This amazing book gives evidence of the importance not only of 'being relational', a core concept in CAT and in our work with young people. It is a systemic reflection on the wider meaning of being in a relation with a client and with ourselves as human beings and professionals, the relation with services and community/society as a whole. It touches on core questions such as 'how do we create relationships, keep and develop them without getting overwhelmed'; 'how do we create within these therapeutic relationships space for learning, modelling and changing'; and 'how do we create hope for this age group – 12-25 – still being attached, but trying to quit, finding new attachments in the process of their development into adulthood in an ever changing, threatened world. This book is not only a dialogue between clinicians; there is hope for promoting change in connection with and relating to young people and the wider communities and systems around them."

Marie-Anne Bernardy-Arbuz
Clinical psychologist, psychotherapist and CAT practitioner

"Cognitive Analytic Therapy offers the tools and ideas to work with young people and their relationships with themselves and the world around them. This wonderful book brings together the voices and methods of those working at the creative edge of helping and empowering young people. Read and discover new ways of working and new ways of relating."

Steve Potter
Psychotherapist, supervisor and author.

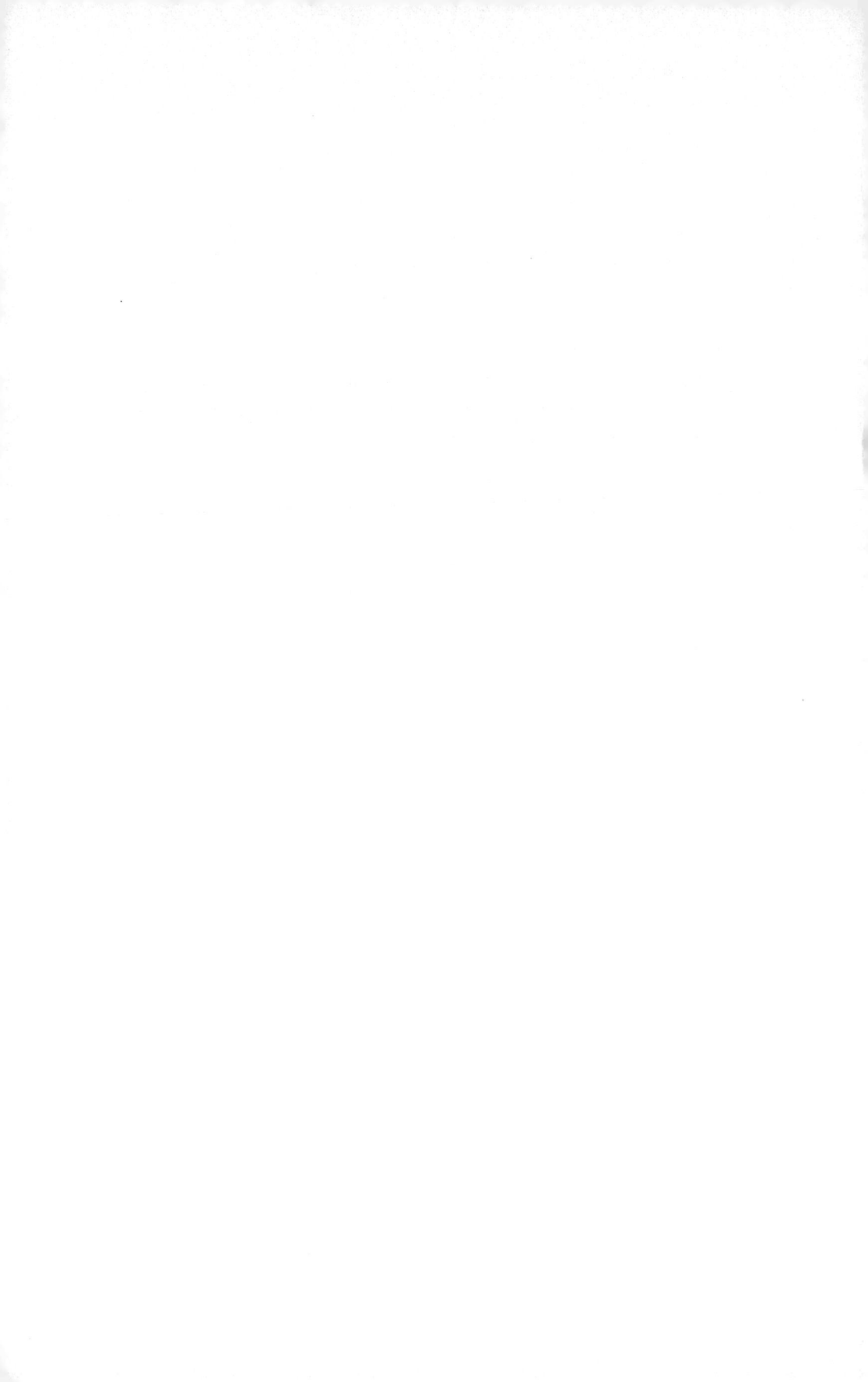

Contents

Series preface
Foreword
About the editors
Acknowledgements
Contributors

Introduction 15

Chapter 1: Being with and belonging – an introduction
to a relational approach to working with young people
 Lee Crothers and Nick Barnes 17

**PART 1: Relational approaches to working alongside
young people** 31

Chapter 2: 'If all you ever see is an eating disorder...'
– a relational understanding and approach to working
with young people with eating disorders
 Lee Crothers and Melissa Keller-Tuberg 33

Chapter 3: Using CAT for neurodivergent young people –
working with intellectual disability and autism
 Jo Varela 47

Chapter 4: Relational practice is inclusive practice – working
alongside LGBTQA + young people
 Victoria Ryall 63

Chapter 5: The power of an embodied approach to CAT
with young adults
 Caroline Greenwood Dower 77

Chapter 6: A relationally informed model of care for young
people living with personality disorder
 Louise K. McCutcheon, Jessica O'Connell, Ben McKechnie
 and Andrew M. Chanen 93

Case Study 1: Being on both sides – reflections by a young
person with lived experience of being diagnosed with Borderline
Personality Disorder
 Brede 109

PART 2: Relational approaches to working with parents, families and groups 115

Chapter 7: A house of mirrors – a role for parent CAT
Clare Young 117

Chapter 8: Bringing CAT into the family and beyond – a systemic approach to CAT when working alongside families and their wider networks
Debbra Mortlock 135

Chapter 9: Using CAT – a relational approach in groups with young people
Cat McKenzie 151

Case Study 2: 'A Game of Two Halves' – CAT in the world of football
Nick Barnes... 165

PART 3: Relational approaches to service provision and the workplace.. 169

Chapter 10: Relationships matter – a case for CAT in an Early Intervention Service
Wendy Giovanelli and Kiara Wickremasinghe 171

Chapter 11: Creating 'just enough' space – setting up a new psychotherapy service in Chennai
Sivakami Suresh Prabalkumari... 185

Chapter 12: Can you even relate? Invitations to think and work relationally in Out of Home Care
Katherine Monson and Kiera Kauler 199

Chapter 13: Burning out and bullying – the need for working relationally within the workplace
Nick Barnes and Lee Crothers 213

Chapter 14: CAT in education – reflections on the spaces between the 'cogs in the machine'
Claire Regan and Leah O'Toole 223

Case study 3: Excluded, disengaged and on the outside – reconnecting through 'Learning to Learn'
Donna Lockett 235

PART 4: Relational approaches to communities and society 243

Chapter 15: From Hellblade to Game Group – relating and connecting in digital spaces

Alex Bretherton and Nick Barnes 245

Chapter 16: Dear Planet Earth – the climate and ecological emergency through a relational lens

Angie Phong, Reem Ramadan and Nick Barnes........................... 261

Chapter 17: Dancing in the spaces between – reflections on proximity and power when working alongside communities

Nick Barnes and Rhona Brown 275

Case Study 4: Shifting the gaze – creativity for Recovery and Emotional Well-being (CREW)

Nick Barnes and Jon Hall 289

Conclusion 293

Chapter 18: Closing thoughts – common threads

Nick Barnes and Lee Crothers... 295

References

Glossary

Series preface

The *Innovations in Cognitive Analytic Therapy* book series aims to offer helpful but also challenging accounts by practitioners in various fields of theoretical development and clinical work based on Cognitive Analytic Therapy (CAT). The editors and contributors are experts in their fields who have undertaken innovative and exploratory work using the CAT approach – the presentation of which, in our view, is long overdue. We hope that these books will make important and compassionate contributions to our understanding of and approaches to a range of clinical and other problems and presentations – contributions that will be helpful and thought-provoking not only for colleagues already familiar with CAT, but also for many others. The series builds on and complements previous overviews by the late Anthony Ryle, creator of the CAT model, and other wide-scope multi-author volumes.

A distinctive feature is a predominantly relational and socio-cultural conceptualisation of mental health problems, or of distress and 'disorder', and correspondingly of therapeutic approaches to them. A fundamental emphasis throughout, based on understandings derived from years of psychotherapy outcome research, Vygotskian activity theory and more recent research in infant psychology, is the importance of a (genuinely) collaborative and co-creative approach to treatment. This long-standing emphasis in CAT will be evident in, for example, descriptions of the co-creative process of reformulation, both written and diagrammatic ('mapping'). These in turn will emphasise recognising and working on enactments of internalised early relational patterns ('reciprocal roles') in life generally, but also between both clinicians and clients. They will also emphasise the gradual internalisation of new, more benign relational experience. This is regrettably far from being the case for many individuals currently in therapy or, especially, undergoing treatment within public health services, despite its recognised importance as a key 'common factor' in outcomes.

As well as offering practically helpful accounts of developing and innovative work in often challenging clinical fields, we aspire for these books also to contribute to the ongoing development of the CAT model, including as a general framework for understanding and treating mental health problems. This will be important for its own validity and vitality as well as more generally to advance the field of mental health. Anthony Ryle, who created the CAT model during a long and avowedly integrative evolutionary process, certainly always welcomed such developments. We look forward to the *Innovations in Cognitive Analytic Therapy* series promoting productive debate, and being part of an open, creative dialogue between practitioners of CAT and colleagues from other approaches and disciplines in support of a versatile, integrative and relational approach to mental health in general.

Ian. B. Kerr and Steve Potter
Series Editors

Foreword

"World is crazier and more of it than we think. Incorrigibly plural."
                                                            Louis MacNeice[1]

Thirty years ago, I was fortunate enough, while training as a counselling psychologist, to be introduced to the novel ideas of Cognitive Analytic Therapy through my supervisor, who had trained with Tony Ryle. I was grappling with the question of how to work meaningfully and at depth with clients in a world where there was limited time and a tendency to focus on what was apparent and measurable. CAT provided the answer, marrying psychodynamic, constructivist and cognitive approaches in a practical way. What is more, the ideas were to be shared with clients and formulations jointly developed, not kept to the rarefied realms of supervision and academia.

Over the last thirty-five years, CAT has flourished; it has continued to grow in the UK as is does internationally, with associations established in countries such as Finland, Australia and New Zealand, Ireland, Greece, Spain, Italy and India. It has developed theoretically, most notably integrating a dialogical perspective on the self – using our ability to imagine and inhabit various positions in our internal and external dialogues. CAT's application with distinct client groups across various settings has also evolved. Because of its relational understanding and accessibility, one of the most significant applications has been in the context of teams and systems, where CAT offers a common language for formulation and helps team members to reflect on enactments occurring between staff, patients and systems. And the evidence base for CAT has grown too. It straddles both practice-based studies of routine clinical care and controlled clinical trials, with analysis concluding that CAT is effective for a diverse range of presenting problems (Calvert & Kellett, 2014). Moreover, their systematic review highlights how CAT is both acceptable to and tolerable for patients.

As the current Chair of the International Cognitive Analytic Therapy Association, I am excited to mark this new milestone – an exposition on working relationally with young people using the cognitive analytic

---
1   Macneice, L. (1967) *The Collected Poems of Louis Macneice*. Oxford University Press

approach. Generally, young people tend to be seen as a problem; they are seen as either the cause *of* trouble or *in* trouble. The conversation in society is deficit-focused, with young people's behaviour and struggles being increasingly pathologised and medicated. In putting together this collection of work, Nick Barnes and Lee Crothers, practitioners and contributors themselves, are clearly challenging how young people are being positioned, particularly in the microcosm of clinical practice. So often today, the words 'complex needs' are used to excuse the refusal of services to a young person. Needs are not complex, however – although the process of meeting a young person's needs may be, complicated by the experience and expectation brought to the relationship by all parties to the conversation. By eschewing the idea that complexity is located in the individual young person, while giving the reader the tools to map and navigate the relationship, this book will give confidence to practitioners who engage with complexity and hold risk. What Barnes and Crothers have succeeded in doing is demonstrating, across a range of settings, how CAT and relational working can build the relational intelligence necessary to engage in and steer a course through this complex process to beneficial effect.

Relationships are at the heart of what it is to be human. This book demonstrates that by focusing on the young person's relational landscape, this approach not only bears witness to their story but also scaffolds growth and change. This book will convince readers of the need to widen the lens and locate ourselves in that landscape. To ensure that our interventions are helpful, practitioners must go beyond self-awareness to relational awareness and think about questions like, "Who I am when I am with this young person?" and "Who am I to them?" Chapter after chapter describes relational awareness in action, and how it is used to keep relationships healthy and affirming.

Young people are not a homogeneous group; they are differently positioned in society based on their class, gender, ethnicity, sexuality and ability. Anyone who is serious about engaging with the lives of young people must engage with the politics of their social position and identity. This book illustrates how the CAT model provides a way of thinking about identity that is neither binary nor static; a framework that recognises the variety of positions we can inhabit in the experience of being human and in the work of staying human. This is critical now more than ever, because current discourses on such matters as truth and identity are polarising and attack the idea of truth as a collective endeavour, founded on dialogue and putting our heads together.

While it addresses such critical matters as identity and current existential threats to humanity, I can assure you that this book is neither esoteric nor abstract. Chapter after chapter provides substantial accounts of how the task of developing a shared understanding of the young person's internal and relational landscape is achieved. From the chapter on working with young people with eating difficulties to the one about using the game of football to develop relational awareness, the accounts sing with clarity, none so much as the passages written by young people with lived experiences of services themselves.

This book does not ask you to discard what you have already learned and know to be effective; it is a transdiagnostic approach to working with young people which anchors interventions in a relational framework. It acknowledges and validates the uncertainty that we feel when we try to move into a helpful space with a young person, especially where there is risk and complexity; doubtless our clients feel this too. This book gives us the wherewithal to tolerate the uncertainty and explore, not to foreclose or retreat.

Barnes and Crothers approached the task of bringing together this collection with remarkable humility. What they have given us is expansive, full of curiosity and affirming.

It fills me with hope.

Elaine Martin
Chair, International Cognitive Analytic Therapy Association (ICATA)

About the editors

Nick Barnes (he/him)

Nick has worked within Child and Adolescent Mental Health services for over twenty-five years, practicing in Cognitive Analytic Therapy (CAT) and in child and adolescent psychiatry, as well as being actively involved in service development and transformation.

For the majority of his clinical practice, Nick has been based in London, focusing much of his energy on working alongside young people for who struggle to access mainstream education as well as statutory services and support. As articulated in this book, there are many young people who do not wish to engage with mental health support, or who may feel unable to do so for a multiplicity of reasons, reinforcing the profound health inequalities that exist across communities within the UK – inequalities that are further sustained by experiences of trauma and marked social injustice. As a result, Nick has often found himself often working on the edge of services, seeking to connect with young people in youth clubs, on the streets, or in community settings that feel safer and more accessible to them and/or their families.

Through academic posts (Honorary Associate Professor at University College London, and Honorary Senior Lecturer at the University of Aberdeen) Nick has been keen to explore the evidence for overcoming social injustices and health inequalities through approaches that prioritise peer support and may involve being outdoors, accessing green and blue spaces. This work is further promoted through his role as Sustainability Champion for the Royal College of Psychiatrists, and co-lead of the ecoCAMHS network, enabling training and teaching about the impact of the climate and ecological emergency on children and young people, and why nature-based practice, alongside the involvement of young people, has become so integral to the development of greener support and services – enabling young people to have a sense of hope and agency for their futures.

Lee Crothers (she/her)

Lee is a Melbourne-based occupational therapist, psychotherapist and Cognitive Analytic Therapy (CAT) practitioner, supervisor and trainer. She has worked in mental health for over twenty-five years, many of them as a specialist in youth mental health. She is passionate about supporting young people, and the communities around them, who find it hard to engage in the traditional office-based therapy.

Lee is a founder of In Dialogue (www.indialogue.com.au), a private practice that provides therapy, supervision, training and consultation using the relational framework of CAT. Lee was one of the first CAT-trained practitioners in Australia, a result of much huddling around a teleconference phone at extreme times of day with a dedicated UK-based CAT supervisor. Lee learned CAT when working in an outreach team seeing young people who were seen as 'complex and high risk'. She found CAT so helpful in working with young people that she went on to help develop, at Orygen, the first CAT course in Australia.

These days, alongside her work as a therapist, Lee teaches CAT and relational thinking through In Dialogue. Central to her teaching is a project called Relate and Reflect (www.relateandreflect.com.au) that provides, to private and government services and organisations, the relational framework that encourages reflection and collaboration. Lee also works as a national advisor around complexity in youth mental health with the highly-regarded headspace, Australia's National Youth Mental Health Foundation (www.headspace.org.au). In addition, she regularly consults to teams such as a university counselling service, youth mental health services and child protection services.

Acknowledgements

First and foremost, our thanks and acknowledgements go to all the young people and families that we, and our fellow contributors, have had the privilege to work alongside in our professional roles. None of the work outlined in this book would have been possible without so many young people and their families, carers and networks trusting in all of us to offer an approach and intervention that is meaningful, accessible and helpful.

However, in writing this book, we also wanted to ensure that we heard the voices of young people and their experiences, especially given the current pressures on services and support. Hence, we are particularly keen to show our respect to all those young people who contributed to or co-authored chapters within this book. Some have chosen to be named, while others asked to remain anonymous, but all are valid and valuable.

As we note in our introductory chapters, we have invited contributors from across the CAT community and beyond to share their work, practice and personal reflections on the importance of offering a relational approach to children and young people's difficulties and distress. We are hugely grateful to every contributor for their generosity and patience in supporting this project, recognising that much time passes from when we send an exploratory email to when they finally see the fruits of their labour in print. We are indebted to you all.

The generosity of our contributors is mirrored by that of the CAT community – a community that has also been welcoming and supportive of all. Many members of this community across the globe have helped in the development and evolution of this book, and we have been humbled by the encouragement and support that has been offered – whether it be for proof reading, offering sound-bite reviews or, not least, writing a Foreword to the book.

This book has also looked to reach out beyond the CAT community, and to offer a window onto relational working through many different constructs – be that education, social care, or wider community engagement and connection. Hence our thanks and appreciation need to reach out to all those parties who have helped to inspire and motivate us, as editors, to ensure that this way of working reaches as many as possible. After all, it takes a village to raise a child.

But more specifically we, as the editors of this book, need to thank the series editors Steve Potter and Ian Kerr, who have been the guiding light and drivers behind this *Innovations in CAT* series. We were very touched when we were invited to pull together this book, and honoured that we had been entrusted to do so by colleagues that we hold with such huge respect. We can only hope that we have repaid their faith in us. Likewise, the publishing team, most notably Darren Reed, have been truly amazing in their support and embracing of this project. They have been enormously tolerant of all our requests, and patient with all our delays, and we are hugely thankful to Darren and his team for all they have done in getting us from a proposal to a published book.

There must also be a note of thanks and acknowledgement for Anthony Ryle. Through his development of the model that is now recognised as CAT, he wanted to create an approach to support that was accessible and effective within a social context – one that acknowledged the complexities and demands of western democratic societies and their resulting inequalities. His conceptualisation of reciprocal roles offered a relational understanding that could allow us to consider the world within, between and around – acknowledging its complexity, but allowing there to be clarity amongst multiple truths. Anthony Ryle was a pioneer, but also a reformer, and it is this radical and reformist zeal that we hope we have captured when seeking to share this book with others.

Lastly, we finish on a note of respect of place, as we acknowledge the traditional custodians of the lands on which we live and work and where this book was written, be this in Australia or the Highlands of Scotland. Parts of this book were written on the lands of the Wurundjeri People of the Kulin Nation, and we wish to pay respect to their Elders past, present and emerging.

Contributors

Brede (she/they) is an early career Registered Music Therapist. Brede draws upon her lived experience of multiple health conditions in her work with young people in Naarm/Melbourne and in her broader advocacy for disability justice. She intends for her work to contribute to the ongoing development of inclusive, collaborative, and creative approaches that expand the boundaries of healthcare.

Alex Bretherton is a Senior Peer Support Worker, a mental health survivor of schizophrenia, depression, paranoia and more, and has been working in the NHS for four years as an Expert by Experience and Peer Support Worker, using his lived experience to help others. He is also a novelist and poet.

Rhona Brown is a CAT practitioner and clinical psychologist. Working clinically with adults from Manchester's diverse communities over many years, she worked towards bridging statutory services with community and third sector organisations. She currently provides psychological support to NHS staff, alongside various roles with Catalyse and ACAT supporting public engagement.

Andrew Chanen is a consultant psychiatrist, professor and director of personality disorder research at the Centre for Youth Mental Health, University of Melbourne; and chief of clinical practice at Orygen. He co-founded the Helping Young People Early (HYPE) program, an early intervention programme for young people with severe personality disorder in Melbourne Australia.

Wendy Giovanelli is a social worker, CAT psychotherapist and supervisor with Barnet, Enfield and Haringey Mental Health Trust. She has worked in the NHS and community mental health for more than thirty years, and she is also trained in Peer-Supported Open Dialogue. She is currently the CAT lead in Haringey.

Caroline Greenwood Dower is an Integrative Psychotherapist with training backgrounds in CAT, Integrative Psychotherapy and Developmental Somatic Psychotherapy. She is a former NHS Consultant

Psychotherapist, the former Head of Counselling and Mental Health Services at Durham University, and an Adjunct Faculty Member at the Center for Somatic Studies in New York.

Jon Hall is a Nordoff-Robbins trained music therapist and founder of Outsider Music (https://www.outsidermusic.org.uk/music-therapy). After training at the Royal Scottish Academy of Music, Jon went on to be a successful artist and record producer. Jon brings together all his skills to work with a range of clients in mental health settings.

Kiera Kauler (she/her) is a community services practitioner who grew up in out of home care. During her final years in care, Kiera began engaging in systemic advocacy to improve the out of home care system, and studies community services and youth services in order to participate in different ways in the system.

Mel Keller-Tuberg (she/her) is a youth mental health advocate, peer worker, speaker, writer and researcher. Her work is based in her lived experience of eating disorders and co-occurring mental health issues as a teenager; the care that was helpful, unhelpful and what would have helped her the most. She believes that the mental health system must give those it seeks to serve a voice in order for programmes to work.

Donna Lockett is a specialist teacher with a broad range of experience in education. She has worked in inner London provisions for thirty years, holding various leadership roles in different settings. Donna is currently leading a provision for young people with anxiety related disorders and complex learning needs.

Cat McKenzie is an Accredited Mental Health Social Worker and Creative Arts Therapist, with experience working in the public and private youth mental health sector and an interest in how we can integrate the arts, mental health, and group work to promote connection, wellbeing, and community care.

Louise McCutcheon is a clinical psychologist, a CAT practitioner and trainer, and a clinical associate professor at the Centre for Youth Mental Health, University of Melbourne. She co-founded the Helping Young People Early (HYPE) program, an early intervention programme for young people with severe personality disorder in Melbourne, Australia.

Ben McKechnie is a clinical psychologist, CAT practitioner, supervisor and family therapist who works as the clinical stream leader of the Helping Young People Early (HYPE) program, an early intervention programme for young people with severe personality disorder in Melbourne, Australia.

Katherine Monson (she/her) is a mental health social worker and family therapist working in Wurundjeri Country – (Melbourne, Australia). For most of her career, Katherine has worked at Orygen, a young people's mental health service in a range of roles including case management, family therapy and mental health consultation to other providers. She also has the privilege of working at the Victorian Aboriginal Health Service.

Debbra Mortlock is a NHS clinical psychologist and CAT Supervisor. She has worked in generic, inpatient and forensic CAMHS and services for families within Children's Social Care. Debbra is experienced in working with children and young people with complex psychosocial needs, as well as with their parents, carers and networks.

Jessica O'Connell is a senior clinical psychologist, CAT practitioner and supervisor working in the Helping Young People Early (HYPE) clinic at Orygen, providing early intervention for young people living with features of severe personality disorder in Melbourne, Australia. Jess is completing her PhD at the University of Melbourne.

Leah O'Toole is Assistant Professor in Early Childhood Education in Maynooth University, Ireland. Located in the broad fields of psychology and education, her work explores relational pedagogy, the role of parents and communities in education, constructions of children and accessing the voices of our youngest citizens from birth.

Angie Phong (she/her) is a Chinese-Vietnamese Australian and strong advocate for climate justice, youth empowerment and the prevention of mental distress. She has a background in psychology and public health, with a commitment to using her experiences to ensure equitable outcomes for young people and diverse communities. She currently works in mental health policy, strengthening the prevention system for mental wellbeing.

Sivakami Suresh Prabalkumari is a Consultant Psychiatrist and accredited CAT Practitioner. She runs a Psychotherapy service in Chennai, India. She has developed the use of the CAT model, working with different age groups, within her context. She is also involved in developing a training programme in Cognitive Analytic Therapy in India.

Reem Ramadan is a clinical psychologist who has worked in public mental health services in the UK and Melbourne. She has worked in youth mental health services for more than ten years. Reem is also a passionate advocate for environmental and social justice issues and a dedicated climate activist.

Claire Regan is a Principal Clinical Psychologist Specialist in talking therapies and a CAT Practitioner, Supervisor and Trainer. She has worked in the HSE Adult Mental Health services in Ireland for eighteen years and is currently co-leading the implementation of the new national Model of Care for Talking Therapies in AMH services in Waterford.

Victoria Ryall has extensive experience in youth mental health, having been trained in a range of different therapies. She has vast leadership experience and is currently the Executive Director Clinical Practice at headspace National in Australia. Vikki is a strong advocate of LGBTIQA+ inclusion, youth participation and family inclusion.

Jo Varela is a Consultant Clinical Psychologist, CAT practitioner and Approved Clinician. She is interested in supporting people who may attract unhelpful, stigmatising labels such as 'challenging', and in assisting those who help them to formulate compassionate narratives that are trauma informed.

Clare Young is a Consultant Clinical Psychologist and Lead for Psychology and Psychological Therapies for Dorset CAMHS. She was previously Clinical Lead for Looked After Children's Services in Peterborough. Clare is passionate about collaborating with parents across her work in children's services, with a strong belief that parents are vital in working towards positive and long-term change for children.

Kiara Wickremasinghe is a PhD candidate in Anthropology at the School of Oriental and African Studies (SOAS) University of London, and is connected to the Anthropological Study Peer-supported Open Dialogue (APOD) research team. She is also a peer support worker and Open Dialogue practitioner within the NHS.

Introduction

Chapter 1: Being with and belonging – an introduction to a relational approach to working with young people

Lee Crothers and Nick Barnes

"If the future is to remain open and free, we need people who can tolerate the unknown, who will not need the support of completely worked out systems or traditional blueprints from the past."
Margaret Mead, US anthropologist

"Perhaps the energy and commendable commitment of those now using and developing the model, and relational approaches in general, may serve to address and challenge this pessimism and to offer some clinical and political hope for the future."
Tony Ryle, founder of CAT

What does it mean to be relational?

What does it mean to be relational? Well, when it comes to Cognitive Analytic Therapy (CAT), it means reflecting on how we relate to others and how they, in turn, relate to us. Moreover, it's about recognising how experiences in our historical relationships – be they of a personal or professional nature – influence our feelings, thoughts, attitudes and actions when it comes to current relationships.

Exploring relational approaches in health, education, social care and well-being settings might seem a luxury at a time when we are still wrestling with the impact of the COVID-19 pandemic, the existential threats of biodiversity loss and climate change, multiple wars and conflicts across the globe and a combative, social media-driven culture which seems to permit the weaponisation of difference, reinforcing a polarisation of stances across communities, rather than celebrating the plurality of our differences and diversity. But relational thinking – on which CAT is built – goes to the heart of who we are as people, and how we navigate the world. It's anything but a luxury. As Ryle and Kerr (2020, p2) suggest, CAT is a model that places the relational understanding – one that guides the way we are when working with people, and the way we understand their behaviour and motivations – above any particular technique or application.

Working in a more compassionate and relational way

Working with young people (defined in this book as 12 to 25-year-olds) using a relational approach is, we believe, a step towards a more compassionate or relational world; one in which we reflect on the kind of relationships we engender as professionals and see how much influence reflective and respectful relating have on people, systems and cultures. Unfortunately, such an approach is not as common as it might be in youth mental health or other predominantly statutory settings, such as schools and social care, where resources and staffing are stretched beyond their limits, as in so many other areas of health-service provision. Given decades of paucity in mental-health funding, especially when compared to other areas of the health system (Rathod *et al*, 2017), this simply reinforces further inequalities of care and experience of support.

As a consequence, in the name of efficiency, and often reinforced by the economics of austerity, a more individualised and reductionistic approach to understanding young people has been commonly adopted across healthcare systems, particularly within the neoliberal economies of the West (Moncreiff, 2022). The CAT model, developed by Tony Ryle in the 1970s and 80s, emerged and evolved in an age of rising neoliberalism, reliant on a celebration of the individual above and beyond the collective, influencing an increasingly alienating and consumerist perspective within the delivery of care models in these countries (Esposito & Perez, 2014). After all, this was the time that former UK prime minister Margaret Thatcher declared there was "no such thing as society" (Thatcher, 1987). And yet, as these countries have experienced profound threats and challenges, a dialogue has emerged within that questions the power and patriarchs that have sustained and perpetuated the social injustices and inequalities that define the lived experience of our worlds. After all, is it any accident that movements such as #MeToo or #BlackLivesMatters have emerged in recent years?

All these services for young people work within a socio-political paradigm that relies upon competition and consumption in order to maintain economic growth, but then result in the individual experiencing a greater sense of alienation and disconnect, within a society that reinforces further inequality and profound social injustice (United Nations, 2020). Tony Ryle, originally trained as a GP, was acutely aware of the need to find an approach to care and support that was meaningful for the many rather than just the few, drawing on the influence of his father as he noted the need to "study the ultimate as well as the intimate causes of disease" (Ryle, 1998)

While some might argue that this more standardised approach is more professional and clinically valid, young people, in our experience, often see it differently. To them, a clinical therapist, though well-intentioned, may seem cold, distant and disconnected. Responding to young people in a more manualised and professionally distant way is often seen to be just ticking boxes, rather than genuinely being curious and seeking to understand, and this may implicitly send a message that this is what one must do, as adults, to get ahead or to be professional, in the world. A relational approach informed by CAT, by contrast, is steeped in the theory that, not only are we social beings who want and need to relate, but that people can better heal through relating.

The emerging crisis in Children and Young People's mental health

Regardless of country, we are currently facing a profound crisis in Children and Young People's Mental Health (Benton *et al*, 2021). Undoubtably, this crisis is reinforced and stoked by the recognition of such uncertain and challenging times. The traumas of the COVID-19 pandemic, the escalating costs of the living crisis, the devastation of the wars in countries such as Ukraine, Syria or Sudan, and the existential threats of the Climate and Ecological Crisis all impact on how we perceive and understand the world around and between us, and all have had a profound impact on children and young people (WHO, 2022). For, fundamentally, it is upon children and young people that the burden of awareness falls most heavily. How do you perceive your future when you remain uncertain about opportunities for jobs, housing, connections with land, or even our very existence?

These are profound and important questions, but perhaps questions that we are struggling to even ask, as we find ourselves in markedly polarised positions, often reinforced by our social media echo-chambers, and focusing on how we can dismiss or disregard the other, rather than think about ourselves as together. We have been drawn into disputes over truths and fake news, and yet fail to appreciate that the truth lies in the spaces between us, for "Truth is not born, found inside the head of an individual person, it is born between people collectively searching for truth, in the process of their dialogic interaction" (Bakhtin, 1987).

In effect, we are exploring what this relational model, informed by CAT, may be able to offer in a world where we need to decolonise our thinking and enable an equity of experience through an authentically relational and collaborative connection between us. By focusing on being relational, CAT has offered a model that allows for "doing with", rather than "doing to", and perhaps, as we journey through such challenging times, both now and with what lies ahead, could this relational working allow for recognition and validation of experience, and enable an opportunity to explore "being with" and, as a result, our belonging"?

Risks of repetition

This book was born out of the observation (and frustration) that young people with significant distress are sometimes treated as "complex cases", especially in a busy and stressed health or education system and, being considered too difficult, are told to go elsewhere (Heads Up Report, 2022). The message they may often receive is that they are burdensome and, what's more, only have themselves to blame. The young person may feel displaced and othered, even from their first point of contact with services, while the service may seek to use complexity as its shield against engagement. This feeling of being 'too much' for the system is, we fear, being taken on by young people, and consequently, it is hard for them to find hope. Of course, this also has an impact on the worker. To think in a truly relational way, when a young person we are working with is too much, it can mean, implicitly, that we are *too little* or *not enough*. The CAT model helps us consider how we may, in our work with young people, unwittingly repeat unhelpful relationships that contribute to someone's sense of self as hopeless, and as being beyond help.

The evolution of Cognitive Analytic Theory and its therapeutic model

Relational thinking is one of the core tenets of CAT, the principles of which underpin this book. A coming together of psychoanalytic theory and cognitive theory, CAT – founded by English general practitioner Tony Ryle – is a collaborative and time-limited therapy. And, yes, a relational one, too. After years as a GP with a key eye on social medicine, his role as Head of Student Health at the University of Sussex gave him a close interest in the therapeutic and mental health needs of young people and led to his dissatisfaction with the prevailing psychoanalytic approaches which he sought to make more accessible. Bringing the influence of Mikael Leiman (2023), a Finnish psychologist who brought the ideas of social formation of mind theory from Lev Vygotsky (1978), and the dialogic self from Mikhael Bakhtin (Holquist, 1990), to his developing theory, Ryle imagined a therapy model that could bridge the cognitive and analytic worlds, thereby finding a common language for these psychotherapies and a more accessible psychodynamic approach for professionals and those they work alongside.

Ryle considered both the social formation of mind theory and the concept of dialogic self to encompass a developmental perspective in CAT; one that forwarded the idea that human beings develop a sense of self and well-being through early care relationships (Trevarthen, 2017). Importantly, Ryle recognised the central value of the zone of proximal development (ZPD)[2] as key to a relational understanding of development. The ZPD consists of two important components: the learner's potential development and the role of interaction with others. This developmental construct was further reinforced by the concept of scaffolding as a tool for growth. Learners complete small, manageable steps in order to reach their goals. Working in collaboration with another (teacher, mentor, therapist or more knowledgeable peers), the learner may then make connections between concepts.

As learners grow within their ZPD and become more confident, they practice new tasks with the social support that surrounds them. Vygotsky maintained that learning occurs through purposeful, meaningful interactions with

---

2 "the gap between what a child is able to do alone and what he/she/they could learn to do with the provision of appropriate help from a more competent other, who may be teacher, parent or peer" (Ryle & Kerr, 2002)

others, and Ryle embraced this understanding in the evolution of the CAT model. Additionally, Ryle recognised that we learn how to communicate and be with others with the help of shared signs/tools that carry relational meaning from our various cultures. For instance, smiling and the meeting of eyes is a sign of love and connection in most cultures.

CAT has added to object relations theory with the idea that we develop a 'good enough' sense of self through 'good enough' caring relationships, acknowledging the role of Donald Winnicott in describing the "good enough mother [parent]" (Winnicott, 1973) who's conscious and unconscious physical attunement to her baby adapts as the child's development needs change and the baby grows. Within these relationships, we internalise both poles (and thus, the whole) of a relationship; that is, both the *doing* part and the *done* to part. When we experience relationships in which the overriding behaviours are repeated often enough (such as caring), we implicitly learn the caring part, from feeling cared for, we are able to take on the other role attached to the cared for and be the carer. Ryle articulated this internalisation of both poles of a relationship as reciprocal roles (Ryle, 1985) – now, possibly the bedrock to all CAT practice, and, we would argue, a useful scaffold for all relational working.

This repetition of being in a caring and cared-for relationship is strengthened when we adopt a repertoire of coping mechanisms that moves us towards yet more confirmatory caring relationships. We also adopt the same relational stances that are familiar to us. We are more able to relate to ourselves, treat ourselves well, and believe that we are deserving if we have been cared for many times in the past. Of course, on the flip side, we can adopt rigid and unhelpful relational stances more readily when the most familiar or repeated relationships we've experienced have been harsh and uncaring.

So it is that many of our beliefs, thoughts and actions are attached to – almost to the point of being hardwired – what we might call our relationship template. It is our understanding that this template becomes our way to locate ourselves, and when we are younger and still developing, when things are being set down more firmly, this growing sense of individual self can be more easily influenced and impacted.

Repeating relational templates and learning to better care for ourselves and others

When someone experiences mental distress, CAT's relational model helps us see that this person is often repeating, or getting caught in, restricted or split-off relationships, ones that are often defined by criticism, neglect and/or abandonment. The distressed and traumatised person might not only feel stuck, but feel that they can do little to unstick themselves. When more helpful relational states are not internalised from our earlier relationships, it becomes harder to move into more flexible and caring relationship patterns. Certain relationship states have become so familiar to us through experience that our reactions and responses become almost automatic. It's like when we drive somewhere so familiar that, upon arrival, we wonder how we got there. It's as if we were on autopilot.

Exploring how a young person experiences and understands their distress and articulating this understanding through reciprocal roles (RRs), we have often found to be one of the most valuable and illuminating moments when working alongside a young person. Noticing that they don't hold just one place (state), but move from state to state, and that even within one state, they can end up hovering (and shimmering) (Potter, 2020) between both poles, can often be experienced as a significant breakthrough by many young people, who are so overwhelmed by their distress. The sudden realisation that their sense of feeling attacked all the time by others may also be connected to their own potential for attacking – either to self or to others (be that through self-harm or through violence/aggression) – can allow the space between to become a genuine opportunity for change.

CAT's relational model encourages a developmental way of looking at this problem. It posits that a person's difficulties in relating (to themselves and others) can be changed through providing them, in therapeutic/well-being work, with a different, more helpful relationship model (repeated often week to week or by many different people). Over time, the person can learn not only how to be in this kind of relationship, but how to be the instigator of relationships that are more affirming. A safe relational space with supportive professionals not only helps a young person feel calm and accepted, but it also helps them learn to be in both parts of a relationship, so that they can become the calm carer to themselves and also to others.

Most of the ensuing chapters were written by clinicians, teachers and therapists who have studied and now employ CAT in their daily work. Some have been written by young people who promote a more relational response in youth-based services. As they have found, and as we have outlined above, the actions we engage in have relational meaning, and they have been learned through either getting our interpersonal or intrapersonal needs met. Or not met. This is one of CAT's central principles and is demonstrated throughout the book. We all seek to know ourselves through relationships, and often act in ways that elicit the common relationships we know, be they helpful or not. We can also take on roles in relationships that we do not intend, as this is what is expected by and familiar to the other person.

The role of mapping

A big part of CAT is mapping out, (usually) on paper, with the young person, their relationship patterns (www.mapandtalk.com). This helps us to formulate these patterns or provide a clearer picture of how they may be playing out in the young person's working relationships. It is in doing this that we see the emergence of stories showing how often they have felt to be in certain restricted relationships, and how that young person has adapted to cope. It is a slowing down of the autopilot we talked about – knowing how we got somewhere familiar may also help us have the space to consider a different route.

But the mapping process itself often allows for a safer and more accessible way of exploring relationship patterns. For many young people, the prospect of being stuck in a therapy room with an older mental health professional can feel frightening enough – but the prospect of then opening up and talking to them about their intimate world can be simply a step too far. Mapping allows for the relational therapeutic encounter to be less about the need for face-to-face work, embracing the opportunity for being more alongside, triangulating the relational working through the active doing, on paper, in the space between.

Formulating through mapping also helps the professional know what kinds of relational responses the young person is expecting. The young person might then start to wonder out loud, often referring to the shared map, if they were playing out one part of the relationship – a hurtful part, say – that is common to them. By doing so, they invite in a chance to repair or observe together with the therapist rather than re-engage in stuck or inflexible ways.

A relational approach aided by mapping, or by sharing relational understanding, is often applied in individual work, supervision and to group and systems-based work as a way to locate ourselves, as workers, in the dynamics and therefore plan a way out of not repeating things through developing greater relational awareness. Throughout all the chapters offered in this book, you will find many examples of how mapping can offer a good enough observation and understanding that allows for an opportunity for change.

For many mental health, welfare and education workers, CAT has provided a way of exploring the complexity that is shared between them, the young person they are seeing, and the surrounding systems. CAT, through mapping and understanding relational patterns, offers a way of embracing complexity, not exploiting it as an opportunity for dismissal, without needing to become overwhelmed by the complexity (Balmain *et al*, 2021). This acceptance of complexity recognises the potential for uncertainty and gives permission for there to be an expression of ambivalence and fluidity. The mapping process allows us to appreciate the dynamic, offering a degree of clarity within the complexity, without resorting to a false promise of simplicity.

Moreover, it provides a way of thinking that both looks at their clients' unrevised relationship patterns and the cognitions and emotions that piggyback on these and keep them stuck. At the same time, it helps these clinicians and therapists consider their own ways of relating, and how, out of familiarity with the client, they may get pulled in to enact certain ways of relating that are ultimately not helpful. We have had this experience ourselves, where the intention to appear caring and supportive has been seen by the young person client as controlling. This sets off for them a familiar chain of events where they feel controlled, yell or push out. This leads to more control from ourselves, or others, exacerbating the problem. Then we say: thank goodness we have a relational model such as CAT with which to reflect on how we may have stepped into a repeat of a relationship experience that could be unhelpful or even damaging, and it has given us the way of formulating how we got there and then the words to negotiate with the young person, or with the system around them.

Likewise, we also need to be mindful of the trap that we can often fall into ourselves, as therapists and helpers, where we may seek to create the "perfect map" – the map that fully understands the needs of the young person, and illuminates through its very creation the exits needed for recovery and change. We run the risk of finding ourselves stuck in the reciprocal role (relational pattern) of "striving for perfection – feeling like it is never good enough", articulating a lack of confidence in our own mapping skills, when we need to recognise that the perfect map is perhaps only located in an idealised and imagined place. Rather, our task as the CAT practitioner, or any other relational practitioner, is to ensure that, however a map evolves in the space between, it is created collaboratively and feels good enough to the young person.

Allowing young people to make mistakes

A relational approach can help us notice and sometimes predict some of these relational landmines that lie beneath the surface. Young people, with their developmental needs for independence and connection, require as much flexibility in the way we relate to them as the flexibility we expect of them. Being an adolescent or young person can feel bewildering and exciting. It's a time for experimentation, of getting to know ourselves and the world. Fundamentally, it is a time for taking risks, and learning how to self-assess risk, and yet how ironic it is that the services they are often asked to engage with are so profoundly risk-averse (Markham, 2019). When young people experience professionals as being cold and detached, how often could this be due to the pages of risk assessment forms they are expected to complete – not by the choice of the clinician, but by the demands of the service? Further, how does this need for assessing risk fall into a reciprocation between the service which often resorts to being "controlling", with the young person then feeling "controlled" – perhaps repeating earlier harmful relational experiences? A relational approach, including a relational approach to risk, in which the reflection is on the dynamics or interplay of these patterns, offers the possibility of a more nuanced, humane and compassionate approach.

Our scaffold for this book

We have dreams of this book promoting and enabling change, of helping professionals who want to connect with and relate to young people they are working alongside, and possibly in the wider communities and systems around young people. Likewise, we hope that this book might encourage those that work with young people, from all backgrounds and disciplines, to reflect on and consider the where, when, how and by whom this relational working is offered if we are to enable individual and/or wider social change. For this is not only about considering the distance between ourselves and the young person in the therapeutic space, but also about considering the wider "social distance between us", and how the gulfs between services and communities, between politicians and the represented electorate, have become so vast that they fail to enable change that feels meaningful and offer agency on the ground (McGarvey, 2022).

This book is about acknowledging the complexity in human relationships rather than placing that complexity solely on the shoulders of the person seeking help. Within these pages, we aim to describe, and provide real examples of, the practical use of the relational approach of CAT with young people. We hope to expand on the possibilities of relating to someone when things feel stuck and restricted, acknowledging that we, too, as workers, feel the pull or the 'compulsion to repeat' the relationships a young person is familiar with. We as workers/therapists have some responsibility in reflecting on and creating a more helpful working relationship, especially when things are feeling 'too much'. CAT being not only a therapy, but a model of understanding self and systems, means many of the authors in this book write about how they have applied this relational approach to settings such as education and workplace consultation, as well as considering the challenges that young people who are questioning (or being questioned about) their gender, sexuality, culture.

We have invited many practitioners from across the CAT community and beyond, as well as many young people, to share their understanding of working relationally with young people, and their experience of this working, to help the reader capture an understanding of the possibilities and opportunities of working within this space. While the views of the contributors are their own and may not always align with others in the field, they have been invited to contribute because of their experience and expertise. Moreover, we believe they share our belief in the need for a more relational and dialogical understanding of our world and, most importantly, of the lives of young people.

The book has been written not only for the CAT therapists and practitioners, but also for the CAT curious, and for those that look to work in a more relational way with young people. This is therefore not a book just talking to clinical practice, but which also seeks to be accessible to all professionals who work alongside young people – and, hopefully, some sections may be helpful to young people themselves. For the CAT-informed community, we should warn you that this book will not offer you a greater understanding of CAT developmental theory that you can't access in other books, and we do deliberately look to step aside from some of our own CAT language (jargon). But what we hope is that, for any person who picks up this book – CAT-trained or not – they will read something that will help them think further about the how, where, when and with whom they work.

The structure of the book

The book looks to contextualise how working relationally with young people can move between many different places: from the personal to the systemic, from the social to the political, from the local to the global, and many spaces in between.

Following this introductory chapter, the first few chapters of the book look to explore ways of working alongside young people at a more individual, one to one level, often directed by specific (diagnostic) needs, such as young people with eating difficulties, with neurodevelopmental and learning needs, or through services such as the HYPE (helping young people early) model, pioneered in Australia. We have also included a chapter in this section that encourages us to take a more embodied approach when we look to engage young people in dialogue. But, alongside these quite specific areas of need, we also looked to include a dialogue about themes that are becoming increasingly concerning, and distressing, for young people, recognising the considerable needs of young people from within LGBTQ+ communities.

We then look to offer contributions from authors providing a much more systemic perspective of relational working, where practitioners can share their experiences of working with parents, within families, and in groups, recognising the need for thinking around the young person, either to complement or to replace working alongside.

This more systemic perspective is then developed further in the third section, when we reflect on the need for a more relational approach when exploring service development and the context of that delivery. This section allows to value the need for relational work within services that focus specific experiences of distress, including working with those that experience hearing voices. But as well as articulating how CAT has been utilised as a scaffold for setting up a new psychotherapy service (in Chennai, India) this section also allows us the space for a relational approach within education, schools and care settings.

But we have also included in this section a chapter that voices a note of caution, with a chapter on Burn Out and Bullying. This chapter speaks to the risks of overstretching ourselves, or seeking to rescue, and failing to recognise the toll this can have on us as professionals and practitioners, and how easy it can be for people to fall into positions of bullying and intimidation, particularly at times of stress and heightened demand. If there is one thing that the COVID-19 pandemic has taught us, it is that we need not only to be kind to each other, but also kind to ourselves, if we are to cope and deliver meaningful work – to be able to connect and work relationally with young people, we need to be connecting with our selves, as well as connecting with each other.

Lastly, in the final section, we were looking to explore CAT in wider settings and contexts, looking at a role for a relational approach within and across communities. This section offers a perspective from different communities who may struggle to find support through more traditional services, such as gaming communities. We also felt the need for a space where the realities of the existential threats facing young people through the effects of biodiversity loss and the climate crisis were heard and validated, offering a relational and ecological understanding to some of the drivers of the escalating pressures and stresses being placed on future generations. But this emphasis on community-based working also needs us to consider how we might support relational working within this context, allowing the need for relationships to be at the heart of any work that seeks to overcome systemic social injustices and entrenched inequalities.

Our closing chapter (Closing Thoughts: Common Threads) allows for a pulling together and integrating of the themes that have emerged throughout all the chapters, looking at what might be specific to CAT and its evolving model, and what might be relevant, when thinking about compassionate care and relational working across all services, agencies and systems.

Throughout each of the sections, we have looked to include the voices of young people – and especially those with a lived experience of support and services. Sometimes, these voices are challenging, where support has not been helpful or responsive, but mostly they reinforce our conviction that it is only through relational working that we will enable the change that is needed – not just for the individual young person, but for societies and communities across the globe. We have drawn on the CAT community (and beyond) from many different countries and looked to offer an international perspective of relational working, and therefore hope that the ideas and ways of working proposed translate to other languages, cultures and contexts.

Challenging enough

We hope you enjoy and are challenged, in a good way, reading this book (yes, it is our intention to be challenging enough). We have found the relational approach helps us zoom up and out from the individual to the wider world, with all the spaces between offering opportunities for change. This approach has helped us acknowledge and use the relating that is happening between us, so we can start to change the part we play, allowing relational repair. We know that the young person's practitioner, be they youth worker, school well-being coordinator, social worker, teacher or psychologist, knows that the working relationship is the key to change, but the task is to create a space that will allow this to occur. For it is in the space between that lies the opportunity for change.

It is our hope that this book provides the space for others to feel inspired and/or sufficiently supported to continue to develop this important work. After all, we believe this was an initial aspiration of Tony Ryle's work, allowing for the continuing evolution of an integrative model of relational (intimate) practice (Ryle *et al*, 2014). We all seek to understand who we are, our sense of being, by being with and developing a sense of belonging, separateness and healthy interaction. Relational working enables young people to explore the possibility for change, supporting the development of an awareness of 'being with and belonging'.

PART 1: Relational approaches to working alongside young people

Chapter 2:
'If all you ever see is an eating disorder…' – a relational understanding and approach to working with young people with eating disorders

Lee Crothers and Melissa Keller-Tuberg

This chapter is written with some of the theory and purpose of a relational approach influenced by Cognitive Analytic Therapy (CAT), interspersed with some personal reflections by and dialogue between the authors. This represents a therapist/clinician and a lived experience perspective learning from each other throughout this process, and hopeful for a future in which clinicians and people with lived and living experience can navigate the tensions and conflicts that often arise in treatment in a more responsive, compassionate and collaborative way. To understand the stories and relational components of eating disorders, we need to hear from as wide a range of voices and perspectives as possible in academic, clinical and peer discourses, particularly from those whose voices often go unheard. By focusing on the dynamics between individuals and their sociocultural contexts, a relational approach fundamentally brings intersections between gender, sexuality, culture, religion and the ongoing impacts of minority stress to the forefront of understanding eating disorders, and the availability of culturally affirming care or lack thereof.

The authors would like to acknowledge the voices not represented in this chapter. To minimise the risks associated with being over-reliant on a small number of experts with unique lived/living and professional experiences, we state our commitment to listening and learning from people from culturally and linguistically diverse backgrounds, including people from the LGBTQIA+ community, indigenous people and people living with a physical disability.

Introduction

Eating disorder (ED) presentations in adolescents and young people have increased in many Western countries since the start of the COVID-19 pandemic. For instance, presentations have doubled in the UK (Solmi *et al*, 2021), with a similar rate occurring in Australia (Springall *et al*, 2021). The social consequences of the pandemic have been particularly impactful on adolescents and young people. They are in a fast-paced and foundational time of development, one in which peer and social opportunities are important for establishing a sense of self and independence. Despite this, there has been little emphasis on socially or relationally considered approaches to understanding and treating young people with EDs. Holmes (2018) writes that the sociocultural elements of EDs are studied and visible but not so their treatment. If a relational (and, implicitly, a wider social) approach is adopted in eating disorder treatment, then the care system may be less likely to focus on just one dimension of treatment – that of the young person eating again – often at the expense of all other developmental goals. A relational understanding and approach provide a shared appreciation that people do things to relate better, and that real change is not limited to simply stopping a behaviour such as food restriction. Eating disorders are understood together through the relational theory and tools of CAT, where co-creation of mapping and letters allows for a sharing of this understanding. These can then be easily referred to, in and outside therapy, allowing recognition of any possible re-enactment of previous relational patterns.

Early intervention treatments can adopt or subsume the relational understanding and approach that CAT can bring. As "relationships are the currency of change" (Perry & Winfrey, 2021), a relational approach can help the professional avoid re-enacting the controlling and, at times, punitive care that the eating disorder may bring, as well as help the young person to understand themselves in a compassionate and all-encompassing way needed for their recovery[3].

---

3   Here, recovery is not defined solely as having no symptoms, but is rather how the person sees recovery, such as it being an ongoing process but living a functional or meaningful life.

CAT as a model for understanding and treating eating disorders

CAT has relationships at the heart of everything. CAT was a recommended intervention for anorexia nervosa (AN) in previous NICE guidelines, but was recently dropped as it lacked comparable research evidence (NICE consultation comments, 2017). However, we recommend that CAT's fundamental construct of reciprocal relationships – often replayed within ourselves and others, and becoming powerful in their repetition in self formation, makes it a helpful model in eating disorder treatment, particularly in formulating what has led to and keeps the ED problematic. With CAT being an integrative model, it allows in other often-needed aspects of treatment such as weighing, food monitoring and exposure work (Wicksteed, 2016).

CAT practitioners believe that people are fundamentally relational beings; we not only need to feel a sense of belonging and connection for our well-being, but our sense of self is formed in and through relationships (Ryle & Kerr, 2020). This means that change and healing often come first through healthy relating with others. This, in turn, influences our ways of relating to self and providing self-care. Food has always played a big role in how we connect and communicate with each other (Lester, 2019). The giving and accepting of food are universal gestures of care. These so-called caring or compassionate gestures are internalised and become the structure to our own caring for others and self. For instance, children who are pre-verbal share food with friends who need soothing and are able to gesture that they are hungry and want a certain food. These ways of caring (or not caring) often get replayed within us and in our interactions with others. Our external parenting voice becomes our *internal* parenting voice. The way we nurture ourselves, through food or other means, can be symbolic of our past relational history. To someone with an ED, food can become a symbol of control or greed rather than of care, and hence, the meaning of such gestures as "re-feeding" in eating disorder care can seem punitive and controlling if not explored. CAT's relational understanding encompasses this theory of self-functioning and is shared with the young person, how their early relationships led to their unique ways of relating that seemed to initially work but now are often circular and confirmatory of difficulties or problem states. "Cognitive analytic therapy (in eating disorders) differs from the education therapy as it integrates psychodynamic factors with behavioural ones and focuses on interpersonal and transference issues" (Treasure *et al*, 1994, p365).

A relational understanding or reformulation in eating disorders

A collaborative and shared formulation of ED and its relational function (see Ryle & Kerr, 2020) allows for a more humanistic space for professionals, families and young people. In CAT this relational understanding (or formulation), when co-created with the client, is called a reformulation as most people have a fixed narrative about their issues, conscious or not, prior to therapy. A shared relational understanding helps young people observe themselves more compassionately as they start to understand they were trying to get their relational needs met, creating more space for change. Newell (2012), writing about using CAT with people with AN, identifies common relationship patterns around food restriction, such as being caught up in idealised care/neglected/criticised/dominated (control)/admired states. These patterns of relating are identified with the young person as understandable, adaptive patterns established in early life that are now more fixed and do not allow for growth and connection. This revised story is a new and more humane way of looking at themselves, fitting with Allen's work (2016), which found that written formulations, when working with adults with eating disorders, were no more useful than no formulation. Rather, it was the respectful and reflective tone of the formulation that helped engage people in treatment.

> **Personal reflections**
>
> **Lee:** Consider a young person with restricting type anorexia nervosa who grew up in a big, boisterous family where both parents worked full time. Through a CBT-E formulation, the young person recognises that their perfectionistic thinking keeps them in a loop of always trying to be a low weight and being underweight keeps this thinking rigid and over-valued. A shared relational understanding, alongside a CBT-E one, acknowledges their past experiences of not feeling emotionally seen in a big family, and of adopting perfectionistic thinking to be noticed, so as to remain close to loved ones.
>
> **Mel:** So many young people can relate to this story. We often grow up in environments that teach us that striving to be 'perfect', 'in control', of meeting every milestone with flying colours, of achieving or impressing in society's eyes, makes us more loveable. When this way of thinking is extended to our relationship with food, bodies and exercise, it can unfortunately spiral into an eating disorder. →

Lee: A shared relational understanding would look upon this strategy of using perfectionism to connect as an adaptive response, a survival strategy, to feelings of not being seen. We would consider how this may have worked well in the past, but is now leading to the young person feeling constantly inadequate and being stuck in a closed circuit of trying to move out of it and confirming it at the same time.

Mel: Maybe that young person felt the most familial love, care and emotional attention when they got their perfect report card back. Maybe they were the target of, or witnessed, appearance-based bullying and teasing at school, and they learned that being safe and accepted by their peers is to control their food and body.

Lee: A shared relational understanding provides a bit more story around our humanness and can inform what might get in the way of the working relationship, too. For instance, when the young person has a more compassionate or relational understanding of the roots of their perfectionism, it is easier for the worker and young person to keep an eye out for this strategy and how it may thwart some of the therapeutic goals. That is, they may expect themselves to be the 'perfect client' in the 'perfect therapy' and how this pressure may lead to them feeling disappointed and not attend. The worker can also be alert to the dynamic of wanting to provide perfect care and can use this relational understanding to address this more effectively by recognising that perfectionism may be something they both fall into, rather than placing it in the one person.

Mel: I remember one of the most powerful things a clinician said to me when I was very unwell. They said, "We can see how determined and goal-oriented you are, and [how hard you are trying to be discharged]". They explained to me that it's not a bad thing; it's something powerful that I could learn to channel for good outside of my eating disorder, and it will be something I could learn through recovery.

Sharing the relational understanding with family and professionals

A shared relational understanding or reformulation, incorporated into the treatment and care of young people with AN, can be hugely helpful in leading to change. In our practice and experience, AN is the eating disorder that seems to have the most relational consequences for young people, and it's where professionals, young people and their families seem the most divided. Interpersonal difficulties can predispose one to AN and perpetuate the illness (Treasure *et al*, 2020). The interpersonal relationships AN elicits, such as greater control, mistrust and forced care, are at odds with what young people often want and need to individuate, to develop their own sense of self separate from their family, and to belong with peers. Having a relational understanding, often in the form of a diagram or map of the main dynamics at play (what is referred to as sequential diagrammatic reformulation [SDR] in CAT), can be a valuable supervision tool for a worker to help them recognise when enactments are interfering with therapy when working with people with ED (Wicksteed, 2016). A relational understanding and approach allow for these recurring patterns of controlling care to be spoken about in ways that help everyone involved to recognise these patterns of relating, helping the young person to "feel empathically understood" and "to contain both patient and therapist anxiety" (Tanner & Connan, 2003, p283). This can create space in which to take up alternative avenues of relating together.

Personal reflections

Mel: From the stories I've heard, young people's turning points and 'A-ha! moments' tend to occur when the dynamic shifts from the tough or firm 'whatever it takes' role adopted by the clinician/family and the 'defend and combat' reaction of the young person. This shift in dynamics is represented by the clinician slowing down, speaking with gentleness and curiosity, and trying to collaborate with a young person, even if just to build mutual understanding.

Lee: Yes, it's often helpful if the professional can take a relational approach. This could involve them articulating the dilemma they face of wanting to be seen as caring but then looking like they are being controlling, such as when they weigh the young person. If the professional talks about how easily they could get into a controlling relationship with the young person, it is some acknowledgement that the professional wants to be relating differently, more collaboratively. The idea is that, if the young person feels more cared for, more respected, then they are more likely to be able to do this for themselves around their eating disorder.   →

> **Mel:** A clinician once said to me, "I forgot how hard being weighed is for you. I'm sorry. Let's talk about some ways it might feel a little easier." This confused my eating disorder ("I thought they were against me? Why are they being so kind?") and challenged the idea that recovery was unsafe or threatening. Their vulnerability made them seem more human and trustworthy.

From a shared relational understanding comes a relational approach

The main treatment options for adolescents and young people with AN are Family-Based Therapy (FBT), if under 18 years old, or Cognitive Behaviour Therapy-Enhanced (CBT-E) if over 18 years (NICE guidelines, 2017). These interventions are quite rightly recommended as they currently have the most evidence. When strictly applied, these interventions can be experienced by some young people as controlling and dismissive, and they understandably push against them – often perpetuating a controlling to controlled (or out of control) loop of health care. A battle ensues, with parents and carers feeling they need to hold firm and take control on behalf of their young person. But this is all occurring at a time when adolescents and young people are learning how to individuate, to become their own person and step away from the child role within their family. What if the eating disorder has been a part of their pushing against boundaries or search for individuation? The family's response might feel like an attack on their more independent self.

> ### Personal reflections
> **Lee:** It is hard to see the battles for control between family members, the young person and the system. The distress of trying to keep someone alive can understandably lead to very reactive and controlling ways. I find a relational approach helps families talk about this 'stuckness' in the relationship, that they feel they are repeating a relationship that contributes to the problem. The real issue, or what CAT calls the target problem, is at the centre of a relational formulation. It is not the eating disorder itself but rather this state of not belonging, being out of control or trapped that a young person is trying to manage. →

> **Mel:** My feeling is that recovery and self-exploration need to happen in parallel. As a peer worker, I often hear young people talk about "missing their eating disorder". As I understand it, that refers to their feelings of missing the space the eating disorder took up in their life.
>
> For years, the torment of an eating disorder hides the fact that they may not have had a life that had fulfilled and preoccupied them enough, or that they liked enough. For me, I only stopped missing my eating disorder when I started to develop my own sense of self, community and identity. For me, this meant exploring fresh ways of moving (I tried gardening in line with nutritional/exercise advice), creating (I joined a drawing from nature art class), and connecting to community and purpose (learning to safely share my story with peers with similar experiences). You need support to recover from an eating disorder but also room from others to safely trust you to explore why recovery is actually worth it.

Parents and families engaging with services are often left feeling torn between professional recommendations and their desire to provide a less controlled environment for their adolescent whose peers are being given increasing freedom. As a result of taking on firm and controlling stances, there is a risk that the treatment unwittingly repeats the relationships the adolescents are often trying to avoid, ones of being controlled or seen in a limited way; a child that cannot be trusted with their own care. The response to this kind of controlling relationship is often to shut down, to take on more control. Wufong *et al* (2019) write about the absence of the voice of the 40% of parents whose adolescents experience ongoing psychological distress despite weight restoration. On interviewing a small sample, Wufong found there may be a risk of overlooking the psychological distress of adolescents and their families if a more formal behavioural approach is taken as the first line treatment for children and adolescents. A relational formulation shared by all parties provides this interpersonal and developmentally appropriate understanding, as well as an empathy that can complement the more fixed aspects of the behavioural intervention and speak to the pushes and pulls that parents experience as they navigate their young person's needs.

Eating disorder teams can consider the relational formulation when using other interventions, such as CBT-E, reminding their teammates if they or the system are replaying or being invited to repeat the very relationships that contributed to an ED for the young person. They can acknowledge that the way they relate to the young person and family as a professional and a service is just as important as following the next step in the therapeutic intervention manual. It can be both liberating and empowering for the professional and team to recognise the use of relating as a therapeutic tool. Helping a team to have space to consider this is harder in a climate where research and KPIs are prioritised. It takes leaders and then the team to stand by what we all know, that the way treatment is provided is just as important as the intervention or treatment modality itself. Protecting reflective spaces where the team and individuals can talk about their own relational responses and normalising these responses is a starting point for thinking about what kind of relationships these young people need in order to become more able to look after themselves. A relational approach, such as one informed by CAT, can provide a shared language that teams can use no matter what their preferred or mandated intervention is.

Personal reflections

Lee: I see many young people who are grateful for their eating disorder teams helping them regain their physical health (through weight restoration), but they are often left with much distress caused by feeling overcontrolled and overpowered. I have seen people feel broken by a system that is designed to care.

Mel: During a time that I was very unwell, I requested some time outdoors (after weeks spent inside and on bedrest). I was told that my brain was malnourished and that my thoughts were not trustworthy (perhaps my request was interpreted as a strategy for movement to lose weight).

The lack of freedom, autonomy and respect I experienced left me feeling highly distressed, frustrated and disbelieving that the treating team had my best interests at heart. Ironically, during these times, more than ever, it felt like the eating disorder was my only source of autonomy and safety, and I was in an exhausting cycle of defending and holding on to it, supercharged by my environment. This treatment made my physical symptoms better and my eating disorder much worse – a recipe for 'revolving door' admissions.

When young people are restricting and are very low weight, there is clearly a requirement to attend to the physical parameters of their condition, but it can then feel like there is no time or space to consider how the young person may be mentally and emotionally affected. A busy and under-resourced health system that has been directed to mostly use CBT models is often not given permission, the framework or time to think about the more psychodynamic or relational past of the young people, let alone how this medical/psychiatric event may affect the young person's developmental trajectory. However, by looking to ensure there is a relational approach underpinning the engagement and provision of care, we would argue, ensures the long-term consequences to people's development are considered.

> ## Personal reflections
>
> **Mel:** I've spoken to hundreds of people of many ages, genders, diagnoses and experiences in my advocacy, and one thing that I hear from everyone is a call for more compassion at all levels of acuity in the mental health system. When I was very unwell, a youth worker said to me, "I look at you and see someone who isn't happy. Do you remember the last time you felt happy?" Happiness, in myself, others, or the world around me, as a thing that had ever existed, hadn't crossed my mind in months. It was like someone teaching me a new word. I felt refreshed and calmed by the human connection and was momentarily wholly present with the emotional impact of my eating disorder. I would constantly ask for that youth worker, because I craved those moments of understanding and connection so deeply.
>
> **Lee:** It is clear to me that, on some level, young people who seem medically compromised remember the relational quality of care they received when very unwell, where the professionals can observe and comment on how they may be re-enacting a relationship that seems harmful or uncaring.
>
> **Mel:** It's interesting that I feel a need to prove to the reader that I was 'well enough' (AKA, medically restored enough) to have been capable of the experiences and understandings I write about. It's a sign of how tenuous the human connections, trust and shared understandings can be in eating disorder care. This is fundamental; we won't be able to move forward easily without it.

A shared relational understanding leads to a more integrated self

Having a shared relational understanding includes exploring the relational function of an ED with a young person which can be useful in helping them feel more empowered to address it. Often, behavioural approaches position AN as a separate entity from the young person. This 'othering' of anorexia, and the need to stand firm and fight against it, can offer a narrative that protects the adolescent from being blamed, and allows the family to come together in 'fighting the good fight'. But this can also go against the developmental needs of the adolescent as they seek to integrate the different aspects of themselves, and yet are being encouraged to disregard, and split off, some features at the same time. The young person is being encouraged to take a very binary position ('eating good, restriction bad') at the very time when they might be seeking to explore a more fluid and dynamic sense of self in other areas of their developing selves.

Personal reflections

Mel: Unanticipated recovery experiences I hear from a lot of young people (ones not frequently talked about) include: hearing "Oh, you're doing amazing!" while crumbling internally; wanting to be fully recovered and back to their worst simultaneously; feeling like everything gets worse before it gets better; missing their sick body or identity while being afraid of relapse; not knowing how to fill all their free time without eating disorder behaviours; being afraid of not knowing or liking who they are outside of their eating disorder. It's clear that overly simple binary thinking around recovery is unlikely to set people up for a meaningful, satisfying or stable journey, as people are more likely to turn back to their eating disorder as a way of coping with the challenges of life.

Lee: The rigid and concrete thinking often associated with anorexia supports a model that responds in a rigid and concrete way, but this may be counterintuitive to how the young person may be exploring ideas of gender, sexuality, culture or even belonging.

Mel: The strong focus on behavioural and medical symptoms in my eating disorder care meant that all conversations I had in treatment were about my weight, eating and exercise behaviours outside of the role they played in my inner and relational world. I find it ironic, →

> that in some ways the conversations I was having in treatment mirrored my internal obsession and hyper fixation with food, weight and shape. I literally remember thinking, "If all you ever see me as is an eating disorder, well that's all I will be".

A shared relational understanding helps the young person develop a benevolent and caring voice so they can relate to themselves compassionately, and not in such a split-off manner. A relational understanding or reformulation that in CAT is verbalised (often written as a narrative in letter form and then more simply with a map (see Potter, 2022), assists in the growth of this emerging and eventually overarching voice. It's one that can bring into dialogue the childish or needy parts of ourselves while recognising that a more neutral and caring response may be needed.

> ### Personal reflections
> **Mel:** I dropped out of many treatment programs, but my true recovery and self-motivated weight restoration started when I was able to make small choices in my treatment. For example, I actively complied in taking liquid supplements after I was able to choose the supplement (with approval from my nutritionist). My choice was 'safer' (non-processed) in the eyes of my eating disorder at the time, but was, in my opinion, a realistic, reasonable and HUGE first step, which set the tone to confront more nuanced eating disorder thinking around food flexibility later down the track.

Conclusion

Treating eating disorders has always been challenging. We believe, however, that psychological, emotional and physical change in treating AN, that leads to so-called normal development, is most likely when the young person, family and treating team have developed a shared relational understanding. This fosters a more compassionate and developmentally led collaboration between all involved, including the young person's family. A relational approach allowing for curiosity and reflection on the kind of dynamics that are commonly enacted between families, professionals and young people – rather than an approach in which one person or party carries responsibility – creates more collaborative and developmentally appropriate relationships.

A shared relational understanding also creates space for the young person to understand themselves in a way that provides an interpersonal perspective rather than just an intrapersonal one. In other words, they can understand their eating disorder as a way to keep relating to others, not just as a means to maintain a self-image. Along with a relational language, a shared relational understanding keeps the working alliance strong as it both acknowledges the resilience of a person who wants to connect, as well as how hard it is for them to change when an eating disorder has served these relational needs in the past.

The collaborative nature of reformulating with the young person while being in a curious, co-creating stance is a reparative and helpful process, recognising their growing autonomy. It is a way to pre-emptively recognise what may relationally play out in the therapeutic work, and it provides the language to recognise and negotiate this together. We encourage the kind of relational understanding provided by CAT's reformulation. It aids engagement, and avoids repeating relational harm to the young person, family and professionals, thereby creating the space for real change.

Chapter 3: Using CAT for neurodivergent young people – working with intellectual disability and autism

Jo Varela

Introduction

This chapter addresses the application of Cognitive Analytic Therapy (CAT) to working with young people with intellectual disabilities and/or autism. CAT is a model that can help us understand the cognitive differences and relational struggles that are experienced by autistic young people or those with intellectual disability, and how they may be repeated by professionals, families and society. As an integrated model, CAT can also be used to facilitate relational attunement or repair for a young person with these labels and experiences and those who love and care for them.

Language and diversity

Intellectual disabilities – also referred to as learning disabilities in the UK – describes significant difficulties across a range of cognitive skills, including reasoning, problem solving, planning, memory, understanding, thinking and communicating. These difficulties impact the development of daily living skills and the ability to self-care across a range of areas of functioning. Autism is a lifelong difference in the way people think, understand and communicate, in and with the social world around them. This diversity or difference in thinking and perception is now better understood as being 'neurodiverse', compared to most of the population being 'neurotypical'. Being in a social and physical environment designed for neurotypical people, not designed for a neurodiverse young person, places additional demands on them, often leading to anxiety and distress. This is particularly so for young people with intellectual disability.

How is CAT different for young people with intellectual disabilities?

"At a fundamental level, working with a person with an intellectual disability in psychotherapy is the same as working with anyone else, and as different. They are often not seen as suitable for treatment, but here it is psychotherapy that is handicapped."
(Linington, 2002)

In writing this chapter, the author considered how CAT as an individual therapy might be different for young people with an intellectual disability or autism. In many ways, it is not. Practitioners working with the range of developmental abilities in young people will be used to making adaptations to support a child to access a concept or mode of working. There is more reliance on the use of visual aids, play, emphasis on mapping-while-talking, or 'sculpting' such as using and arranging objects to represent mental or abstract concepts (see Varela (2016) and Bork & Varela (in press). It is important to simplify concepts and use adapted communication such as pictures instead of words, break ideas down into smaller components until they are assimilated and understood, go at a slower pace or contract additional sessions (24 rather than 16 sessions, for example), and work with the dyad of carer and child in the therapy room. The use of mapping in CAT as a 'navigational aid' may be more salient for a young person with intellectual disability. These maps hold core constructs of CAT-based ideas about relationships and how we internalise them from the thinking of Bakhtin, Trevarthen and Vygotsky. The maps hold familiar ideas to CAT practitioners, but they really come into their own when working with young people with intellectual disabilities, co-creating and mediating meaning using signs and symbols.

Learning to have a learning disability

Much of the literature on working with or for young people starts with a definition of the 'disorder', followed by a warning that they are more likely to have associated vulnerabilities such as mental health difficulties

(Emerson & Hatton, 2007) and challenging behaviour (Nicholls *et al*, 2023) and are disproportionately more likely to experience traumatic events and relationships including restraint and assault (ICARS, 2023). Narratives in the press are likely to reflect 'difference', as eugenics has in the past, reinforcing the need to classify these young people as 'other', which remains a live issue in current discussions about gene editing and abortion. This background generates a narrative that growing up with and parenting a young person with learning disability is a difficult path. However, this is not necessarily true, and it does not need to be this way. Parent advocates describe the joy, love and pride with which they accompany their loved one on their journey to adulthood, and protest about the barriers they face from the system and wider society. People with intellectual disabilities advocate for inclusion and being valued, calling for a change in relational stance from others rather than a change in their self (see Salman, 2020).

Literature on 'goodness of fit' between parent and child suggests that the more attuned and able to scaffold the parent is within an individual dyad, the better the outcome for the child (Newland & Crnic, 2017). In understanding the issue of disability and difference as a relational one rather than as a deficit in the young person, it becomes easier to find a relational understanding and solutions to support the development of a positive, autonomous identity.

We learn to be who we are through being with others. We also learn how to care for ourselves through the style in which others care for us. A child or young person with additional intellectual disabilities and their carers may find that the weight of a history of othering, exclusion and fear affects acceptance and support from the society around them. The isolation, lack of resources and fear of being taken away and placed 'in care', far from home and family, or in a 'special' school away from other children, is still all too frequent. In Kegan-Bull's autobiography (2022), he shares his story as a man with intellectual disabilities with a loving and warm family, but, heartbreakingly, has experiences of entry and acceptance into the world that are mixed. Even on the first page, he describes that he may not have a place in the world and how his family are advised to "put (him) away".

Relational labels, relational positions

The terminology of intellectual disability has never been one of self-determination. It is an uncomfortable story with its roots in eugenics, and it is curious how, as we change the terms (we are moving towards 'intellectual disability'), each past iteration has needed to change after becoming a term of abuse. These labels are then used to subject the person to relationships based on rejection, othering, belittling and jeering (Sinason,1992). 'Mental deficient' is replaced by 'mental retardation', which is rebranded as 'mental handicap'. The wheel is turning again as 'learning disability' morphs into 'intellectual disability'. Suddenly, something that should only be a part of who the person is (cognitive difficulties) becomes a slur on the whole self. Societal supports for young people also have their roots in uncomfortable relational positions of exclusion and control (see Series (2022) and Skull (2017) for an overview).

This historical and social context makes young people doubly vulnerable, not just to difficulties in thinking, understanding and planning, but to abuse, exclusion and neglect from a wider society that may not value and support them (e.g. Nicolle, 2023), and asserts a position of superiority and othering.

We do not have to re-enact these historical roles, but we do need to be mindful of their capacity to unwittingly invite the same relational frame. For example, self- and parent-advocates warn that, although the names have changed, little has changed in the care given. Segregation and exclusion still occur, on a system level (with separate 'special' and residential schools) and within schools (in euphemistically named 'calm' rooms). Restriction and restraint are also widespread, as well as physical holding as a treatment if young people do not conform. All of these are 'rebranded' interventions that would have been found in institutions 50 or 100 years ago and serve no care or therapeutic purpose. Once we recognise the relational dynamic (controlling-to-controlled, punishing-to-punished, excluding-to-excluded), we can appraise practices from the young person's point of view and challenge them wherever they occur.

What is it like growing up with an intellectual disability?

When working with young people with intellectual disabilities, it is important to have a model that understands and supports their *neurocognitive* difficulties and differences (the 'C' or cognitive part of CAT) as well as the *relational* dynamics (often represented by the 'A' or analytic part of CAT) that young people may experience growing up. These challenges include those faced by their families, the wider societal relationships, political strategy and funding (or the lack thereof) as suggested by Bancroft *et al* (2008). It is worth considering this question in the application of CAT for young people with intellectual disabilities in terms of the relational ripples stemming from the initial difficulties they have.

1) The 'C' in CAT

As described above, young people with intellectual disabilities have difficulties with the thinking skills that are integral to negotiating their own experience and the world around them. CAT has a number of conceptual frameworks that may be drawn upon to help children and young people become effective agents of change through reflecting on their thinking in the world. Procedural sequences (the 'arrows' on a diagram) are based on a cognitive model of the world which, if mapped out, can accommodate and structure learning skills, or support difficulties in thinking within a young person's 'zone of proximal development'. This concept was initially developed to explore how a child learns, then borrowed by CAT to scaffold the pace of therapy effectively.

As an example, Lizzie, 12, was frequently distressed in school, and spent significant periods engaging in 'challenging' or 'stereotyped' behaviour. On assessment, it was apparent that this behaviour occurred as a way of soothing and occupying herself. Independent observations in the classroom showed that, before the 'behaviour', Lizzie would get distracted, 'zone out', become inattentive or appear increasingly anxious. There appeared to be a direct link between these behaviours and the complexity and demands of schoolwork. Lizzie struggled to understand instructions, made an error that she struggled to rectify or became shamed, distressed and overwhelmed. This resulted in ('self-to-self') soothing or self-occupying 'behaviours' as a coping mechanism.

Figure 3.1 draws out the patterns that show cognitive difficulties as procedures or cognitive strategies often used to cope with or move out of a relational state, such as feeling shamed or othered.

Figure 3.1: Cognitive difficulties or cognitive strategies

State – I feel… Lizzie was often in a shamed state

Aim – I intend/want/need/am expected to… Lizzie's intention was to soothe herself from this relational state of feeling shamed

Appraisal – I think/assume/predict/expect… Lizzie predicted 'zoning out' would be an efficient way of coping

Define task – I will soothe myself by zoning out

Plan – I remember/sequence/plot/set out how/compare with before

Execute – I do… Lizzie zones out

Evaluate – did this meet my intended aim? This aim can be discussed more with Lizzie after going through the above steps and validating how understandable and clever it is to choose zoning out to cope with shame.

2) The 'A' in CAT – Mapping the relational experience of having an intellectual disability

The experience of growing up with an intellectual disability or autism may be very different from neurotypical people, and the experience may be more impactful than the actual 'brain difference' itself. The therapist should be aware of the dynamics and experiences common to many people with these labels. Consider the language we use. I live in my own home. A person with an intellectual disability lives in a *residential* home. What does the additional word 'residential' add to your understanding of where we both live? The key difference is that I live with people I love: friends and family. Residential means, oddly, not a place to live but conveys the meaning that the other is not like 'normal' people. The other lives away from those they may choose to, and with people who share a similar label. The word 'residential' in this context carries a certain relational stance to someone with an intellectual disability. We treat them differently. By taking a relationally curious stance to this type of language, we can ask ourselves why this is and what impact it has.

When freed from the medical model's emphasis on deficit, and remediation as treatment, it is possible to have a relational understanding of identity and cognitive functioning where the disability occurs within a relationship or is understood between others. Disability and difference may then be experienced and accepted by either individual and can be explored between therapist and patient. Acceptance of disability as relational (and a transient characteristic of the therapist, or anyone for that matter, at times when we struggle with understanding or communication), may help the therapist work effectively at times when they feel they do not understand, feel disempowered or cannot think due to the pain or enormity of an experience.

In order to support Lizzie (in the example above) to successfully engage at school, it is important to consider not only what the caregiver is helping with (the task of learning) but also to construe the problem as more than a cognitive deficit (inability to learn) located within the young person. Rather, like the procedural map above, it is a different way of responding to feeling shamed. In being curious and considering that the issue as a 'relational rupture' in understanding the needs of the other, it is possible to adapt how the caregiver is helping (the relationship). CAT allows us to map the nuances of a helping relationship that may be needed at different times. A relational lens also allows for a different kind of curiosity about the young person's needs. Usually, the question about what the young person 'needs' when they have an intellectual disability is answered behaviourally: they need to 'stop inattention' or need to 'be on task'. This, in turn, is more likely to be responded to by 'teaching' (thereby potentially increasing demand and perpetuating the problem) or behavioural approaches, which are often punitive in nature, and perpetuate unhelpful experiences.

When considered relationally, the question 'what is going on for Lizzie?' results in an invitation to be attuned to her experience, resulting in an answer that allows the young person to thrive and feel included. Lizzie may need a variety of helping relationships, from showing, structuring and controlling (this is how you do it) through to attentive and curious (How are you? What is happening for you? Why are you struggling?), and encouraging, soothing and regulating her anxiety and shame.

Bruce Perry's work on trauma (Perry, 2022) is helpful here as he articulates the need to go through a variety of relational processes to support a young person to be an effective thinker and problem solver. He postulates that a young person needs help to regulate distress, then to engage and relate, before they can reason effectively. A CAT map can help Lizzie and the therapist locate that distress. Hughes and Baylin (2012) also construe care relationships as both relational and neurological in nature in their book *Brain-Based Parenting*, focusing on development as a dyadic, relational feedback system where child and parent mutually construe each other's behaviour and respond to promote healthy development and learning. CAT is a method of mapping for the individual these theoretical ideas, allowing a more personalised understanding of the problematic procedures and reciprocal roles for the young person.

3) Relational experiences of growing up as a child with intellectual disabilities

Psaila and Crowley (2006) looked at the common reciprocal roles experienced by people with intellectual disabilities. They found that people with intellectual disabilities had fewer relational roles and hypothesised that this may be linked to dependence and trauma. Commonly occurring roles were found to include:

- abusing-to-abused
- damaging-to-damaged
- rejecting-to-rejected
- abandoning-to-abandoned
- blaming-to-blamed
- overwhelming-to-overwhelmed
- rescuing/caring-to-rescued/cared for
- special/perfect-to-intellectual disabled
- controlling-to-controlled (and fragile)

The assumptions of others influence how we relate to them and ourselves. A young person may grow up with the expectation that they cannot do things and will always need care. They are less likely to be invited into relating equally or with mastery. They may not be encouraged to appraise and reflect, so, relationally, are not invited into opportunities to change problematic patterns impacting on them. This lack of trust in the young person's ability to appraise for themselves becomes a problematic pattern in its own right. A young person's struggles with learning also impact on mastery. Experiences of mastery allow for the possibility of *active participation* in change and interaction, as Ryle originally invited us to do (Ryle, 1991). The young person with intellectual disabilities will often be expected to passively occupy the 'done to' position in a relationship and not an active one.

Young people with intellectual disabilities will have more experience with paid carers as a proportion of their relationships than neurotypical peers. Paid or professional carers are defined by 'doing to'. They are a carer and therefore need to have someone to care for. The young person is expected to take the passive position of 'cared for', reinforcing a power differential. Wilberforce (2014) finds professional helping relationships to have an uncomfortable problem at their core. Wilberforce poses the question, "if we (professionals) are here to help, what it is the 'patient' here for, in relation to us?" He links this with being invited to feel helpless and unable to help themselves, since, otherwise, the relationship as it is constructed cannot exist.

Other, more natural relationships may be pathologised in the professional care relationship. The potential for love and friendship or equal relationships where a dyad negotiates caring and loving to cared for and loved at different times is less available in a relational field dominated by professional care.

CAT may not be as accessible as traditional one-to-one psychotherapy for some young people because of their disability. This chapter invites the reader not only to offer CAT as an individual therapy if funded and appropriate, but also to use CAT concepts as a way to expand relational thinking out of the therapy room and into day-to-day relationships for the young person. For this group of young people, it is important to consider how to give them a voice so they can go on to articulate their needs and experiences to others. To enable carers to alter their thinking of what they have been taught about this group of young people, the CAT reformulation is shared, with consent from the young person. To see them not as challenging, complex or special (all terms used to other and exclude), but more compassionately and inclusively as whole and trying to relate like any other person. This helps a team to do with rather than to do to.

This is where the role of the CAT letter, which provides a reformulation, may be different. In a typical therapy, the letter may be understood as a way for the therapist to convey directly to the young person a hopeful and compassionate understanding of their story – one that invites hope and possibility for change. While this also remains true for the young person with intellectual disabilities, it may additionally serve the function of integrating and amplifying the young person's voice for others. It can be seen as a way of encapsulating stories of social injustice, repeated in past and present relationships, that may have roots in a century of paternalistic and exclusory care models, and narrating how these have impacted on the young person in the context that is unique to them. It may allow for the therapist-young person dyad to call for change from others and find a way of engendering not just hope, but reflection in others who purport to care for the young person.

Challenging behaviour

Up to 15% of people with intellectual disabilities have been described at some point as being challenging (NICE, 2015). The term 'challenging behaviour' is essentially a relational construct (Varela, 2014). It is used to describe behaviour that we don't understand, gets in the way of our ordered way of seeing the world, and causes us distress. The labelling of another person as 'challenging' is interesting from a relational perspective. We are less questioning of why and how we are challenged and put the onus for change on the young person, rather than consider how we may move from feeling challenged. Once labelled as challenging, there is quickly an expectation that the young person 'stops' the behaviour, otherwise they could be excluded. The definition of challenging behaviour has historically been a curiously relational battle. Initially labelled as 'antisocial', 'maladaptive' etc, there was an attempt to relationally redefine it as challenging to us (behaviour that challenges), but the term has quickly been wrestled back into line as 'challenging behaviour' (NICE, 2015; RCP, 2016). Challenging behaviour is now construed as communication to others of a need or distress. However, the predominant model for people with neurodevelopmental disorders such as intellectual disabilities and autism has historically been behavioural, again, the focus being one of changing the person's behaviour rather than their environment, task, expectation or the person caring or relating with them.

Today, behaviourism remains the single most popular and commonly used model of support for these children, whether it be dressed up as Positive Behaviour Support (Nicholls, G et al 2023; CQC, 2017; NICE, 2015) or 'school rules' that are based on debunked 'token economy' type methodology. However, the majority of behavioural interventions are not delivered by trained professionals but are devised by support staff seemingly re-enacting parent-child relationships when they were children themselves: for example, adults in their lives telling them they would cut pocket money, ban TV time or ground them as consequences for their behaviour.

In order to be practised ethically, it can be argued that any behavioural intervention should be delivered through a relational frame, which explicitly sets out to articulate both the beliefs and aims of the (challenged) appraiser as well as of the (challenging) young person. It should also set out to develop a relational map of the problematic interaction and exits that seek not to 'eliminate' the behaviour but to set out how the relational and behavioural dance will be more mutually beneficial in the future.

'It's behavioural': problem behaviour and the problem with behaviourism

It is a basic truism that all relational behaviour at the heart of CAT is essentially stimulus-response (Bancroft *et al*, 2008). Taking a radically relational approach to supporting children with intellectual disability helps to expose ethical and functional flaws in the application of behaviour analysis. It also helps us to understand that behavioural approaches such as punishment are many times more powerfully reinforcing for the punisher (adult) than the punished (young person).

Figure 3.2: Power and problems in working with challenging behaviour

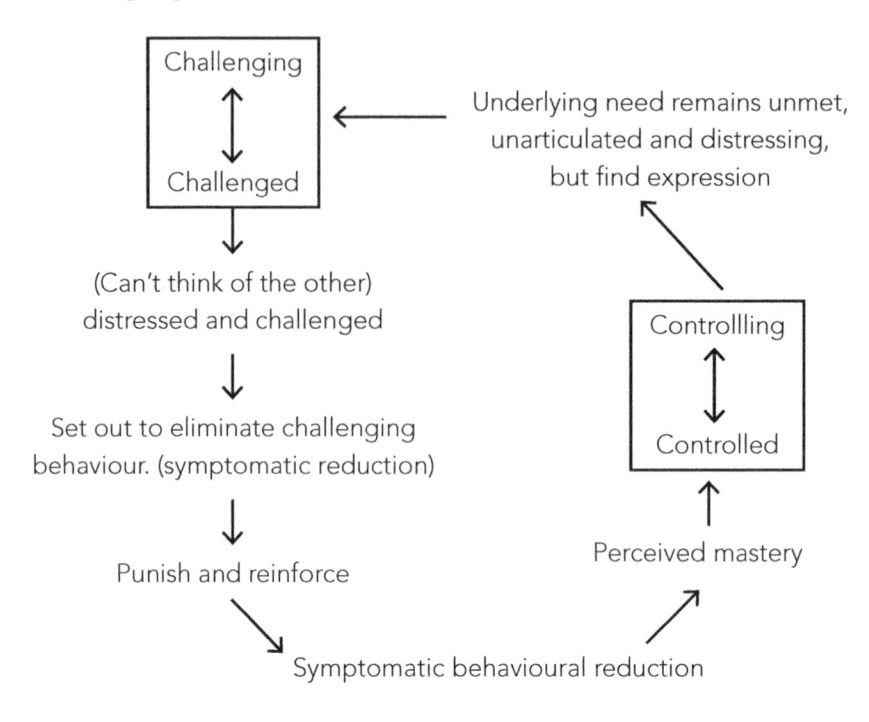

```
    Challenging
        ↕               ←——— Underlying need remains unmet,
    Challenged                unarticulated and distressing,
        ↓                     but find expression
                                              ↖
  (Can't think of the other)
  distressed and challenged          Controlling
        ↓                                 ↕
  Set out to eliminate challenging    Controlled
  behaviour. (symptomatic reduction)      ↑
        ↓                          Perceived mastery
  Punish and reinforce                   ↗
         ↘  Symptomatic behavioural reduction
```

In this scenario, the 'punisher' is highly unlikely to elicit from the young person with significant intellectual disabilities, the desired response of learning a new way of being and problem-solving. CAT enables us to articulate that, only through co-learning, with the adult sculpting, scaffolding and shaping, can the child develop their own adult self and start to explore self and agency independently.

CAT offers us the opportunity to *reformulate*, starting with exploring the world through the lens of the adult and validating their experiences, understandings, frustrations and attempts at solutions while also holding in mind the effects of these on the young person. Without doing so, it is difficult to form a working alliance. Behavioural techniques and tools may be integrated successfully into CAT (Varela, 2014).

The little monster formulation

Lee was 11 when he was referred to me. He was accompanied by a label of 'moderate intellectual disability' and a list of sins. He attended with his father with an air of bemusement as if floating or blundering through a world he did not fully understand. His father did not mince his words. I was informed that his son was a 'little monster' who made every attempt to thwart the parenting interventions of the whole family and caused general chaos. It was challenging. Lee was challenging. He needed sorting. He had been brought to psychology for 'sorting out' – I was going to 'sort him out'. I started with a general assessment, getting to know him and his world a little more. Attempts at making tentative links with the impact of an intellectual disability on Lee and various traumatic family events were cast aside, with a firm assertion from Lee's father of the initial formulation. He was just a 'little monster'. Getting nowhere fast with various attempts at inviting a different formulation, we drew the current one.

Figure 3.3: The little monster formulation

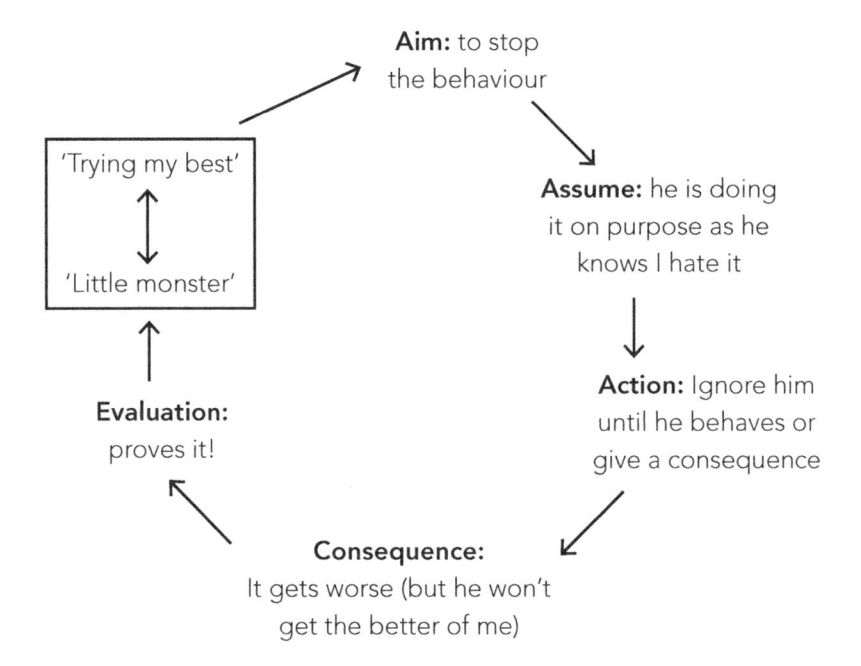

'Trying my best' ↕ 'Little monster'

Aim: to stop the behaviour

Assume: he is doing it on purpose as he knows I hate it

Action: Ignore him until he behaves or give a consequence

Consequence: It gets worse (but he won't get the better of me)

Evaluation: proves it!

Once this was completed and acknowledged as a way of understanding, we looked at whether it was helpful and agreed that it was not, as it was not changing the status quo. Mindful that we needed to work within the ZPD of the family, I was able to introduce some behavioural ideas, such as functional analysis, to check the validity of our formulation. Functional analysis is an observational method that invites a different stance to the 'problem'. It involves an active, structured curiosity that attempts to review what wider factors, such as interoceptive skills as well as relational, may be impacting patterns of behaviour. In this case, it opened up the possibility that Lee's behaviour was used by him to communicate something other than a wish for 'mischief at whatever cost'. Lee's behaviour was an attempt at communication to relate, and once functional patterns had been mapped, it was clear that he was communicating a need for attuned support so that he was not overwhelmed by a demanding world. It was easier when reformulated to find exits that were accessible and more relationally helpful to Lee and his family: being attentive to the need to support someone struggling in a challenging world.

Figure 3.4: The little monster reformulation

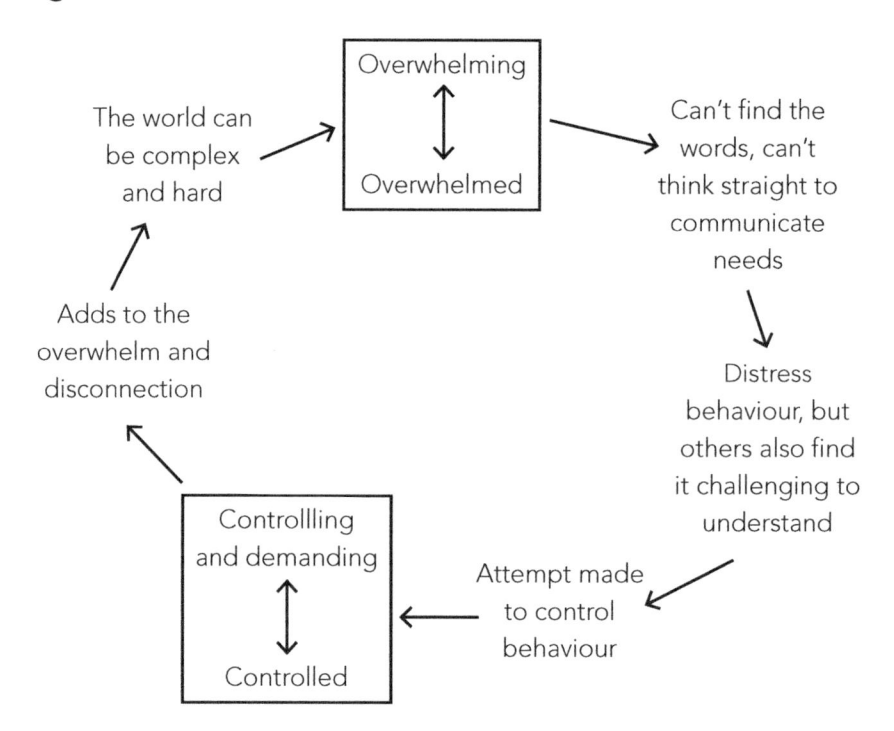

The world can be complex and hard → Overwhelming ⇅ Overwhelmed → Can't find the words, can't think straight to communicate needs ↓ Distress behaviour, but others also find it challenging to understand → Attempt made to control behaviour → Controlling and demanding ⇅ Controlled ↖ Adds to the overwhelm and disconnection

CAT and working with young autistic people: who is struggling to understand who?

Research suggests that emotional health difficulties are much more common in autistic young people. "Up to 70% of 10–14-year-olds have at least one other psychiatric disorder and 41% have two or more" (BPS, 2021). Autistic people are shown to have high levels of thwarted belonging, one of the possible causes of emotional distress (Mitchel et al, 2021).

Despite initial conceptualisations of autism as a disorder that is identifiable by a deficit in empathy, communication and understanding of others, a more recent frame considers autism to be a central identity, neurodivergence being something that should be accepted and accommodated by others and which places difficulties in the arena of interpersonal relations. Understanding others is thought to be mutual and transactional. It follows that deficit does not reside in an autistic individual but in 'double empathy' difficulties (Milton, 2012). CAT procedural sequences can be used to explore assumptions and relational patterns of self and others. Mapping is a helpful tool in formulating how these patterns keep being repeated and navigating the interpersonal world more effectively. Because of difficulties in understanding abstract social material, autistic individuals may struggle to imagine future scenarios and predict how they and others will feel and respond and may be highly anxious. CAT maps offer a literal 'road script' or map with which to approach scenarios (Murphy, 2008). Developing co-constructed relational maps helps autistic people see the bigger picture rather than focus on details or literal iterations of patterns. Being a highly visual therapy can also be of aid (Victoria, 2015).

A common way of coping with expectations and confusion in the social arena for autistic young people is to camouflage and mask. When working using the collaborative, reformulation and relational approach of CAT, supporting autistic people to understand problematic cycles as between people rather than within them, places their distress in the context of the belief and assumptions and reactions of others, and in language that validates their experience. Distress is then understood as being a product of being isolated, placed under pressure, misunderstood, controlled or rejected and is within the scope of human experience, rather than seen as some sort of deficit peculiar to them. Maps of these repeating patterns and their exits can be developed to explore other ways of coping and being, including embodying the authentic self without the need to engage in masking as a way of coping.

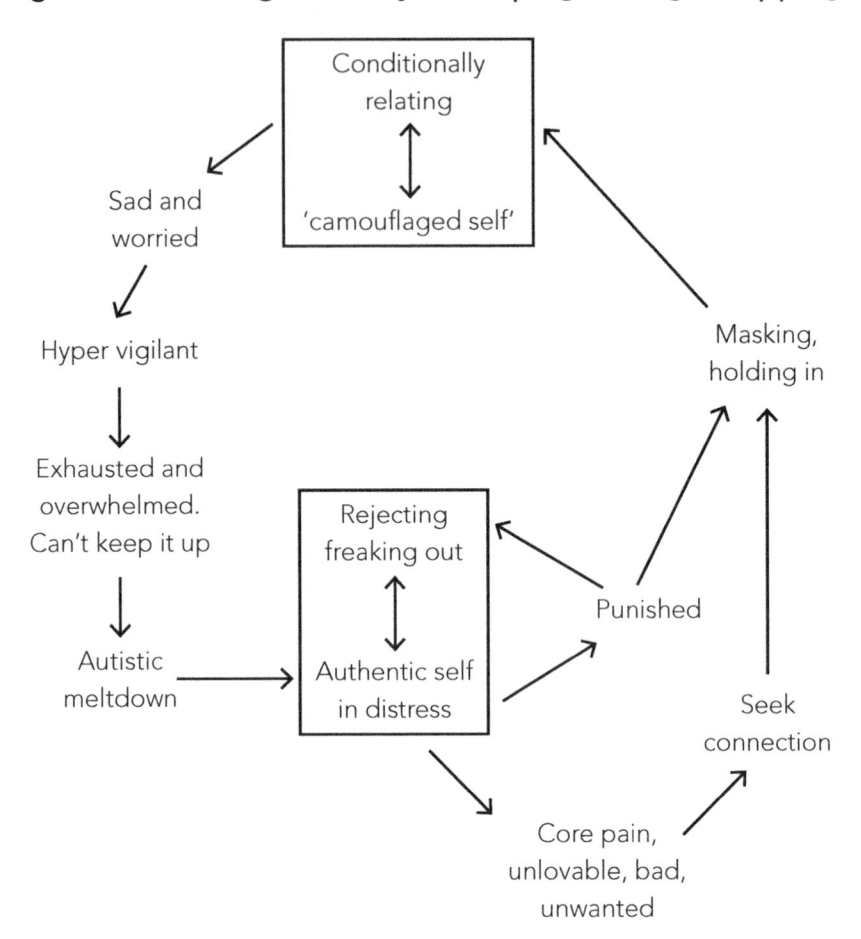

Figure 3.5: Finding new ways of coping through mapping

```
         Conditionally
           relating
              ↕
        'camouflaged self'
```

Sad and worried

Hyper vigilant

Exhausted and overwhelmed. Can't keep it up

Autistic meltdown

Rejecting freaking out
↕
Authentic self in distress

Masking, holding in

Punished

Seek connection

Core pain, unlovable, bad, unwanted

Conclusion

Neurodiverse young people and young people with intellectual disability may benefit from a relational and curious approach as an alternative to behavioural approaches steeped in a problematic past. CAT can invite relational understandings of their experiences rather than viewing them through a lens of deficit, allowing us as professionals and helpers to be curious about language and roles that have historically invited control and manipulation as a substitute for care. It also encourages us to question our assumptions about what young people would like to communicate to us about their hopes and needs.

Chapter 4:
Relational practice is inclusive practice – working alongside LGBTQA+ young people

Victoria Ryall

Introduction

This chapter is intended to help service providers to offer a safe and appropriate experience for lesbian, gay, bisexual, trans and gender diverse, queer, asexual plus (LGBTQA+ [4, 5]) young people through adopting a relational approach. Such an approach is more likely to enable open discussion about gender and sexuality and improve access to care and help-seeking (Australian Institute of Family Studies, 2022).

A relational approach to working with LGBTQA+ youth offers a framing that supports and builds a space that allows for a young person to safely explore their identity – and thus individuate or develop a separate but connected sense of self – one of the main tasks of adolescence. A relational approach described by Cognitive Analytic Therapy (CAT) states that we develop and maintain who we are through social interactions which occur within broader cultural contexts (Ryle & Kerr, 2002). CAT is both a psychological therapy, used to support individuals, and an understanding of the development of the self being created socially or in relation to other people (Lloyd & Pollard, 2019). CAT can also be useful for gaining a macro-level understanding. It acknowledges that experiences are

---
4   Variations of the acronym LGBTQA+ exist: the most commonly used with young people is LGBTQIA+. For this discussion, I have removed 'I' given that this discussion does not include reference to young people with intersex variation, though I acknowledge their unique experience and encourage readers to undertake an understanding of the experience of people with intersex variations (Carman *et al*, 2020).
5   LGBTQA+ comprises a hugely diverse group of people and communities, each with distinct experiences, needs and backgrounds. This chapter is a brief discussion. It does not seek to represent the full range of identities and intersections that comprise LGBTQA+ people.

impacted by the societies we live in, and by our class, race, gender identity and sexual orientation (Lloyd & Pollard, 2019). A relational approach therefore not only provides a socio-cultural context, but also a guide for the worker on how to work with someone who is exploring identity and self in a world that can feel restricted or closed. This approach not only seeks to understand how people develop in relationships and culture, but also informs how we can use the helping relationship to promote change or growth, through new relational experiences such as acceptance and curiosity.

In Australia, like many other countries, people who identify as LBTIQA+ have been and continue to be discriminated against or 'othered' (Ferfolja & Ullman, 2020). Mental health problems including suicide and self-harm are statistically higher for the LGBTQA+ community. However, it is often not clarified that continued experiences of discrimination – not gender or sexual identities – leave LGBTQA+ people with poorer health outcomes in comparison to non LGBTQA+ young people (Hill *et al*, 2020). The problem is relational and so a relational approach is required to support the well-being of LGBTQA+ youth.

As a result of gradual social change, achieved through collective action and increased representation on social media and television, LGBTQA+ communities have become more accepted in some countries (Ferfolja & Ullman, 2020). However, significant discrimination and prejudice continue where LGBTQA+ people remain "objects of loathing" (Ferfolja & Ullman, 2020). The experience of being othered or 'hated' is reinforced when events such as anti-trans or anti-gay activism occurs. The relational effects of discrimination and feeling unsafe or unaccepted in the community have severe negative effects on mental health. A relational framework helps workers and young people not only consider how being related to as 'other' can negatively affect their development, but also help identify ways of relating within a working relationship that allows for exploration and the acceptance of diversity and difference.

Language, gender and sexuality

A brief understanding of the language associated with the journey of gender and sexual identity development is important to any discussion exploring LGBTQA+ communities (Australian Institute of Family Studies, 2022). Discussion about language and past and current identity development offers insights into the present social-cultural context of LGBTQA+ youth. From a relational perspective, this is an important consideration as the language we use signals to others how open and informed we are. This openness, or curious stance, often represented through language, allows young people the space to be more openly and authentically themselves.

Words hold relational and cultural meanings, and terminology used by LGBTQIA+ young people may include words that are understood differently among community members and others outside the community. Further, the language around gender and sexuality is rapidly evolving (Carman *et al*, 2020). The evolution of language is likely a reflection of societal changes in our understanding of gender and sexuality (Ruberg & Ruelos, 2020). There is growing recognition that language, gender and sexuality are becoming increasingly multiracial, intersectional, queer and trans-inclusive (Calder, 2020). However, there is room for improvement around language use. *Free to be… yet?* surveys young people aged 13-18 across Australian schools. The report notes that homophobic language is a weekly if not daily occurrence for respondents (Ullman, 2021). An alarming 93% of LGBTQA+ students had heard homophobic language at schools, whereas only 6% reported that adults intervened to stop such language (Ullman, 2021). While transphobic language was reported slightly less overall (71%), students also noted that adults were less likely to intervene (Ullman, 2021).

'Sexuality' is understood to be the sum of our sexual interests, identity orientation, expressions and desires (Ruberg & Ruelos, 2020). 'Sexual identity' refers to our individual identity in relation to our sexuality. For example, we may identify as bisexual, queer, lesbian etc. 'Sexual orientation' is like 'sexual identity'. It describes a person's sexual and romantic interests. The word 'queer' can be both an umbrella term for those in the LGBTQA+ communities and a description of a person's identity, political positions and experiences related to sexuality and gender. Some views, which are not unanimous, also suggest that queerness resists social norms (Ruberg & Ruelos, 2020).

Gender is conceptualised separately from biologically assigned sex. 'Gender' is understood as a socially and culturally constructed personal identity (Ruberg & Ruelos, 2020). 'Transgender' or 'trans' refers to people whose gender identity does not match the gender they were assigned at birth. 'Cis gender', conversely, refers to individuals whose gender matches the gender they were assigned at birth. 'Nonbinary'[6] refers to individuals who do not identify as either men or women, girls or boys or whose gender identity does not fit within a binary gender construct (Australian Institute of Family Studies, 2022). People may identify as gender fluid if they feel their gender identity is changing or gender questioning, indicating someone who may be unsure which (if any) gender they identify with (Australian Institute of Family Studies, 2022).

The above definitions are further understood to be socially, culturally and time bound. For example, the current dominant heteronormative model of coupled romantic monogamy emerged in the late 1800s and early 1900s (Barker, 2017). Additionally, social and cultural understandings of sex, gender, sexuality and relationships vary across the world. Some cultures do not separate gender and sexuality as predominately white and Western cultures do (Barker, 2017).

Consideration and use of current terminology, its history and its importance to the community, is part of a relational understanding, and it advances the view that the information itself may enable more inclusive care (McDermott et al, 2021). We need inclusive care that not only provides the safety and support any young person requires, but offers a curious and reflective space where the relational effects of being LGBTQA+ are recognised and explored so the young person can move towards feeling supported and OK about who they are, even if it is different to their peers. Further, non-inclusive language raises a relational red flag for a young person indicating that they are (again) in an unsafe situation.

Identity development and relational approach

I have been fortunate to spend almost all of my near thirty-year career working with 'young people', commonly defined in the youth mental health sector in Australia as people between the ages of 12 and 25 years of age. What gives me particular satisfaction is walking alongside young people as they explore their identities. My work, influenced by CAT, helps me develop a curious and reflective relationship with young people

---

[6] While some nonbinary people identify outside of the binary (neither men or women/boys or girls), others may not identify as solely men or women, i.e. they may feel like they sometimes identify as women or men and other times as outside of the binary altogether, and some may not identify with having any gender, which is also known as *agender*.

while they explore who they are without having imposed on them certain pressures or binaries that they may receive from others.

The development of the self from a CAT perspective is viewed as being shaped and maintained through our interactions with others (Ryle & Kerr, 2002). The characteristics that we are born with interact reciprocally with the people immediately around us (in a given culture and at a given time). These interactions (or relational experiences) are internalised, continuing to guide how we relate to ourselves and how we relate to others (Ryle & Kerr, 2002).

Identity development is one of the significant developmental tasks associated with youth. Sexuality and romantic relationships are both important parts of the development of a young person's identity (Bates *et al*, 2020).

Gender identity

Gender identity is our sense of whether we are a man, woman, non-binary, gender queer, agender or genderfluid, or a combination of one or more of these (Australian Institute of Family Studies, 2022). It is recognised that input from the world around us has an enormous influence on what it means to be male or female, and arguably that the world is and should be divided into these binary gender concepts (Wallace, 2015).

Gender identity has, over time, been conceptualised in many ways, including how a person's identity does or doesn't align with physical sex characteristics, how it does or doesn't fit with socially prescribed gender roles, and how people may experience differing degrees of gender dysphoria; distress associated with incongruence between experienced and assigned gender (Steensma *et al*, 2013). Most of these discourses explore gender in a predominantly binary way: female or male. Over the last decade, a less binary, more dimensional and diverse view of gender identity has gained prominence. Gender diversity is now largely understood along a spectrum (Ferfolja & Ullman, 2020). Concurrently, in recent years there has been a sharp increase in young people presenting for support from gender clinics. This increase in presentations may be due to the increased availability of gender care but is also likely affected by changes in social acceptance of gender diversity.

Some individuals' gender identities may not be associated with distress and these young people may not seek treatment and or may not want any medical treatment to change their gender (Steensma et al, 2013). For some young people, their gender identity is part of who they are, and it's not a cause of concern (Steensma et al, 2013). Other trans young people do want access to affirming care, and many report difficulties accessing services with appropriate expertise and specialist knowledge. Unfortunately, many report experiences of discriminatory care and feeling disrespected through their help-seeking journey (Strauss et al, 2022). Further, these access issues are compounded by insufficient accessible services (Strauss et al, 2022).

Several research pieces acknowledge that young people who identify as transgender experience disparities in violence, victimisation, substance use, suicidal risk and other risks when compared with their cis-gendered peers (Johns et al, 2019; Hill et al, 2021).

A relational perspective can help make sense of the varied impact of the range of social and cultural understandings of gender as they may relate to a young person's gender identity. These socio-cultural phenomena impact on young, gender-diverse people and are important to understand in order to provide safe and appropriate support. A relational perspective helps workers position themselves in an informed, curious, open and exploratory way in order to seek to understand a young person's gender identity.

Sexual identity

Sexual identity development is a key aspect of identity formation (Realista et al, 2019). Many young people experience difficulties in the development of a positive sexual identity. LGBTQA+ young people face additional challenges due to social stigma and associated discrimination (Realista et al, 2019).

The last few decades have seen significant cultural and social changes associated with sexuality and gender diversity (Bishop et al, 2020). Many young people who are exploring their identities may be doing so in the context of new understandings about gender and sexuality that go beyond heteronormative and binary concepts (Bishop et al, 2020). These social changes have seen young people 'coming out' earlier in their life and have also necessitated a new understanding of how sexual identity develops (Bishop et al, 2020).

Previous models outlined a more linear, somewhat uniform process, that did not consider interpersonal and sociocultural factors (Bishop *et al*, 2020). This linear model was limited as it did not fit with current sexual identities, which are more continuous and are shaped by social and interpersonal contexts (Bishop *et al*, 2020). 'Milestones' was another model of understanding sexual identity development. It described young people's identity consistently with specific milestones: experiencing attraction, self-identifying, engaging in sexual behaviour and then disclosure of identity (Bishop *et al*, 2020). More appropriate and relevant models acknowledge both the historical timing of the development as well as the life-stage impact of identity formation (Bishop *et al*, 2020). Further, an intersectional perspective considers how various social factors and components of an individual's identity (such as sexuality, race, class and gender) interconnect to influence one's experiences of oppression and privilege. Following this logic, sexuality cannot be considered in isolation and should be understood in the young person's individual social and cultural context (Bishop *et al*, 2020). The life course and intersectional perspectives together enable consideration of a range of contextual influences on sexual identity development which better represents the diversity evident in young people's current identities. These models also align better with a relational perspective on gender and sexual identity.

CAT's relational understanding of the development of the self, incorporating Vygotskian activity theory and Bakhtin dialogism, share some features with social constructionist accounts of sexuality that suggest that people learn to be sexual through both interpersonal and external factors. People pick up cues and information from those around them and the society they live in, which teach them that sex means something, and that particular activities and identities have certain values and meanings. Further, from a relational perspective, how others perceive and respond to a person's expressed sexual identity greatly impacts how they see themselves and their place in the world (McCormack *et al*, 2014).

When working individually with young people from a relational viewpoint, we explore interpersonal relationships, social contexts and macro environments. For LGBTQA+ young people, a relational perspective helps us stand back and consider that person's experiences in the development of their identity and how particular experiences may repeat both macro and interpersonal experiences of being othered or discriminated against. In some parts of the world, LGBTQA+ people face criminalisation and violent repression (Brown, 2019). There is evidence that unequal societies generate more troubled and troubling societies (Brown, 2019). People with non-heterosexual identities were historically classified as having a mental illness. A relational viewpoint recognises that these contextual factors will have had an impact on young people's intra- and interpersonal experiences of their gender and sexuality.

For example, if a young person is of South Indian background and identifies as bisexual, their identity will be explored in the context of how their communities (however defined) have responded or may respond, how their family (however defined) has or may respond, how their peers have or may respond, and how they are thinking and feeling about their identity. This would be different to someone who identifies as bisexual in an Anglo-Saxon, Western family from Melbourne. A relational framework recognises not only the relational effects of feeling different but also how they can be explored in a safe and culturally fitting way. A relational approach provides a guide to discussing this with young people, how they can feel able to relate enough in their world to build on this for more safety and openness later. A relational framework is not prescriptive. Being prescriptive would somehow replay this idea that there is a correct way (or pathway) of being.

The sexuality and gender identity of young LGBTQA+ people are not static nor singular (Ruberg & Ruelos, 2020). Research indicates that our understanding of our sexuality and gender identity is overlapping. For some of us, it's incomplete, and for many it is continuously evolving. That is, young LGBTQA+ identities are highly nuanced, unique, temporal and intersectional (Ruberg & Ruelos, 2020).

Positive relating leads to positive identity development

Many LGBTQA+ people experience loving relationships and a strong sense of connection to their communities (Carman *et al*, 2020). It is noted that positive life experiences can come from challenging norms, finding an authentic expression of identity and consciously creating chosen social networks and communities. Many LGBTQA+ people experience comfort and pleasure in engaging openly with themselves and others about their identity (Carman *et al*, 2020). In *Writing Themselves in 4* (a national survey of health and well-being among LGBTQA+ young people in Australia), over 95% of young people had disclosed their identity to friends and over 71% to their families. Many young people reported having attended an LGBTQA+ group in the previous twelve months, and over 22% accessed health information specific to LGBTQA+ people.

Many young people reported having stood up for the rights of their LGBTQA+ peers. When asked what made them feel good, young people noted the value of social connectivity, romantic relationships, feeling good about themselves from within, being affirmed by others, and positive social change (Hill *et al*, 2021). Having a relational response in a bigger group that is affirming or empowering can help young people explore their own individual identity while feeling hidden enough to do so safely. When people feel isolated, they spend most time looking outwards, and are ready to be criticised or rejected. Groups that young people identify with provide the safety needed for them to say, "I'm different and I belong".

When young people feel accepted, they will have stronger self-esteem and feel safer from psychological distress. This is further improved when young people can disclose their identities in a safe and supportive environment (Realista *et al*, 2019). Evidence suggests that if young people are able to establish a healthy identity their risk factors for other difficulties decrease (Realista *et al*, 2019).

Below are the experiences of two LGBTQA+ young people and an account of how they continue to explore their own identity, and what has helped and what hasn't.

Iz (age 17)

I identify as non-binary (using they/them pronouns), asexual and a lesbian.

I grew up in a very accepting environment, which I'm very grateful for, especially since a lot of LGBT children don't get that. I had several family members and family friends who identified as LGBT in some way. I think I realised I wasn't straight when I was nine or ten, but I wasn't sure what identity fit yet. I remember thinking at some point that I had to have a crush on a boy, because that was the way the kids at my school saw it (many of whom now also identify as LGBT). I often mistook a desire to be friends with another boy I was acquainted with as romantic interest. In Year 6, I remember having several crushes on girls, which was the moment I fully realised that I was gay. →

In Year 7, I found a group of friends who were either LGBT themselves or allies. It made me very glad because I finally had people my age to talk to about being LGBT. One of my close friends in Year 7 identified as bisexual and told me I "should be bi" because then I would have "more options", which I now realise was a problematic thing to say, but then I was 13 and pretty gullible, so I identified as bisexual for about two weeks before I realised it didn't fit me at all.

What I enjoy most about my sexuality and gender identity now is that I'm comfortable in it. I am finally in a place where I feel as if I can be myself around the people I hang out with, and I can talk freely to them about LGBT-related topics. A lot of people in my grade are allies, and although I can't really talk to them about being gay because they aren't, it's good to know that they accept me for who I am.

The most difficult aspect for any LGBT person is obviously homophobia, and considering I go to a Catholic school, there are some days when I feel like I have to hide who I am so I can be accepted, and just to keep myself safe. Despite that, I have a lot of people who I know will accept me, so I don't think about it as much. Another difficult aspect for me was figuring out my identity. My sexuality was easier to figure out, and so were my pronouns, but it took me quite a while to find a gender identity that fit me.

Lu (age 15)

I identify as transgender male, and bisexual with a preference for women. This identity might change in the future, because I am still discovering who I am.

A memorable moment for me occurred when I was around eleven. I heard about something called 'non-binary' and I thought, *That feels right for me, rather than being female.* I changed my name, my hair and my pronouns. I suddenly felt that I had to completely change my appearance in order to 'look trans'. I think this was an expectation represented in the world of queerness because a lot of trans people look different to how they would look as their assigned gender. →

> After about two years of identifying as non-binary, I realised that I was male, and didn't have to look like anything or anyway in particular to be able to identify as a man. I knew that being a heterosexual, cis-gender woman was not the right title for me, so when I changed it, I expected people to be more surprised, but a lot of the time, family and friends seemed to think that this was a teenage attention-seeking thing.
>
> I enjoy finding safe queer spaces, like 4ZZZ FM program Queer Radio, being surrounded by queer youth groups, and being able to relate to other queer and transgender people around me. Another fun aspect of being part of the LGBTQIA+ community is to be able to protest and show homophobes, transphobes, biphobes and all the other... phobes... that they can never take down our community because we are stronger than you think.
>
> It can be difficult, at times, to tell people how I identify without the fear of being dismissed or told that my personal identity is a phase or childish. Or even being judged for the way I dress, and it not matching with what some people think a certain gender should look like.
>
> I have felt like the black sheep in the family when I identified as non-binary, and no one else in the family had expressed any gender dysphoria. Having a queer space with other trans youth and adults is so crucial for a teenager to have, because having a trans role model that you can learn from and relate to is such a great support system. Without finding this support, it's difficult to authentically express who you are and experiment with different identities without being judged for it. It felt scary and different at first, but that feeling never fully went away. But, with help, I can feel comfortable with myself.

Relational practice offers a useful way of ensuring we are aware of ourselves and how we engage with an LGBTQA+ young person. Working relationally supports us to be aware of the experiences a young LGBTQA+ person has had, offering a way of connecting that allows them to continue to openly explore their identity. Here are some suggestions for relational practice:

- Explore and recognise your own experiences and biases related to gender and sexual identity. For instance, my own experience as a bi/pan sexual woman in my early 50s is very different to many young people I have seen in private practice. I need to continue to educate myself about changing language and young people's experiences of their identities.

- Recognise that LGBTQA+ young people are impacted by their social and cultural contexts (as is evident throughout this discussion). These experiences impact young LGBTQA+ people and may result in internalised homo-, trans- or other phobias. Most LGBTQA+ young people live in a context that is cis-heteronormative and therefore are likely to have been 'othered', had erroneous assumptions made about them and/or been discriminated against. Try not to replicate non-inclusive experiences a person may have previously had.

- Take an intersectional approach and recognise that young people's identity is evolving and may change.

- Understand that many LGBTQA+ young people may have experienced trauma associated with hate, prejudice and discrimination. Ask gently about this and ensure you are in a position to provide trauma-informed care (Bendall *et al*, 2018).

- Explore where they can connect with peers. Social media provides LGBTQA+ young people with daily access to a broader social-cultural dialogue that may support them in their exploration of their emerging identity. It may also provide a safe and accepting environment to interact with similar young people across geographic boundaries. Social media can also provide some anonymity (or pseudo anonymity) which may enable expression, disclosure and continued development of a young person's identity as it emerges, changes and shifts over time (Bates *et al*, 2020).

(For more on LGBTQA+, see LGBTQA+ inclusive practice (Stephens *et al*, 2013)).

Services should:

- Ensure the environment you provide for LGBTQA+ young people is overtly inclusive with the use of LGBTQA+ flags, images of LGBTQA+ young people, and self-determined pronouns. LGBTQA+ young people will have experienced exclusion and therefore understandably may be more alert to signs that they are unwelcome in spaces.

- Stay informed about LGBTQA+ issues and language. A useful glossary can be found at https://aifs.gov.au/sites/default/files/publication-

documents/22-02_rs_lgbtiqa_glossary_of_common_terms_0.pdf (accessed August 2023).
- Create and maintain links with local LGBTQA+ organisations.
- Engage young LGBTQA+ people to review all processes and tools ensuring that any feedback they have is heard and, where possible, acted on.

This brief and inherently limited discussion has been an incredible privilege to work on. As a queer, bi or pan sexual-identifying woman currently in a same-sex relationship, it has reminded me of the context I am in, how the world has changed and is changing, and that less binary notions of gender seem to have opened up experiences of sexuality in a way that feels to me both freeing and hopeful. I was reminded that I never really used labels such as 'bisexual', 'queer' or 'lesbian', and of my own experiences of being othered by both the heterosexual and lesbian communities. I recall accusations of my sexuality being 'fashionable' and am saddened that, for Lu (and likely others), this experience continues to occur. A relational framework such as the one supported by CAT can inform us not only how to be curious and supportive, but can also guide us in formulating how the relational effects of being LGBTQA+ in our world, culture, community and family is affecting the young person's identity development (in positive and negative ways). This understanding can inform a plan to help young people find relationships where they are accepted as 'whole' and learn to do this for themselves as adults and pass it on to the next generation.

Chapter 5:
The power of an embodied approach to CAT with young adults

Caroline Greenwood Dower

"We are all in the process of becoming" – Audre Lorde

We are all in the process of becoming. With every breath we take, every move we make, we create an experience of ourselves in the world that goes on to inform the next moment. This is true for all of us throughout life, but there are periods in life when our process of becoming is foreground; changes in our relationships, living situation, occupation, body, bereavement. Sometimes we choose to make the changes. Sometimes they happen anyway. Our becoming is always shaped by changes in the expectations of those around us. In my therapeutic work with young adults, I am struck by the potent combination of changes they are experiencing, and the frustrations they face when there are constraints on the possibility for change. The young adults who present to services are often painfully aware of how they are becoming or how hard it is for them to become the person they want to be, or the person others want them to be.

In this chapter, I describe how my therapeutic experience with young adults has informed, and in parts transformed, my practice of CAT. My intention is twofold:

- For professionals new to CAT, to highlight the features of CAT that make it a containing, flexible and responsive relational model for this particular cohort.
- For CAT professionals seeking to develop their work with young adults, to propose a subtle reorientation of key CAT principles towards an embodied practice to enhance the model's effectiveness.

My contribution rests on a foundation of practice with young adults between the ages of 18 and 25 in higher education, private practice and physical health clinics in the UK's National Health Service. It does not reflect therapeutic practice in in-patient or residential settings, so I welcome a dialogue with those working with young people in those contexts.

I begin with a brief sketch of the key elements of a CAT approach across all life-stages and move on to discuss a perspective on the young adult experience that informs my practice. While embodied approaches are now widespread across psychotherapies and approaches to well-being, I argue that, in places, these also risk an objectification of the body and experience. Phenomenology – as a philosophy and an implied psychotherapeutic method – is proposed as an important counter to these objectifying tendencies, by placing the young person's subjectivity of relational, embodied awareness at the heart of the work. I use a brief composite vignette of the therapeutic process to show how a phenomenologically inflected CAT offers a potent approach. It clarifies, makes sense of and expands the repertoire of relational experience.

Key features of CAT

From its inception, CAT was conceived as a collaborative approach to psychotherapy. Working closely and transparently with the client, CAT aspires to distil the experience of distress into an understanding of how habitual ways of relating to others and to oneself have become limited, and hence problematic. The aim of therapy is to bring these patterns of relating and coping into awareness by exploring both the client's history, their present-day relationships and their relationship with the therapist. A time-limited intervention, CAT illuminates and retains a focus on a core relational theme. Individualised 'reformulations' are narrative and diagrammatic explanations that reflect the highly subjective and contextual nature of the client's distress. The explicit intention of a CAT approach is twofold. First, the focus on an area of distress concentrates attention on identifying new relational possibilities, all the more potent if they arise organically in the therapeutic relationship. Second, the intention is to handover the skills of relational reflection such that, at the end of therapy, the client can offer a similar support to themselves.

As I encountered CAT in the 1990s, three aspects of the CAT model were particularly attractive. First, CAT's time limit was not simply a pragmatic response to service demands; rather, from the outset there was a respect for the autonomy of the client, the desire to offer a potent therapy and to handover the tools for self-support. Second, the model of change felt inclusive and non-aggressive. Change is not transformation, nor personality-overhaul. The idea of change as a collaboratively generated expansion of the relational repertoire, and as a greater capacity for reflection, is a gentler and more respectful stance towards our clients. Third, the model lends itself towards a recognition of the social and political field – the forces that have acted historically and those that act in the present to shape relational possibilities. This contextualisation of distress offers considerable therapeutic support and is a meaningful bulwark to overly individualised or medicalised perspectives.

Key features of the field for young adults

I propose a model that emphasises the subjectivity of our experience of the world, so it would be incongruous to describe the features of young adults as a homogenous group with readily identifiable, shared characteristics. Rather, a more appropriate starting point is to acknowledge the field within which the young adults of my experience (in the UK, presenting for therapeutic support) have lived to date.

The 25 years of my therapeutic practice have been in a culture with increased discourse around psychological or mental well-being. It is rare now to encounter young adults who are not familiar with the language of anxiety, depression or stress, from their families, education settings and the media. De-stigmatisation and psychoeducation have undoubtedly benefitted many. The increase in demand for therapeutic support is in part a positive development, but it has entailed the adoption of simplified explanatory models, self-help workbooks and manualised approaches. For some, these offer a helpful nudge into new ways of thinking, feeling or behaving that suffice. I recognise the challenge to deliver low-cost, high-volume symptomatic relief. There are, however, unintended and unfortunate consequences of these approaches. One powerful consequence is that, in didactic approaches of psychoeducation, when young people are 'taught about' their experience, actual experience can be overlooked in favour of the objectified position handed over in the models, descriptions, or casual use of clinical terms.

The objectification of the self and self-experience may be exacerbated by the media. Passive viewing of idealised body forms or lifestyles has been more widely available through childhood and adolescent formative years. Active engagement with social media encourages a high level of reflection upon oneself and how to present oneself. To be conscious of oneself and to manage one's presentation are enduring human traits; the capacity to 'post' images of oneself and one's life so frequently and widely is a more recent phenomenon.

The wider provision of publicly funded and education-based support services is both a response to, and a possible catalyst for, psychological help-seeking. Again, we can view this as a positive development, but it is important to note that the encouragement to seek support (from families, teachers, peers) can also run counter to the broader developmental project of the shift from situations of dependency and care towards autonomy and individuation. This potentially places young adults in the ambivalent position of both needing and seeking support and simultaneously wanting to push away, to break free and to secure an independent footing in the world.

A further feature of the landscape of young adulthood today is the challenge of securing an independent footing in the world. Across the Western world, housing costs and the overall cost of living are increasing the age at which this is possible for many. In contrast to their parents' experience, many young adults live with their families. Access to independent living may only be possible with additional family financial support. Alongside this sits a growing awareness of the long-existing social and political structures that have inhibited, and continue to inhibit, possibilities.

Young people are well-served when our therapeutic models address the challenges they face. The objectification of the self and experience, encouraged by the discourse around psychological well-being and the media, is countered by approaches that attend deeply to the subjective experience of the self-in-relationship. Ambivalence towards support and independence needs to be actively addressed within the model, or the pushes and pulls will serve as undercurrents to destabilise the work. Finally, the social and political qualities of the world that inhibit agency, and hence the 'possibilities for becoming', are forces that impact the quality of young adult's lives. In our very being as their therapist, we stand in some power relation to the young adult. A model that creates a safe enough space for these forces to be named and experienced deeply offers a depth of therapeutic support not adequately addressed by medical models.

Relational therapies like CAT have the potential to fulfil these needs. I consistently turn to my CAT methods and tools to work with young people. I would go further, though, to acknowledge that my work with young adults has profoundly influenced how I practice CAT. There is a fine balance to be struck between facilitating deeper qualities of experience – supporting subjectivity – and making sense of this experience in ways that leave them feeling that they are not alone. My quest to become more skilful in striking this balance has driven my interest in the embodiment of the pushes and pulls of relational contact and how CAT can help us to make sense of them.

Embodied perspectives

Bodies are everywhere. The past 20 years have seen an explosion of interest in the embodied aspects of our well-being, whether through the burgeoning attention to the impact of trauma or the ubiquitous concept of 'well-being'.

The concept of trauma has extended – often helpfully – from consideration of the impact of particular events towards the cumulative influences of living in prolonged situations of abuse or neglect. Popular writers like Bessel van der Kolk (2014) have introduced these ideas into the mainstream. The language of 'fight, flight and freeze' responses to threat are now widely adopted and it is striking how many clients bring these terms into the consulting room. Trauma-oriented therapies, like Sensorimotor Psychotherapy or EMDR (Eye Movement Desensitisation and Reprocessing) emphasise the imprints left upon the nervous system and aim to address and re-train our capabilities to respond to the environment. These approaches have brought understanding, and some relief, to many. The recognition of a shared experience can itself go some way to restoring a sense of belonging, and hence safety, in the world. CAT has established ways of understanding and mapping how being 'related to' impacts our experience.

Well-being has become a popular concept in recent years, but its roots are deep. Within the mental health movement, there have always been groups championing the need for preventative approaches. Public health messages in the media and in schools, universities and the workplace about the role of sleep, nutrition and exercise in our mental well-being invite us all to pay attention to how we take care of ourselves. In CAT terms, we might think of this as the quality of our self-to-self relationship. How available and willing are we to tune into our own needs and to meet our needs?

Approaches to both trauma and well-being have foregrounded the body in important and helpful ways. Both are congruent with CAT and can be helpfully incorporated into the approach. However, both approaches foreground one aspect of our bodies – the 'object' of the body. We are, of course, blood and bone, complex nervous and digestive systems. The empirical sciences seek to continually refine our understanding of the body as an organism, and our education in this brings undoubted benefit. As a practitioner in physical health and education settings, and a keen yogi, I have first-hand experience of how understanding breath and movement patterns can increase our skillfulness in navigating the challenges of everyday life. Even where there is some element of experiential exercise within the teaching, at heart these are didactic approaches, teaching individuals about their embodied experience and encouraging them to take responsibility for it through their care and attention. In the context of time-limited interventions, or self-help workbooks, it is hard to escape the position of telling people 'how they are' or inviting them to identify and define themselves from a small range of options.

CAT has always sought to escape the powerful position of 'diagnosis'. Rather than telling people how they are or fitting individuals into a rubric, the intention has always been for the understanding to arise organically between the therapist and client. CAT understandings are co-created. They emerge in the dialogue and through careful enquiry.

CAT is hence a natural home for a more phenomenological approach to embodied experience. In the next section, I set out a brief introduction to phenomenology and its potency in work across all client groups, but perhaps particularly so for young people.

Phenomenology 101

Phenomenology as a philosophical tradition counters the idea of the human being as passively receiving the world and reflecting upon the representations they have of it. While the world, other people and the self, exist as entities, these are not experienced as 'objective'. How the world shows up for me is unique to me. There is a rich vein of philosophical thought from Husserl, Heidegger, Merleau-Ponty, Gibson and through to contemporary thinking in enactive theories of cognition. When we see a chair, we do not immediately perceive its objective properties – although we can choose to do so. We could examine it as a series of shapes and textures, joints and assemblages, but our more instinctive and immediate experience of a chair is for the possibilities it offers to us. If we have the embodied capacity to use it as a chair, we will perceive it for the possibility it offers for sitting down. We perceive a tree from our own embodied standpoint. Encountered on a walk, a tree may be something to walk around, but for a physically able and vigorous 12-year-old, it may present itself as a climbing frame. How the world – physical and social – shows up for us is shaped by our bodily capabilities. As complex human beings, we also consciously reflect on our experience, but our primary experience of the world is through our unreflective action in the world.

As therapists, we understand how much our unreflective action is shaped by experience. In CAT, we make use of the idea of internalised relational roles. We internalise (incorporate, bodily and cognitively) how people are with us. The most influential others in our world are those with whom we spend the most time and have the deepest attachment bonds, but we have the capacity to be impacted by every person that we encounter. This is the very basis upon which therapeutic processes are based. What phenomenological approaches bring to the table is the deeper acknowledgement of the subjectivity of our responsiveness to the world and its active role in the creation of the world in which we live. Phenomenology points to the crucial role of the body in these unreflective relational processes.

Phenomenology highlights the dual aspect of embodied experience. On the one hand, we have an 'object body'. How tall I am, how strong I am, how much I can move – the physicality of my body matters, and hence learning about it has its place. But my body is also the seat of my very experience of the world – we have a 'phenomenal' body. It is the prism through which I perceive and take an active part in creating the physical and social world in which I live. Changes in the object body – development, illness, injury – feed into our phenomenal experience, just as changes in our experience (coming to perceive the world as 'safe') feeds into the quality of our object body, through muscle tone, for example.

What is the relevance of this for psychotherapy? At heart, I believe that the aim of psychotherapy, and many other helping interventions, is the clarification of experience. Through bringing to awareness how the world shows up for me, how I experience myself and others in the world, we bring awareness to our framing, and raise the tantalising possibility that it could be otherwise. This awareness is most helpful when it is deeply subjective – not the objectification of psychoeducation, but rather careful enquiry into the uniqueness and the contextual nature of the experience.

The value of phenomenology for young people

Bringing together the strands of this chapter so far, I have highlighted how a CAT approach offers potent support to the processes of becoming for young people today. It addresses current difficulties and hands over the tools for reflection. Change is seen as an expansion of relational repertoire and the model allows for the active acknowledgement and integration of the social and political contexts of distress. Faced with well-intentioned but often 'objectifying' experiences of self and approaches to well-being, CAT orients itself towards the subjectivity of the young person with their unique temperament, background and context. It offers therapeutic support and a space for the ambivalence toward support to be expressed and explicitly worked-with.

A phenomenologically oriented CAT, I would argue, offers additional potency. I think it is both developmentally indicated and therapeutically helpful. Allow me to take each of those in turn.

Phenomenology is developmentally indicated as it has a hovering attention towards, and recognises the interdependency of, the self and the perceived world. As introduced at the outset of this chapter, young people experience profound changes in themselves and their world. There is physical growth, hormonal changes, shifting contexts from school to college or work, and changes in familial and intimate relationships. This is a life stage when it can be tremendously helpful to clarify and contextualise experience. Additionally, it is crucial to build the skills of clarifying experience because it will surely all be changing again after the end of therapy. Phenomenology is further indicated through its focus on the immediacy of the present relational challenge. For older adults, making sense of how things came to be can be a more helpful aspect of therapy. For young adults, the present is larger in consciousness.

Phenomenology is therapeutically helpful for young people given the wider field of 'objectification'. Now more than ever, our relational therapies need to hold a clear space for the development of subjectivity – a willingness to slow down and attend carefully to the moment-by-moment experience, rather than move quickly through time-constrained models or self-help, off-the-shelf solutions. Staying true to my earliest attraction to CAT, retaining a focus on one thing well – deeply, respectfully, attentively, subjectively – can set a foundation of skills to explore a wider range of issues down the line. An attention to the phenomenal body counters the objectification of the body in many of our cultures.

Phenomenology is additionally helpful in its counsel for us as practitioners to avoid collapsing into a didactic role. We can bring attention to how, and investigate why, we find ourselves 'teaching' our clients. Sometimes, this stance is appropriate and embraced, but what might we be avoiding or missing? In response to the distress stirred in us by the predicament of the young person before us, are we steering them towards a certain experience? Is this an appropriate and supportive use of our power? Or a consolation for us, that misses the young person?

Let's turn to how this might look in practice. I offer this composite vignette as a sample of a phenomenologically inflected CAT approach.

	Therapeutic dialogue	Commentary
Client	I'm just, like, I'm a really bad friend. I should have gone out with her, and she was like, "Where were you? I thought you were coming. You always do this."	[I observe her shrinking a little as she describes herself this way – but I do not want to make her self-conscious by naming it. I also remember that she did not come to our previous session and we had talked about it earlier.]
Therapist	You feel like a bad friend. How did you feel when she was talking to you?	[I name the 'objectification' of herself as a bad friend, but rather than explore that, I enquire how the experience was for her.]
Client	Just really shit… you know?	[If I write 'bad' or 'shit' on the map it stays like that – and there may be more to know.]
Therapist	But how – how was it to feel shit? Can you remember how it was?	[I know this happens to her at home, too, but it feels more important to feel it in this moment than to make the links with her history and other relationships – that can come later.]
Client	Not really… I mean, I wanted to disappear, just, like, it was awful…	
Therapist	How did you feel like you wanted to disappear?	[I keep going until she describes something she is doing, rather than what she wants in the future.]

Client	I was, like, getting smaller. Like I could feel myself wanting to pull back, like get out of her way. I didn't want her to see me.	*[So here she names the shrinking that I observed at the start. It is better that she notices than that I do.]*
Therapist	Because…? What was her 'seeing you' like? How was she seeing you?	*[I want to clarify how she perceives her world.]*
Client	It was like she was having a go. Like, really coming at me…	
Therapist	So, if we imagine her moving – what… what was she… sort of coming at you?	*[I gesture here with a hand moving towards myself, so she can see it happening to me.]*
Client	Yeah, she can be quite full-on	*[I don't want to get too caught up in 'how her friend is' – that would objectify her, rather I stay with how the friend is for my client.]*
Therapist	I can hear that, when she talks to you like that, it really feels as if she is coming at you – that feels full-on… And in relation to that – you, what? What is the 'wanting to disappear'? How would that look, in movement?	*[The words 'as if' begin to open other possibilities.]* *[Keeping my hand coming towards me, I repeat the gesture a few times.]*
Client	Well, I… I definitely go back a bit, and get a bit smaller. Yes, I sort of… *[she slumps a little in her chair]*	

Therapist	I can see, yeah. You get a bit smaller. What happens there? Your head drops… what happens to your chest?	[I stay with this, to get a bit more information.]
Client	I drop it a bit, and my chest goes in, yeah, like.	
Therapist	So – yeah – your chest goes in… almost like her coming in has sort of pushed you back and in.	[I move my hand now towards me and rest it on my chest, and repeat.]
Client	It makes me feel like shit… [moment of sadness]	[Perhaps seeing it visually helps her here to stay with the feeling.]
Therapist	It looks like it feels shit, to feel as if pushed down like that… when she talks to you that way. I wonder – does that happen here? How might I push you down?	[I mirror the feeling back in both my gesture, words and in the tone of my voice.] [But it will most helpful if we can get this familiar dynamic in the room between us.]
Client	No, you're alright…	[Clients often want to reassure us that we are not a problem, either to keep us or to avoid the conflict…]
Therapist	Maybe, some of the time… but it still could happen, couldn't it? I might say something or do something that feels like that for you… [leaving space to respond]	[So, I keep open the possibility – I step out of the 'good therapist' position and make it OK for her to feel like that with me… There is likely to be ambivalence around.

Client	Well, you were also giving me a hard time for not coming last week.	[…and, usually, the dynamic will have happened already…]
Therapist	I was giving you a hard time – earlier? When I asked you about last week?	[Of course, in my mind I had not 'given her a hard time' but it felt like that for her, so I acknowledge and do not deny.]
Client	Yeah – it's quite similar. I felt like you were saying, "Where were you? You should have been here – why weren't you here?"	[These were not the actual words I used, but they were her experience – that was the world she perceived, how I showed up for her, and we need to clarify that and respect it, not deny it.]
Therapist	Ah, I see. When I asked about last week it felt just like that – so was I coming in on you? Making you feel shit, feeling smaller…?	[I use the hand again to demonstrate the relation between 'coming in on her' and 'feeling smaller, pushed down, shit.']
Client	Yeah [energy building], but I also feel like, quite cross about that.	[Here she sits up taller in her chair.]
Therapist	Cross? Tell me about cross…	[So I want to know more about that.]
Client	Yeah, 'cos I couldn't come, and you just don't understand, and sometimes I just want to shout, "Why is nobody taking my side?"	[She is becoming animated, taller, sitting forward.]
Therapist	Yes. You do want to shout. This looks like a different place you're in.	[I reflect her increased force in my voice tone. I gesture to show that she seems bigger.]

Client	Hell yeah. I'm not shrinking now!	[She smiles, so I smile back.]
Therapist	You're not! What are you doing?	[I can see, but I want her to describe it, so she knows more fully.]
Client	Right back at you! [stated triumphantly]	
Therapist	Right back at me – how? Like, how are you coming to me?	[Again, I can see and feel it, but it is helpful to get her to describe it.]
Client	I'm coming in on you now. Take that!	[It is important here that I neither shrink nor retaliate by coming back at her.]
Therapist	I feel you coming at me. You really want me to know how unfair it is to be questioned…

So, sometimes you shrink and feel smaller, and maybe sometimes – but not all times – you can get really big and come back on the Other… | [I say this clearly, so she knows that I have heard – and I use the hand gesture to show that the same position is being experienced reciprocally. At a later point, we might explore how it was for her that she expressed herself like that and I did not shrink or retaliate, but for now the priority is for the experience to be clarified.] |
Client	Well, I try not to do that…	
Therapist	Not to come back…	[Clarifying that she is saying that she avoids being the one to 'come in on'.]
Client	No, cos' it just makes things worse, and makes people feel shit.	

Therapist	So, if we get this on the page – there's a place where someone is coming in on someone, and there are two possibilities. Either someone shrinks, feels small and shit, and it sounds like that makes the Other feel bad, too, OR it escalates – you get bigger – feels like maybe you are too big, or too much…? Let's maybe both move between those places… are there any other possibilities…?	*[As I write the words on the page, I also move them as postures… so we can see and feel the felt-difference between the states.* *In encouraging her to move between the states she will feel them more clearly, and this is the foundation for finding another place – a new possibility, shaped by her embodied presence.* *Writing **and** moving are a potent combination.]*

This composite vignette demonstrates the value of staying with a particular relational exchange and exploring it phenomenologically. At several points, I defer from naming the place too quickly and putting it on the page. Early in this exchange, I could have written, 'critical-to-criticised' as a relational role, or 'critical/attacking' to 'bad/feeling shit'. These would not have been wrong, but they also would not have revealed the dynamics of the situation. Attention to embodiment invites a spirit of curiosity and playfulness. We could have explored how the Other feels to her when she is OK and how the Other feels to her when she shrinks. She would come to recognise how much she 'makes' the Other bigger and more powerful, and hence exacerbates the feeling of 'as if coming in on her'. We could play with how to find a place between, like Goldilocks, neither too big nor too small. How can she hold her own and hold her ground, without coming in on the Other? These are new relational possibilities. We can also play by going back to our earlier exchange. How did she experience my enquiry about her non-attendance in the previous session? I may need to acknowledge the power in that situation. How was I for her, and how did she organise herself in response? How could it have been different?

I believe that, especially with young people and young adults, the connection back to the source of these relational roles is often less salient to them. Where young people continue in states of dependency upon care givers, we need to attend to how the relationship may be undermined by our work. When young adults are in the early stages of independence, there is often less interest in looking back towards the early influences on their distress. Acknowledgement and insight have their place, but of greater value is how it lives – in the here-and-now of their worlds as they live, and in the here-and-now of our therapeutic relationship.

CAT therapy, inflected with a commitment to phenomenology and embodied experience, offers potent therapeutic support. We can combine the methods of phenomenology to clarify experience and the tools and therapeutic frame of CAT to both address issues of immediate concern and to handover the tools for ongoing self-support after ending.

Chapter 6:
A relationally informed model of care for young people living with personality disorder

Louise K. McCutcheon, Jessica O'Connell, Ben McKechnie and Andrew M. Chanen

We wish to thank the young people who contributed their personal experiences of referral, engagement and treatment in our programme to this chapter. They have chosen to use initials, a first name or a pseudonym to protect their privacy.

Young people living with a diagnosis of personality disorder (PD) experience incapacitating problems and profound emotional distress, and are at high risk of poor future personal, social and economic outcomes. In this chapter we discuss how the relational, flexible and trans-diagnostic nature of the Cognitive Analytic Therapy (CAT) model supports working with young people with complex and varied needs. We describe the evidence-based Helping Young People Early (HYPE) early detection and treatment program for young people living with personality disorder, which applies CAT to a model called Relational Clinical Care (RCC), and how this improves their outcomes.

Introduction

Personality disorder is defined in the ICD-11 as, "impairments in functioning of aspects of the self (e.g., identity, self-worth, capacity for self-direction) and/or problems in interpersonal functioning (e.g., developing and maintaining close and mutually satisfying relationships, understanding others' perspectives, managing conflict in relationships)"

(WHO, 2022). By its very nature, personality disorder is relational and lends itself well to being understood through the Cognitive Analytic Model. Moreover, this model's understanding of the development of the 'self' facilitates understanding of PD from its developmental origins to its clinical 'onset' in young people.

PD is described on a continuum from mild through to moderate and then severe. This severity continuum also includes reference to "personality difficulty", which indicates pronounced personality characteristics that might be clinically relevant but do not merit a formal diagnosis. Assessment of an individual's personality functioning along this severity continuum constitutes an essential first step a clinician takes in making a diagnosis of PD and planning its treatment. Pragmatically, the term 'severe' PD is interchangeable with the older term 'borderline' PD, which is reflected in the terminology used in this chapter.

The term personality disorder is associated with stigma and discriminatory practices in many healthcare settings, often leading to covert or overt exclusion of young people (and adults) from healthcare services and/ or wider supports. Paradoxically, the healthcare needs of this group are higher than for young people who do not live with PD. We have argued that diagnosis for the purpose of discrimination is unethical and harmful. Rather, diagnosis is an issue of social justice, identifying a highly vulnerable group of young people with high needs, who are also at risk of serious and adverse long-term outcomes. This enables them parity of access to early intervention services. Early intervention for personality disorder (EIPD) programmes should actively promote accessibility, fair allocation of resources, opportunities for young people's participation in their own care, diversity and inclusion, and seek to fairly weigh the principles of 'duty of care' and 'dignity of risk'.

Like other major mental disorders, PD has its clinical onset and peak incidence from puberty to early adulthood (young people) (Chanen, Sharp *et al.* 2022). Robust evidence and international consensus demonstrate that PD can be validly diagnosed during this developmental period, affecting 10% of the population, with the severe presentations occurring in around 3% of young people in the community, and around one fifth of those attending specialist youth mental health services (Schandrin et al. 2022).

PD ranks among the top ten causes of burden of disease in young people and is the fourth leading cause across all age groups. Young people who have features of severe PD diagnosis experience severe and harmful current problems, which have been comprehensively documented elsewhere (Chanen, 2023; Chanen, Sharp, *et al.*, 2022). Briefly, these include extremely poor quality of life, very high levels of distress and psychopathology, worse physical and sexual health, higher rates of drop-out from education, employment and training, and higher rates of interpersonal violence, family violence and non-violent offences. Their families also experience negative caregiving experiences and high levels of distress. PD also increases complexity of clinical presentation and treatment delivery, poorer access to care for other serious problems, high rates of treatment drop out, and worse response to treatment for related problems, such as depression.

Among young people severely affected, PD acts as a 'gateway' to diverse and serious problems later in life (Chanen, 2023; Chanen, Sharp, *et al.*, 2022), including persistent personality difficulties, severe mental disorders, becoming a perpetrator or victim of violence, increased health care costs, and educational and employment outcomes that are among the worst for all mental disorders. Most tragically, the mortality rate among this group is tenfold that of the general population, with life expectancy being reduced by nearly two decades, and suicide risk (up to 10%) is among the highest for any mental disorder.

Despite these persuasive, evidence-based facts, along with good evidence that early intervention can improve these short- and medium-term outcomes (Chanen, Sharp, *et al.*, 2022), in some countries PD remains a controversial diagnosis, especially when applied to young people (Chanen, 2023; Hutsebaut *et al.*, 2023), and notably in the UK (Hartley *et al.*, 2022). We suggest that this is largely because the condition is associated with a high degree of individual clinician and institutional stigma, which has commonly led to inhospitable clinical cultures or ones in which the diagnosis is intentionally avoided or delayed, or substitute diagnoses are used, in the belief that this is in the best interests of young people. This practice risks using ineffective, inappropriate and/or harmful treatments which, in turn, lead to delays in effective treatment, poor outcomes and risks further stigmatising people living with the disorder (Chanen, 2023; Hutsebaut *et al.*, 2023).

For these reasons, the Helping Young People Early (HYPE) program in Melbourne, Australia, has adopted a relational approach in which proactive dialogue is used to counter damaging myths, to address bigotry among colleagues and institutions, and to nurture hope among those living with PD and those who care for and about them. This supports a positive, hopeful, and just clinical culture in which the needs of this marginalized and high-risk group of young people can be directly, honestly, and genuinely met, using evidence-based early intervention for personality disorder (EIPD). In recognition of the relational difficulties at the core of PD, early intervention in HYPE is offered through the model of relational clinical care (RCC) and is described in detail in this chapter.

Early Intervention for Personality Disorder (EIPD)

The term 'early intervention' refers to the stage of the disorder, rather than the age or developmental phase of the young person. The period of transition from childhood to adulthood, 'youth' (defined as from puberty to the middle twenties), is a period of vulnerability, coinciding with the onset of major mental disorders including PD (Chanen, Sharp *et al.*, 2022).

Personality pathology or diagnostic criteria are a 'heuristic device' that identifies a vulnerable group, at significant risk of poor outcomes (Chanen, Sharp *et al.*, 2022). Early intervention programmes acknowledge the heterogeneity of early presentations by setting broad inclusion criteria, with minimal exclusions for co-occurring problems, such as substance use or antisocial behaviour.

Flexible, adaptive and time-limited

Current mental health services for people with PD have largely failed to deliver upon their aims because they are usually oriented to adults and are often inflexible, inaccessible, are developmentally inappropriate for younger individuals, and are rarely funded adequately for the scale of the problem. EIPD programmes should be engaging, 'youth friendly', and responsive and adaptive to young people's needs, such as providing care in their preferred setting (McCutcheon *et al.*, 2019). This allows young people to make more informed choices about care ('informed refusal'). Time limited, episodic treatment acknowledges that young people often move in and out of care, providing an opportunity to build confidence and autonomy and inviting 'shared decision making' in relation to their support. Offering clear timeframes for care prompts early discussion about the goals and expectations of treatment, and regular reviews of progress prevent 'drift', in which both clinician and the young person are unsure about the aims or direction of treatment. The EIPD programme provides a realistic experience of care that is both time limited and caring, and which facilitates normative activities and reduces expectations that the mental health system can or should meet all of the young person's needs.

Maintaining a focus on functional outcomes, rather than 'delivering' psychotherapy

Growing evidence indicates that structured interventions lead to similar outcomes to the specialised individual psychotherapies for PD in both adults and young people, and that individual psychotherapy is neither necessary nor sufficient for good outcomes (Chanen, Sharp *et al.*, 2022). Individuals living with PD report that being able to live satisfying lives is more important to them than symptom reduction (Ng *et al.*, 2019). Even where there is a reduction in distressing symptoms, functioning remains persistently poor for people with PD (Gunderson *et al.*, 2011). Despite this, most PD treatment programs continue to focus almost exclusively on intensive psychotherapy, with little attempt to address practical needs of those experiencing PD (Chanen, Sharp, *et al.*, 2022), leading to a perception that, unless trained in these specialist psychotherapies, clinicians will not have adequate skills to address the needs of those living with PD. As such, ongoing impairments in relationships, educational and vocational functioning and physical health and wellbeing are prolonged. In contrast, EIPD includes a key focus on functional engagement and improvement, where young people are supported to identify and work towards personally meaningful social, occupational and vocational goals. Clinicians with sound youth mental health skills can, and already are likely to be, caring for individuals with PD, and practical EIPD programmes are 'scalable', greatly increasing access to care while still delivering positive outcomes (Chanen, Sharp *et al.*, 2022).

EIPD involves families

Families of young people with PD experience high levels of distress, grief, burden, disempowerment and mental ill-health, and even higher levels of burden than for the families of young people with conditions such as anorexia nervosa or first episode psychosis (Cotton *et al.*, 2022; Seigerman *et al.*, 2020). Almost two thirds (64%) of these families experience moderate to high disadvantage (Betts *et al.*, 2023). Many families of young people living with PD experience their own challenges and distress, along with worry about their loved ones. While many young people have disengaged from their family of origin by age eighteen, most would like these relationships improved (Chanen, Betts, Jackson, Cotton, Gleeson, Davey, Thompson, *et al.*, 2022) and EIPD can support this.

The HYPE approach to EIPD

For over two decades, the Helping Young People Early (HYPE) program in Melbourne, Australia, has offered evidence-based, frontline services to young people aged 15-25 years living with severe personality disorder (Chanen *et al.*, 2014), and it has been further implemented or emulated in the Netherlands, Switzerland, the UK, Germany, and North America (Chanen, Sharp *et al.*, 2022). Relational problems are central to PD; therefore, a relational and reflective framework, underpinned by cognitive analytic therapy (CAT), guides all aspects of the program. Whilst many services for people with a diagnosis of PD offer psychotherapy alone, HYPE provides a comprehensive programme called Relational Clinical Care (RCC). RCC comprises practical clinical case management, psychiatric care, and family work, along with an optional time-limited contract of individual CAT (McCutcheon *et al.*, 2019; Ryle & McCutcheon, 2006). RCC is provided by a multidisciplinary team, in which case managers (clinical psychologists, social workers, occupational therapists and psychiatric nurses) and psychiatrists work collaboratively with psychosocial services, including vocational specialists whenever possible.

Young people are offered a defined period of care (e.g., six months) or number of sessions, which helps to keep everyone focused and 'on track'. As with any front-line service, some young people do not engage, or drop out of care unexpectedly. Sometimes the mental health or psychosocial difficulties they most need assistance with are what gets in the way (e.g., substance use). Where possible young people are assertively followed up for six weeks, with attempts to re-engage them through letters, home visits or online appointments, before informing them that their care has ended, but with an explicit message that they have an open invitation to return.

RCC has four key aims (i) to improve psychosocial functioning, particularly relationships, educational and vocational pathways, (ii) to reduce mental health problems and distress, (iii) to improve capacity to effectively seek care from others, and (iv) to increase the young person's health, wellbeing and sense of agency.

The principles of Relational Clinical Care (RCC): Collaborative assessment, feedback and psychoeducation

Careful, collaborative assessment is at the core of good treatment, and is necessary for the development of the shared formulation and the design of interventions. A comprehensive biopsychosocial assessment is conducted. Whilst identification of severe PD features (previously operationalised as DSM-5 borderline personality disorder (BPD) features) is the 'ticket' into the HYPE programme, rigid adherence to DSM diagnosis is not the goal. Ideally assessment will also include family members or significant others, and early relational hypotheses are explored and tested with the young person and those involved.

RCC takes a non-judgemental, open and honest approach to diagnosis and psychoeducation, and talks in a practical, no-nonsense and open way about PD. We acknowledge and inform young people about the stigmatising attitudes that they might encounter, especially online. Our experience over two decades and with thousands of young people is that that realistic, hopeful, tailored psychoeducation that addresses the young person's difficulties is almost universally welcomed, validating, and often a relief.

> *"Things were really bad: everything was going wrong, and I couldn't take it anymore. I read about BPD, but I was told I couldn't have it. It wasn't possible because I was only 17… I felt like no one listened or cared enough. I had to keep showing them how bad I felt inside… It was such a relief to finally talk to someone who knew what BPD was and could explain it and talk with me about what I needed to do about it."*
> Young person, 18

Establishing a collaborative working relationship

The relational model emphasises taking a curious, collaborative approach, in which everyone's ideas and expertise are respected, and which focuses upon changes to make life better. Most young people with PD have had few respectful and mutual relationships with adults. A clinician's invitation to take a more active or equitable role in the treatment can be welcomed, but is often initially responded to with suspicion or confusion. RCC clinicians therefore need to demonstrate that they are trustworthy, rather than make assumptions. This might mean being willing to acknowledge what we do not know, or when we get things wrong.

Engaging in a respectful, collaborative relationship from the outset might mean signalling that we are keen to understand the young person's perspective, rather than assuming we understand, making judgements about them, or engaging in problematic relational patterns. RCC invites a discussion about one's own and the young person's expectations about the sessions (length, frequency, location and cancellations), setting a collaborative tone rather than providing a list of rules or a written attendance contract. In setting up the expectations of both parties, there is an undertone of a more equal relationship from the beginning.

RCC acknowledges that working with young people with interpersonal difficulties and complex needs will inevitably involve some ruptures and tensions in the working relationship, disagreements about goals, difficulty maintaining motivation, and misunderstandings. The relational model provides tools and processes for working through these.

The Zone of Proximal Development (ZPD)

The concept of the *Zone of Proximal Development* provides an understanding of the young person's capacity to engage in and use treatment. It invites the clinician to actively engage the young person in a way that maximises their potential for change, and to work in a way that assists the young person to see things from a new perspective and to explore change at a pace that is optimal for them. It might involve using tools to scaffold the learning (such as diagrams to aid reflection on one's own patterns), or it might involve the clinician adapting common techniques to better suit a particular individual (using special interest areas to tailor therapeutic metaphors). RCC appreciates that much of a young person's communication is nonverbal, and that they might have limited capacity to negotiate or report feeling distressed or overwhelmed. Importantly, we are aware that the ZPD, and therefore the capacity to engage helpfully, will shift and change from day to day or even within a session. Actively considering the young person's ZPD throughout the treatment allows the clinician to better anticipate possible challenges, such as self-state shifts that might suddenly affect what is possible to achieve in a session.

> "The relationship that I had with my clinician in HYPE was very different to any relationship that I had previously. There was a focus on not controlling me and instead collaborating with me. In my life, the only way that I was able to see that people cared about me was when they controlled me, took things away from me, or pushed me to do things. At the start I found it super uncomfortable that I wasn't being controlled; it felt like the team didn't care enough. I still did some dangerous things and pushed boundaries to see when I would be controlled. Through slowing things down and understanding what was driving this, I started to notice other ways they were trying to care. This meant we could actually work together, set goals, and make plans for when I was in crisis. There were still times when I was angry with them and reacted impulsively. But when the intensity passed, we could discuss and reflect on the issue. I'd never done this with someone before."
> Lia, 19

Developing collaborative management plans

RCC clinicians explore what young people want and support articulating realistic, shared goals for treatment. CAT's explicitly social model emphasises consideration of the whole person within their unique context, leading to exploration of educational and vocational goals, relationships, cultural or spiritual engagement, physical and sexual health, and engagement in meaningful activities.

Importantly, the key focus on functional goals and living a life of meaning to the young person is prioritised, both when they are engaging in an individual contract of CAT and when they are not. While some young people can articulate their goals, many struggle to imagine change. Negotiation, especially about self-defeating or self-damaging goals (such as when someone wants to lose an unhealthy amount of weight) requires time and patience – but might also require action if the young person cannot disengage from harmful goals. Remembering that all relational patterns have emerged as attempts to solve past difficult situations can allow clinicians to take a more reflective stance while exploring them, and recognises that a young person is less likely to give up any coping strategy if it is at least partially working and offering some sense of relief.

RCC clinicians help young people to identify the function of particular ways of being or acting, and to consider more effective ways of getting their needs met. Regular reviews allow acknowledgement and celebration of a young person's engagement and achievements as well as identification and consideration when progress is not as optimal, ensuring that any necessary changes to the management plan are made in a timely way.

Relational formulations and optional CAT contracts

RCC clinicians aim to develop a relational formulation for every young person accepted into the programme, including those who do not go on to engage in a contract of individual CAT. Ideally this is developed collaboratively with the young person, with input from their family or others. It provides a narrative that acknowledges the current difficulties and the relational patterns that maintain them. It seeks to give a meaningful explanation of the origins of these patterns in non-blaming language, while creating some hope and space for change. The relational formulation guides the treatment and assists in managing any difficulties that might arise. In most cases, the discussion and tentative testing of ideas with the young person and others involved will start from the first contact. Any early mapping is usually kept simple and helps make the patterns explicit, especially those likely to disrupt engagement.

Generally, after a few sessions it has become clear whether the young person is wanting to and/or is likely to engage in a course of therapy. When providing therapy, the HYPE program usually offers contracts of sixteen CAT sessions, unless there is a specific reason to offer fewer (e.g., if the young person is ambivalent about therapy, or is moving out of the area). Progress is regularly reviewed, and sometimes contracts are reduced by negotiation to allow the young person to experience a tolerable ending rather than drop out. More extensive mapping or writing of letters would usually occur as part of a more formal CAT intervention (see McCutcheon *et al.*, 2019; Ryle & McCutcheon, 2006) and are not covered in this chapter.

Working with the most complex young people living with PD can be taxing, with multiple agencies involved. Despite everyone's best intentions, systems are often pulled into collusive and unhelpful patterns that maintain or exacerbate the young person's difficulties. A relational formulation ('contextual reformulation'), developed jointly with the rest of the system, can promote collaboration, consistency in care and flag ways to resolve differences of opinion (Ryle & Kerr, 2020).

Medical and psychiatric care

Young people living with PD can have complex mental, physical and sexual health care needs. Evidence from systematic reviews does not support the use of pharmacological interventions for the treatment of PD. Yet young people are commonly prescribed psychotropic medication in the absence of clinical indications – sometimes multiple medications and for extended periods of time. In contrast, there is also evidence that when mental state disorders (such as first episode psychosis or mood disorders) co-occur with PD, they are frequently undertreated (Chanen, Sharp *et al.*, 2022). The team carefully reviews any medications, to ensure that harmful or inappropriate prescribing does not occur. The relational model informs all interactions with young people, their families or others in their system, providing consistency in the way that the team responds to demands and challenges, regardless of the discipline of the team member. For example, a conversation with a young person seeking medication can include a discussion about both the young person's need (perhaps to find relief from difficult emotions) as well as the medical practitioner's need to prescribe safely and ethically.

Managing risk and safety planning

Self-harm is common, and understandably causes considerable concern to families and others in the system. RCC takes this seriously and uses structured crisis planning and clear processes of risk management, allowing everyone's expectations of care to be clarified (Chanen *et al.*, 2022). Although most young people describe using self-harm to regulate extreme emotion or to punish themselves, one in four is not able to identify any reason for harming themselves. Ideally, interventions will attempt to explore the function of behaviours and patterns involving self-harm, and to encourage reflection on the systemic responses that might exacerbate or reinforce these. Some young people lack helpful adaptive coping skills, so a clinician might teach these when indicated (Kaess *et al.*, 2020). Brief, goal-directed inpatient admissions can assist in containing acute suicidal crises; however, there is little evidence supporting the use of long episodes of hospital care to manage non-suicidal self-harm (Chanen *et al.*, 2022).

RCC supports collaborative reflection about systemic responses to crises with ongoing risks, especially those that don't seem to be resolving. Increasingly, restrictive practices are common, sometimes inadvertently escalating risk. A common dilemma is how to balance taking over too much responsibility for the young person's safety, potentially reducing their opportunity to learn new skills, versus stepping back too far, often colluding with their prior experience of neglect and increasing risk-taking. RCC's collaborative analysis of contextual patterns can validate the young person and assist the care team and family to support them, working towards finding more adaptive strategies that allow their needs to be met more effectively.

> *"The HYPE treatment, where situations and emotions were mapped out, made tackling the issues confronting us much easier to navigate. However, there was a lot of trial and error. Due to the severe nature of my mental health, I was admitted to a psychiatric hospital against my wishes by my team, and this was a really scary experience for me. We came to learn together though, that such a restrictive method of care was detrimental to my overall mental health. By learning this, it helped us map out better ways to manage acutely distressing situations without relying on what could be perceived as more punitive forms of care."*
> Zac, 24

Managing transitions and endings

For most young people with PD, their experiences of endings are usually abrupt, rejecting, and highly distressing, resulting in sensitivity to transitions during their care. RCC approaches endings in an open and explicit manner that invites the young person and their family or systems to consider the nature of any future support that they might need. RCC acknowledges that these needs will fluctuate, and that a fundamental skill is how to seek and utilise support effectively. Experiencing a 'good enough' ending promotes a hopeful stance and encourages greater autonomy and self-efficacy. Rituals, celebrations, goodbye letters and cards are all helpful in marking an ending for the young person, and can shift the focus from loss to the more hopeful achievements.

Some young people and/or their families will experience an ending as overwhelming, and this might precipitate clinical deterioration. Even when new patterns have been practiced, as the ending draws near, the urge to re-enact old patterns can be strong, which might pull the clinical team to delay the ending. Usually, we find this to be counterproductive, reinforcing that endings are unmanageable, undermining confidence and autonomy. Alternatively, some clinicians become very insistent and rigid about the deadlines, which also represents an enactment of an unhelpful pattern. RCC aims to step back and identify the relational patterns, and to support a more adaptive experience of a shared ending.

> *"Transitioning to the ending was a difficult experience that brought up countless emotions. It was a situation that terrified me from the beginning. It was overwhelming to know that no matter how hard I tried to not be discharged, the ending had to occur. I feared that my life would go back to how it was, and that I could be controlled and misunderstood all over again.*
>
> *"Through reflecting on the ending now, I can see how ending was a really important step. During this care, my identity was based on my mental illness and the ending allowed me to move to a different chapter of my life. The HYPE team had met the very unwell version of me and as a result, I felt like I had to hold onto this part of me, even if I wasn't doing dangerous things. The ending gave me an opportunity to let that part of me go, and to take important steps in my recovery where I was able to grow into a person whose identity wasn't based only on my past experiences."*
> Lia, 19

Including families and friends

Family members and other care-givers report wanting greater involvement in assessment, diagnosis and treatment (Barr et al., 2020), especially if the young person is at risk. RCC includes families whenever possible. However, RCC also respects the emerging autonomy of young people, such as when they express reluctance to involve their family. Rather than force the issue, RCC clinicians indicate a willingness to understand and revisit the issue. Our clinical experience is that family involvement is constructive and has rarely been counterproductive. RCC clinicians can be a go-between for the young person and their family, checking with each what they might share with the other and supporting new ways of relating, improving communication. Rarely, family involvement might be unhelpful (e.g., family violence) and this is managed decisively to protect the young person. Where possible, family perspectives are included in the development of the relational formulation, allowing for a richer understanding of the strengths and origin of difficulties. RCC clinicians can respectfully acknowledge trans-generational experiences of adversity, trauma or abuse, whilst assisting families to reflect on their own part in unhelpful relational patterns. Remaining curious helps to ease any expectations that they will be blamed for the current situation. Occasionally, families with entrenched difficulties require referral to specialist family services.

> *"What I also found to be vital, while fighting poor mental health, was strong collaboration with my family. A strong network of support at home was essential for me and my capacity to recover. From a place of fear, my family was often only capable of helping me by calling emergency services, which often led to traumatic interventions. Through family sessions, I was able to improve relationships with my parents, which led to a home environment where I could communicate my problems and feel heard and understood. This has led to a much healthier home life."*
> Zac, 24

Supervision

Self-defeating patterns of behaviour and rapid 'state shifts' (swings between extreme relational positions like Demanding to Angry/Abusing to Defeated/Helpless) are an inevitable accompaniment to working with young people with PD. RCC is supported by more expert supervision, usually by supervisors with formal CAT training, to assist clinicians to understand and respond helpfully to state shifts, and use moments of rupture in the therapeutic relationship as useful opportunities to model how to notice, name and repair such tensions. Other challenges such as missed sessions and difficulties with self-management can be managed more effectively when clinicians are assisted to think relationally, identify their own patterns and practice addressing these challenges in a straight-forward and open manner (McCutcheon *et al.* 2016; Ryle & McCutcheon, 2006).

Conclusions

Early Intervention for Personality Disorder (EIPD) is supported by two decades of research. However, implementation in clinical practice is in its early stages. The Helping Young People Early (HYPE) model demonstrates that EIPD can be based on a straightforward, scalable model, comprising commonly available clinical skills, delivered through a relational lens. The CAT model underpins Relational Clinical Care (RCC), providing a framework that explains the origins, the complexity and heterogeneity of the disorder. It is sympathetic to the developmental processes that young people experience, and provides a respectful, humane, collaborative and just way of understanding developmental disruption and the transition to adulthood. The CAT model is flexible and trans-syndromal, providing a framework for all aspects of care, and is offered as a time-limited contract of individual psychotherapy, should the young person choose this. Finally, it provides a model for reflecting on team dynamics and systems interactions that allows a building of capacity in all who work with young people living with PD.

Case Study 1: Being on both sides – reflections by a young person with lived experience of being diagnosed with Borderline Personality Disorder

Brede

Living with a BPD Diagnosis

I felt relief and validation when I was first diagnosed with BPD – the diagnostic criteria covered many of the things I struggled with that couldn't be explained by my existing mental health diagnoses. It also served as an explanation for why certain medications hadn't worked for me, and directed me towards therapeutic approaches that might be more relevant. Interpreting myself through a BPD framework validated a lot of my experiences. I felt solidarity talking with BPD friends and reading about people's experiences of BPD. It became easier to articulate some of the things I struggled with, because they were so neatly summarised in the DSM. Importantly, these struggles were no longer personal 'failures' or 'bad behaviour' – they fitted into a recognised set of symptoms/characteristics.

BPD can also be a heavy diagnosis to hold. My earlier diagnoses of depression and anxiety were a lot for a child to comprehend, but they were presented to me as conditions that could be temporary; conditions I could 'recover' from with the help of therapeutic supports. This sense of hope and recovery was absent from BPD narratives. Rather than a condition I was experiencing, BPD was a disorder I embodied. Accordingly, the focus of my therapeutic supports shifted toward mitigating the impact of an enduring cluster of personal deficits. This shift gave me a new set of reactions to question and behaviours to police. For example, I had already learnt to limit negative reactions from others by repressing my emotions, but the criterion of 'Inappropriate, intense anger or difficulty controlling anger' meant I became even more diligent in making sure I didn't acknowledge or express anger. Rather than aiding my capacity to understand, process and hold difficult feelings and emotions; I found myself over-intellectualising my reactions and experiences, so that everything remained in my head rather than being anchored in my body. I moved further from a place where I could 'feel my feelings', nullifying any sense of interoception.

I wasn't ashamed of the diagnosis, but I was always anxious disclosing it. In health settings, the stigma surrounding BPD meant that some professionals would not work with me. Others refused to acknowledge my diagnosis, or to respond to my questions and comments about BPD – potentially due to broader debates regarding the legitimacy of BPD as a diagnosis. In social settings, disclosure typically meant hastily trying to counter someone's existing negative assumptions, or giving a 'crash course' BPD overview before they began their own search and inevitably came across the overwhelmingly negative portrayals of BPD in media and literature.

Despite my efforts, the label became a scapegoat for some people. My BPD seemed to make it easier for people to absolve themselves of any need to reflect on their own biases or behaviours. Any relationship problems were bound to be my fault because I had BPD. My efforts to communicate and connect were undermined with comments like: "Don't trust her – she's got BPD, so she'll manipulate you without even realising she's doing it" and "People with BPD have abandonment issues, so they'll do anything to make you like them." It also became easier for people to gaslight me – they could question whether something actually happened, or whether my memories were being influenced by experiences associated with BPD such as dissociation, paranoia, or identity disturbance. If I became upset, this was often written off as a 'BPD overreaction'. Experiences like these further reduced my sense of self-worth and distorted my identity. I questioned the validity of my reactions and emotions, and struggled to trust my own opinions and memories. Ironically, this led me to think and act in ways that even more closely resembled BPD; and to further identify with the diagnosis.

When my BPD was eventually determined to be a misdiagnosis, this served to highlight broader issues related to the power held by individual clinicians – and the general ambiguity in mental health spaces.

Diagnostic ambiguity

A BPD diagnosis requires you to meet at least five of nine diagnostic criteria. This means that there are two hundred and fifty-six combinations of diagnostic criterion that may lead to a BPD diagnosis, and two people who share a BPD diagnosis may have only one criterion in common (Antoine, 2023). BPD also shares many symptoms and characteristics with other mental health and neurodevelopmental conditions, with considerable overlap between the external presentation of BPD symptoms and the ways in which people respond to traumatic experiences.

This means that a clinician's speciality and the perspectives developed through their life experiences can heavily influence whether a cluster of 'symptoms' is recognised as BPD or something else. In my case, it's also relevant to know three things: firstly, that BPD is over-diagnosed in women[7]; secondly, that the alternate conditions I was later diagnosed with are generally under-diagnosed in women; and thirdly, that individual clinics and clinicians may differ in the range of diagnoses they can assess for. As a young person seeking mental health support, I could only access services if they were free or heavily subsidised. These services did not have capacity to provide the assessments required for my current diagnoses.

The psychiatrists who diagnosed me with BPD assessed me during particularly traumatic periods of my life. As the most defining traumas I've experienced were heavily gendered, implicit bias may have prevented these men from recognising my experiences as traumatic. This would make it easier to mistake my discrete trauma responses for enduring BPD symptoms. My observable actions and reactions during the times when I was diagnosed and re-diagnosed with BPD did align with the diagnostic formulation of someone with BPD, but they could also be interpreted as understandable ways of responding to trauma, or indicators of other conditions.

---

7   I recognise gender is a spectrum, not a binary. I'm using binary terms here because there is currently not as much information about how this relates to other genders.

Diagnostic labels

Diagnostic labels can provide validation and may generate guidance and recommendations on therapeutic approaches or medical interventions to relieve distress and improve quality of life. But diagnostic labels are unable to provide a complete understanding of an individual's needs, social circumstances, or potential strengths and resources. So it seems limiting to treat people with shared diagnoses as a homogenous group. The symptoms and experiences of two people with the same diagnosis can vary so significantly, especially when considering other influential factors such as race, disability, gender and class. This highlights a need for mental health diagnoses to be reviewed as relevant clinical and societal understandings and contexts change over time.

It is also important to recognise that there are many reasons why people will continue to identify with a specific diagnosis, even if alternate explanations may be more valid. For example: a diagnosis may offer a good-enough explanation for their current circumstances; it can feel more concrete and comfortable to have a recognised diagnostic label rather than a cluster of uncertainty; societal stigma or personal history can make other more 'accurate' diagnoses feel more confronting; the legal or financial ramifications of receiving a specific diagnosis may outweigh the benefits of accessing more relevant healthcare; the hierarchical power dynamic of 'expert' and 'patient' may discourage people from questioning a diagnosis; and/or insufficient resources and general barriers to healthcare can prevent people from seeking a second opinion.

Personally, I only received more accurate diagnoses after reaching circumstances that aren't available to everyone. I began working and studying in healthcare fields, making it easier to learn more about BPD and alternate conditions. I had space and support to begin processing the influence of trauma on my daily experiences, and improved financial circumstances gave me access to more comprehensive diagnostic assessments. As my situation improved, I became more able to make informed decisions about my own healthcare. This also enabled me to reflect on past healthcare – acknowledging the ways in which it supported my critical thinking and saved my life in the short-term, while also recognising the ways in which it guided me towards internalising negative stereotypes and harmful beliefs about myself and my identity.

Despite the widely accepted links between BPD and trauma, this was not an explicit focus of the healthcare I received post-diagnosis. Curiosity and questioning from my therapists generally took a tone of "What are *your* negative thought patterns?", "How do they influence your actions and reactions?", "How can *you* deal with that?", and "How can *you* manage your behaviour and emotions?" Acknowledging current circumstances is often a relevant precursor to changing or accepting those circumstances, but without context this can place unnecessary blame and burden on the individual by centring them as the 'problem'.

Regardless of my overall diagnosis, if BPD thought patterns were wired into me through trauma, wouldn't it make sense to critically assess that trauma and its influence? This might have been approached through questions like: "What have you experienced?", "How have circumstances beyond your control influenced the way you move through the world today – and what can we do about that now?" or "How can we recognise the influence of these external factors, so that you have more autonomy to shape your circumstances in future?"

Summary

Diagnostic labels can be useful clinical tools, but they can also be harmfully inaccurate and based on incomplete or outdated information. It's essential for clinicians to remain curious and critical about the ways in which diagnostic information informs their practice. Curiosity can uncover relevant factors that were missed in earlier assessments, and critical thinking can help clinicians to utilise, alter, or avoid remaining rigidly focused on 'best practice' methods for certain diagnoses based on individual circumstances. This is not to dismiss or reject 'best practice' but rather to encourage the clinician to think about the bigger picture of a person's presenting circumstances and context before deferring to checklists of signs and symptoms. In other words, to interpret the individual through what they have experienced, rather than what is 'wrong' with them. Ultimately, my experiences of identifying with BPD highlighted the solidarity, hope, and strife that can accompany different diagnostic labels. My story also reinforces how essential it is that these labels, and the preceding diagnostic formulations, are informed by the unique narrative of an individual's personal and interpersonal history, and considerate of the ever-changing context of societal and clinical understanding.

PART 2: Relational approaches to working with parents, families and groups

Chapter 7:
A house of mirrors – a role for parent CAT

Clare Young

"My child needs help."
"There is something wrong with my child."
"The child has X/Y/Z problems."

How often do we hear things like this in our health, education and social care services? There are additional statements that describe the problems, distress and difficulties a child may be experiencing – so often stated by the adults *about* the child: parents, teachers, doctors, social workers… the list goes on. I am a clinician, and I am also a parent of three young children. Everything my children do affects me, and everything I do affects them, to some degree. Dr Tony Ryle, the originator of Cognitive Analytic Therapy (CAT), would argue that everything we do is relational – there is usually a cause and an effect based on meeting our own or others' relationship needs, but it can also often be selective. As parents, we can celebrate and take pride in the achievements and successes of our children, often having instilled within our children the constructs of perseverance, hard work and ambition. Parents often like to be seen and related to as 'good parents'. Conversely, if our child self-harms, how do we (as parents) make sense of our role in this, how we relate to ourselves and how people will relate to us, and where do we locate the pain we feel? As parents, we may live in a house of mirrors and choose to divert the critical gaze to enable approval or to project disapproval to protect a certain way in which we relate to ourselves as parents. Can we separate the pain a child feels from the pain a parent feels if they are seen as not a good enough parent and vice versa? My argument would be not, but as a parent, we may struggle to be aware of the relational dilemmas we find ourselves in so we can continue to feel OK in a role that most parents value the most.

> *"If a community values its children, it must cherish their parent."*
> (Bowlby, 1988)

CAT is an open and versatile model and has a great deal to offer parenting due to its emphasis on the 'relational' core difficulties, as shown by the work of Jenaway (2018) in her blog 'Parenting the Middle Way'. Jenaway argues that psychoeducation programmes delivered in CAMHs are often processed (by parent attendees) 'in the head', struggling to reach the parents on an emotional level when parenting is often about tuning into emotions, our own as a parent, and the child's. CAT with parents enables an exploration of underpinning, and often unseen, relational patterns that the parent has experienced as a child and is re-enacting by/with the child, and in so doing enabling a shift towards learning 'from the heart' and healing from not repeating history.

Being a parent is, by its definition, being relational. The Latin word for parent is 'parentim' meaning 'father, mother or ancestor', and the participle is 'to bring forth'. The term 'parent' is a concept that embodies a multitude of experiences and voices. If you have worked with parents, or you are a parent, then there is also a child who is 'brought forward'. This child takes two forms:

1. The child *of* the parent – the visible child that we can see.
2. The inner child *in* the parent – held within (and so often overlooked by services).

When we look in the mirror, which child do we see? This chapter is about the hidden child in us all and how CAT offers a way to find and connect with them and help them parent while holding in mind their own inner child.

A house of mirrors: the reflections of parent CAT

A 'house of mirrors' is a maze with mirrored obstacles and glass panes that prevent access to other parts of the maze. Sometimes the mirrors curve to offer a distorted image, giving the observer an unusual and confusing reflected image of themselves; sometimes humorous, other times frightening.

A house of mirrors provides a striking parallel to the work we can do with parents as we too provide different reflections and note that there is not just one way of seeing or relating to ourselves and others. All the mirrors are real and true and have a part to play in the experience. They may reflect a distorted image of ourselves, but they also reflect our multifaceted selves. In CAT, everyone's perspective is valuable and of interest, and as Mikhail Bakhtin would propose (1981), meaning is not contained by words and utterances but is found only in the dialogue between them and their context; wherever there is meaning there is more than one voice at play.

When working with a parent, we must therefore think not only about their role with their own 'outer' child, but also the child within; their experiences of being parented, and the meaning that this brings to their relationship with their child. Many parents are unaware of how much their inner child's experiences are 'brought forward' when they become a parent, and this lack of conscious awareness can be reflected in the system that works with parents whose children are referred to services because something is 'wrong' with the child. This is not to suggest that for every child needing support there is a parent who has unconscious needs behind their child's presentation but, in some situations, this may be true and support for the child may meet a need for the parent.

It is important to employ a compassionate perspective that Ryle adopted when working with people in distress who act and react in many ways; on some level their actions and reactions all makes sense (e.g. Ryle, 2021). Focusing specifically on working alongside parents is truly wonderful, deeper-level work; undoubtedly a house of mirrors, with multiple ways of seeing and making meaning, and remaining so important for professionals – who might be connecting with parents in schools, social care or health settings – to hold in mind.

In Dorset Child and Adolescent Mental Health Service (CAMHS), we wanted to actively promote the role of the parent in health, social care and education services as important in understanding, stabilising and managing distress experienced by children and young people. I would go so far as to state that working with parents is one of the main roads to promoting health and well-being in children. I was told once that, as a parent, you are only ever as happy as your least happy child. I would also suggest that children are only as happy as their least happy parent. This isn't a chicken or egg scenario; it is about both. But the chicken can tell the story of the egg, and that is often the key to understanding what is happening between them.

Our aim was to create a safe enough space that offered the opportunity for the parent or carer to re-connect with their inner child – directly, compassionately and curiously, through an experience of CAT. We wanted to help identify the early relational patterns and procedures of the parent that may contribute to their child's presenting 'problems'. This was not simply offering CAT to parents, in the same way you might offer CAT within an adult service. We were explicitly supporting parents to explore how their own relational patterns, their traps, dilemmas and snags, articulated through the psychotherapy file (see Glossary) and which had developed from their own childhood experiences, may (re)present in their current parent-child to child relationships. Instead of adult CAT, we were offering parent CAT:

Figure 7.1: Working with the unseen and seen child

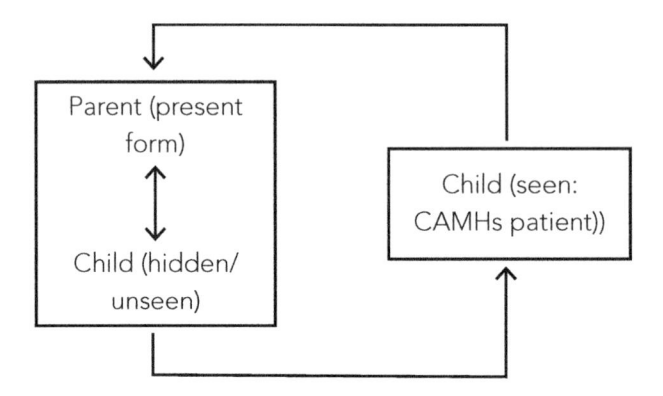

```
         ↓
┌─────────────────┐
│ Parent (present │
│     form)       │
│       ↑         │──────────┐
│       ↓         │    ┌─────────────────┐
│ Child (hidden/  │    │  Child (seen:   │
│    unseen)      │    │ CAMHs patient)) │
└─────────────────┘    └─────────────────┘
         │                      ↑
         └──────────────────────┘
```

Some parents have embraced the CAT space; others have been suspicious, cautious, mistrusting and blatantly resistant to the offer of space for CAT for themselves as parents – and we have worked with all. Many parents spoke of childhood experiences of feeling invisible, excluded, overlooked and dismissed – we can re-enact this (unwittingly) in services by focusing on the child (CAMHs patient). Through offering CAT to parents, we intended to embody an exit to these earlier experiences.

Mirroring stories

The use of stories, pictures and narratives within this work has been particularly helpful and seems to have provided space for safe reflection (a playful mirroring) and recognition with parents. By way of modelling the use of creative narratives I have chosen two well-known fictional parent figures who we have met, in different forms, of course, in our clinical work: the Wicked Stepmother and The Fairy Godmother from Cinderella (recognising that any gender may take on these roles). Of course, these are metaphors, but we have worked with parents who have experienced similar challenges in their roles as parent.

The Wicked Stepmother is portrayed as a critical, contemptuous and demanding parent, and professionals can get pulled into a dance where they are left feeling criticised and overwhelmed by them. This may be such a powerful reciprocal role that we stop being curious: why is the Wicked Stepmother so wicked? The same happens with The Fairy Godmother who is so happy to please, and we (as professionals) fall under their/his/her spell, forgetting to be curious again: why does the Fairy Godmother live their life ensuring that others have all that they desire to the sacrifice of what they truly need?

In Cinderella, the story is almost exclusively focused on the child, and yet the parent figures in the story have significant parts to play; their stories are as valid and important. Hence the need to find a way to work alongside parents to understand why they are so vulnerable to being stuck in past, present and repeating patterns that are now becoming a narrative of their child.

Working alongside parents and connecting with the system around the child

An attempt at understanding the behaviours and needs of a child in a manner that does not routinely explore the role of and relationship between the child and primary adult (parent/carer) will be woefully inadequate. In the same context, understanding the needs of an adult without exploring their childhood experiences is akin to trying to fathom a novel after starting it halfway through. Services for children and adults must think flexibly and fluidly across the age continuum and be informed by the family story as a whole. Unquestionably, this is never more needed than in services for children, where the notion of working exclusively with the child in a manner that positions them as distinct or disconnected from the relational source that created and cares for them makes little sense.

A child's behaviour therefore offers us clues to solving the mystery of whatever the child is inviting or needing the adults around them to be attentive of. In health services, for example, a child presenting with symptoms indicative of social anxiety or depression can be treated for these diagnoses, but if these were symptoms or reciprocal role procedures (activities that have a relational aim) of something that might be hidden from consciousness (in both the family and the professional) then you could reasonably predict that the symptoms will return. When we are trying to understand the problem, we must be curious about the origin and the family story it exists within, else we shall fail to treat the cause. The reflection you see as a parent and professional can often depend on where you are looking (and what you are asking); the image can be distorted.

As mentioned, it is often the case in children's services that the adults make requests for help and support for their child but are really asking for support in how to parent and meet the needs of their child. Regardless of the concerns raised by a network around a child, it can be the case that the child is not willing to engage in support/treatment, and this position needs to be respected. Therapy is about being collaborative and enabling trusting and trusted relationships to inform opportunities for change, especially for those children where difficulties with relationships, such as trauma or loss, have contributed to their distress.

If the young person declines therapy, there is still much that can be done to work alongside the parents and within the systems around the child and their family. After all, even if the child is not opening up in their own individual space, they are still communicating what may be going on within through their actions in relationships, between and around. For example, if a young person is angry and lashing out, and being reprimanded as a result, then we need to ask what may be occurring with the reciprocated experiences of others, of those around the young person. Is there a need they are asking to be attended to but which is being overlooked repeatedly because the behaviour is overshadowing it?

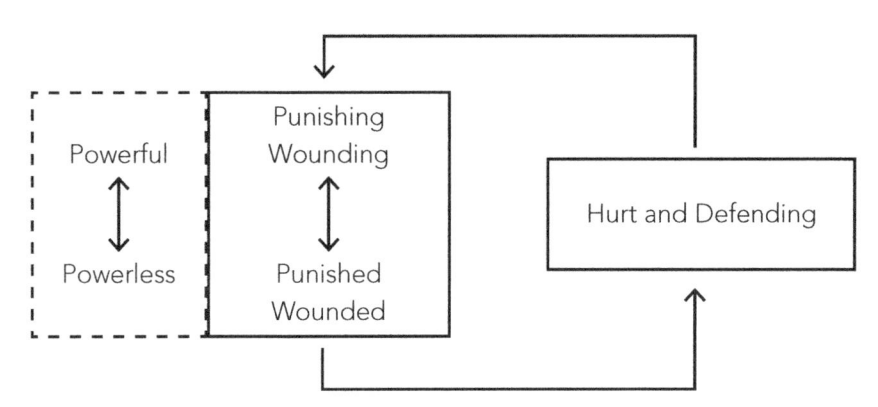

Figure 7.2: Seeing beyond the behaviour

```
          ┌─────────────────────────────────────┐
          ↓                                     │
┌ ─ ─ ─ ─ ─ ─┬──────────┐                       │
            │ Punishing │                       │
│ Powerful  │ Wounding  │      ┌──────────────────┐
    ↑       │    ↑      │      │                  │
│   ↓       │    ↓      │─────→│ Hurt and Defending│
  Powerless │ Punished  │      │                  │
│           │ Wounded   │      └──────────────────┘
└ ─ ─ ─ ─ ─ ┴──────────┘              ↑
          │                           │
          └───────────────────────────┘
```

Mapping these patterns with parents and/or with the systems around the young person helps offer a relational understanding of behaviours and resulting feelings that allows for a shifting of the gaze upon the child – a different reflection – and allows new ways of exploring help and support. For the child that might be angry and/or lashing out, this might be understood as a way to feel closer to the parent (they can see me enough so therefore I am safe), helping the parent to learn not to lash back, allowing room for change and learning in the relationship between parent and child.

A conversation with parents to help them reformulate their child's emotional challenges as a relational issue (be it with themselves or the wider system), and therefore allowing this to become understandable, can be powerful. To support parents in being able to see beyond the more overt behaviours to the origins of the symptoms as a representation of past or present relational difficulties is valuable work, illustrating the power of relationships and, perhaps, for parents who may be inadvertently contributing to or maintaining the distress, this new knowledge and framing of relational understanding opens windows to change.

Working directly with parents to understand the child within: a place for parent CAT

In my work with children and young people, there are many cases in which the child's distress is a legacy of earlier parent/family pain that does not solely belong to the child. There is a wealth of research on epigenetics and intergenerational trauma offering accounts of how this experience of trauma can span generations (e.g. McGowan, 2009; Bale,

2015). When trying to understand the mental health challenges of the children and young people we meet today, we should be mindful not just to ask "What have you been through?", but also to be curious as to "What has your family been through?" This latter question widens the lens and relocates the problem away from the person who is carrying or bearing the hallmarks and scars of events that happened in generations past.

> *"We repeat what we don't repair"*
> (Christine Langley-Obaugh, date unknown)

These past stories may be held unconsciously and only when exploration of the wider family story is encouraged, supported and held can the missing pieces of the puzzle be found. Early family trauma can lie dormant within the body and mind until specific life events cause them to become active and alert (Felitti *et al*, 2010; Lange, 2016). One such major life event can be the transition to becoming a parent. If these relational difficulties were potentially part of a process that was either triggered when the adult became a parent or has become more intense as a result of being a parent, then it makes sense to be able to offer an effective and broader therapeutic intervention to the parent.

Our work in Dorset CAMHs through Parent CAT recognised the central role of the parent in cultivating their child's emotional well-being. The therapy enabled parents to explore their own relational stories in the context of their history and present experiences with their inner and outer child. But let us return to Cinderella…

Once upon a time…

The use of stories in CAT is a very helpful therapy tool. Stories are a wonderful way of working with parents and inviting the child (inner and/or outer) into the therapy space. Using fictional stories can provide a safe means by which to talk about parts of the self or others. The use of stories and characters in therapy is not new, having been a frequently used approach for many years (Bergner, 2007), and I shall use stories here to mirror experiences and encounters in my work through Parent CAT.

The Wicked Stepmother and the Fairy Godmother both expressed difficulties in their relationships with Cinderella. The Wicked Stepmother was angry and hurt by Cinderella's indifference to her, while the Fairy Godmother was exhausting herself trying to protect Cinderella and ensure that her life was a fairytale. Both parents were offered Parent CAT.

Chapter 7: A house of mirrors – a role for parent CAT

In Cinderella, we all know the story of the abusive, humiliating, contemptuous stepmother who treated Cinderella so harshly. We know that the Wicked Stepmother only loved her two daughters (the Ugly Sisters) and had completely spoiled and smothered them to the degree that they fawned over and revered their mother, following her everywhere and demanding to be admired and waited on by Cinderella. In the relationship between the Wicked Stepmother and her daughters, there was a need to be revered and adored – with the Ugly Sisters demanding the same from Cinderella. But Cinderella didn't comply, and the Wicked Stepmother became hateful, excluding and abusive.

Figure 7.3: Mapping with the Wicked Stepmother

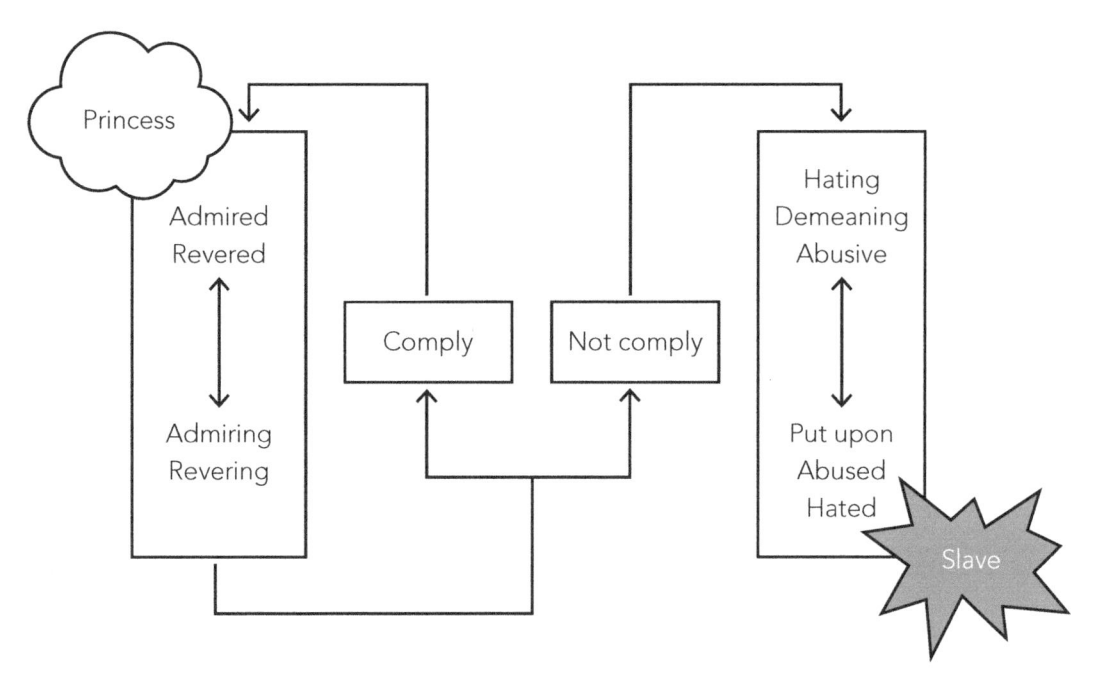

Princess

Admired / Revered ↕ Admiring / Revering

Comply

Not comply

Hating / Demeaning / Abusive ↕ Put upon / Abused / Hated

Slave

125

Reformulating and mapping with the Wicked Stepmother

It didn't begin this way for the Wicked Stepmother. In the family story, she grew up with an unpredictable father who was largely absent and difficult to please. When he was home, he could be volatile and easily angered. Her mother came from a large family with many siblings and little money, so they'd had to learn to 'make do and mend'. Her mother had vowed to only ever have one child and would often tell the Wicked Stepmother that she regretted having a child as she didn't like being a mother. The Wicked Stepmother's mother had a high-powered job and a wide social circle who they would entertain frequently. The Wicked Stepmother was always told to stay out of sight. Both her parents were often too tired or too busy to spend time with her, unless she achieved an award or a top grade, whereupon she would be paraded in front of her parent's friends. The Wicked Stepmother learned that there was little point in going to her parents for help – to earn their time she had to do well. She learned to strive for greatness and be autonomous; character traits her father encouraged as he had needed to do the same as a child. He could be contemptuous of emotions and would become critical and rejecting of the Wicked Stepmother if she ever cried or made a mistake. Her parents did not understand the importance of being emotionally available and believed they were helping her to become self-reliant and successful. She learned that, if she didn't show emotions or ask for anything, she would receive the approval of her father.

In one therapy session, the Wicked Stepmother describes the difficulties she is having with her new stepdaughter, who is not treating her as she has expected:

> **Wicked Stepmother:** She just doesn't love me!
>
> **Therapist:** What makes you believe she doesn't love you?
>
> **Wicked Stepmother:** Well, for a start she spends all her time by herself, and when I ask that she comes and sits with us [Wicked Stepmother and the Ugly Sisters], she says she is busy, as if she has so many better things to do... all she does is read! My girls would never dream of being so rude, they always want to spend time with me.

Therapist: So, when you would like Cinderella to be with you and her stepsisters and she says no, how does that feel?

Wicked Stepmother: I feel angry, like I'm not important.

Therapist: Like you're not important, ok. There is anger there. I'm curious about whether there were other times when you may have felt like you're not important. When you were younger, how would you spend your time with other people in your family, your parents, or siblings?

Wicked Stepmother: We didn't spend time together, my parents worked hard, and they were very busy people with work and friends… I spent most of my time at home by myself, I learned to look after myself.

Therapist: Your parents worked hard – how did it feel that they didn't have time to give you?

Wicked Stepmother: A mix, I admired them … but it did feel lonely, mmm, very lonely… but you can only ask them so many times to do something with you only to be told to stop bothering them, or that they're too busy, can't you? So I stopped asking.

Therapist: Yes, it is understandable that, as a child, you would have stopped asking because it is painful to be dismissed by your parents. I wonder if you want to include Cinderella in a way that you weren't included?

Wicked Stepmother: I do! I've never let my girls feel the way I did, and we have always done absolutely everything together – how dare Cinderella tell me she's too busy, who does she think she is? Well, she wanted to spend time by herself so she will, down in the cellar!

Mapping in the moment (an example in Figure 7.4), we can start to see some parallels between the experiences the Wicked Stepmother is having with Cinderella and her own childhood experiences:

Figure 7.4: Mapping the procedure for the Wicked Stepmother and Cinderella

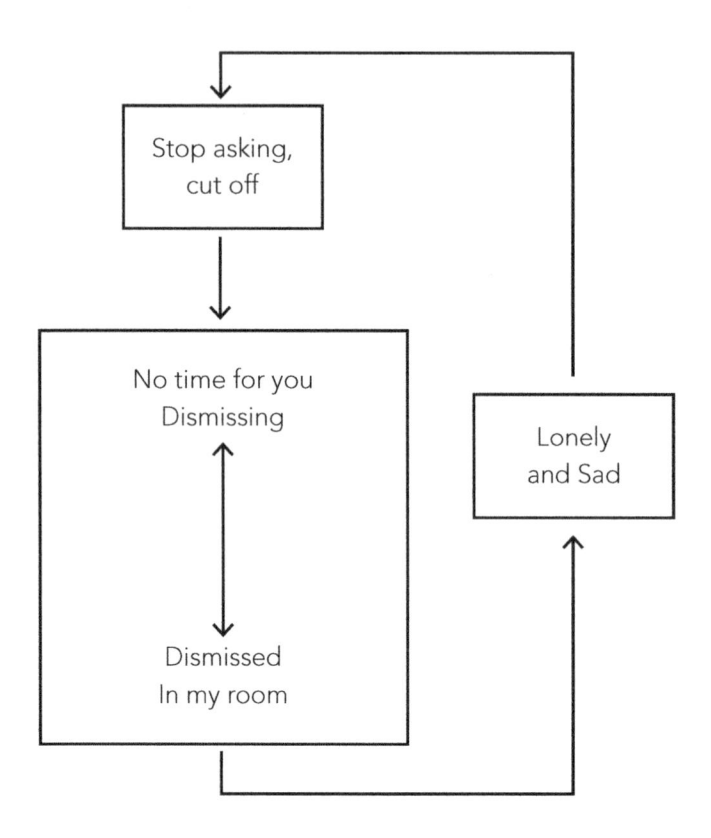

```
         ↓
  ┌─────────────┐
  │ Stop asking,│◄──────────────┐
  │   cut off   │               │
  └─────────────┘               │
         │                      │
         ↓                      │
  ┌───────────────────┐         │
  │  No time for you  │   ┌──────────┐
  │    Dismissing     │   │  Lonely  │
  │         ↑         │   │ and Sad  │
  │         │         │   └──────────┘
  │         │         │         ↑
  │         ↓         │         │
  │     Dismissed     │         │
  │     In my room    │         │
  └───────────────────┘         │
         │                      │
         └──────────────────────┘
```

There is also anger in the descriptions the Wicked Stepmother gives about how she feels towards Cinderella. It is reasonable to hypothesise (and reformulate) that the anger was there before Cinderella. The anger seems to suggest a core pain in the Wicked Stepmother, felt as a child linked to feeling dismissed and unimportant. When Cinderella chooses not to spend time with the Wicked Stepmother, she is re-enacting the (top) role of the Wicked Stepmother's parents ("no time for you") and the anger that was connected to the core pain is shown in a rageful manner towards Cinderella. Cinderella is then angrily banished to the cellar (cut off and invisible – see Figure 7.5).

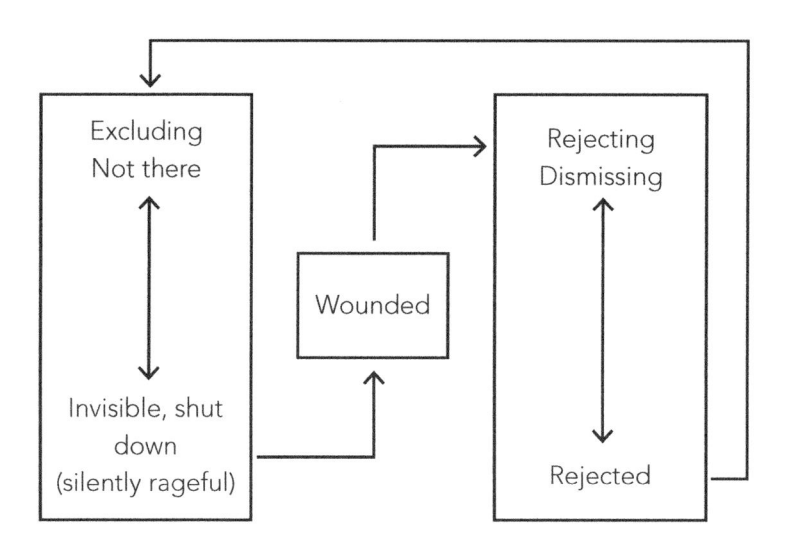

Figure 7.5: Procedural map for the Wicked Stepmother

```
            ┌──────────────────────────────────────────┐
            ↓                                          │
┌──────────────────┐          ┌──────────────────┐    │
│   Excluding      │          │   Rejecting      │    │
│   Not there      │───────→  │   Dismissing     │    │
│        ↕         │          │        ↕         │    │
│                  │  ┌─────┐ │                  │    │
│                  │  │Wound│ │                  │    │
│                  │  │ ed  │ │                  │    │
│   Invisible, shut│  └─────┘ │   Rejected       │    │
│   down           │     ↑    │                  │────┘
│   (silently      │─────┘    │                  │
│   rageful)       │          │                  │
└──────────────────┘          └──────────────────┘
```

At this point in the story, Cinderella begins to fantasise about living a different life to the one she is experiencing, in which she is excluded, denied, demanded of and hidden away. Here, we turn to our second parent figure – the Fairy Godmother.

Reformulating and mapping with the Fairy Godmother

The Fairy Godmother epitomises perfect and ideal care. From an attachment point of view, she is the perfectly caring mother who is completely responsive, sometimes to the point of predicting all of her child's needs. Little, if any, distress can be shown by the child before the Fairy Godmother appears to make it all better. It seems that from the outside, she is perfect, dreamlike, and able to meet the child's every need - to the point that the child never feels wanting. The Fairy Godmother is kind, thoughtful and giving – everything that the Wicked Stepmother is not (on the surface). It all seems ideal. We all sometimes wish we had a Fairy Godmother and we can get lost in the fantasy and wonder of having someone who can wave a magic wand, cast a spell, and turn meaningless objects, like pumpkins, into horse-drawn carriages that will take us towards our true heart's desire. When I gave birth to twins, I frequently fantasised about having a Fairy Godmother who would know – even without me ever saying it – that I needed someone to make it all OK. She never appeared, and I was furious.

In CAT terms, the Fairy Godmother is the perfect carer. She is the dreamlike and idealised place on our map (see Figure 7.6):

Figure 7.6: A primary reciprocal role in the Fairy Godmother's map

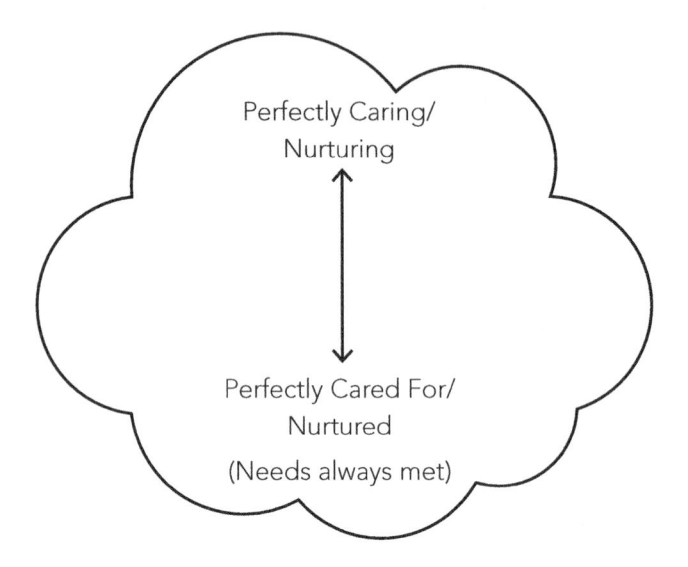

Perfectly Caring/Nurturing
↕
Perfectly Cared For/Nurtured
(Needs always met)

But this can also be smoke and mirrors – as we also know from attachment studies that a parent who seemingly provides perfect care has often found themselves in such a place for a reason (Bowlby, 1988). When I refer to perfect care, I am referring to care that never risks not being there, never risks getting it wrong, never risks letting the child down or disappointing them. In essence, it is the perfect mirage – another mirror that distorts the story. Welcome back to the house of mirrors.

The Fairy Godmother steps into therapy:

Fairy Godmother: I've had a really good week actually!

Therapist: Ok, what has made it a good week?

Fairy Godmother: So, you know I told you about a girl called Cinderella who I've been recently assigned to? Well, I've not really had much to do up until now, but last week her stepmother banished her to the cellar and so now I finally have something I can do!

Therapist: I see, I remember you saying in our last session that you often feel like a no-one?

Fairy Godmother: I did, completely – like, I was told Cinderella needed me and so I've been watching her and actually getting a bit frustrated because she clearly didn't and that's what I do, I come in and make everything wonderful.

Therapist: Yes, and you were saying that this week things had been different for her.

Fairy Godmother: Completely! Her stepmother, the wicked one – she's horrible, mean and so spiteful, and as for her daughters, well, the apple doesn't fall far! Anyway, I don't know what happened, but she shut Cinderella down in the cellar with only a few blankets and some raw potatoes, which is terrible for her because she's been so sad, but brilliant for me because I can take all of that away, with just a wave of my wand!

Therapist: So, is that what you think Cinderella needs from you?

Fairy Godmother: Well, yes, to be perfectly and blissfully happy – I can give her all that her heart desires.

Therapist: And... is that what your heart desires?

Fairy Godmother: [silence] Of course... my purpose is to see her happy again – then I'm happy, I've done something, I've given them their happy back so I'm happy.

In a later session, the therapist and the Fairy Godmother are discussing the procedure of rescuing Cinderella and the goal this serves for the Fairy Godmother:

Therapist: I wonder if we could map that out together – you described feeling like a no-one when Cinderella didn't need anything from you, then she was sad, and you could help her by taking the sadness away and making it all better – then you felt happy too because she was happy?

Fairy Godmother: Yes, that's right – I can't be a Fairy Godmother if I'm not making all the dreams come true – if I wasn't doing that then who would I be?

Therapist: Then who would you be…

Fairy Godmother: Well, either I'm her, or I'm no-one.

Therapist: Then you'd be no-one [writes 'no-one' onto the map]. So, can we write 'make all the dreams come true' over here [writes onto map]… are there any feelings to add into the map over here [points to the 'no-one'] I wonder?

Fairy Godmother: Sadness, loneliness.

Therapist: We've spoken before about the time you needed to be the 'perfect carer' for your mum, making sure she had what she needed, and though you saw how happy it made her, yet the care you needed from her wasn't available.

Fairy Godmother: I don't even know if she ever knew that I needed it, maybe I didn't know I needed it either back then, I just felt better when I could do what she needed and make it all wonderful for her.

Therapist: And you? Who makes it wonderful for you?

Fairy Godmother: That's how it works – either I make it wonderful for everyone else or I am no-one.

Figure 7.7: The dilemma that the Fairy Godmother describes

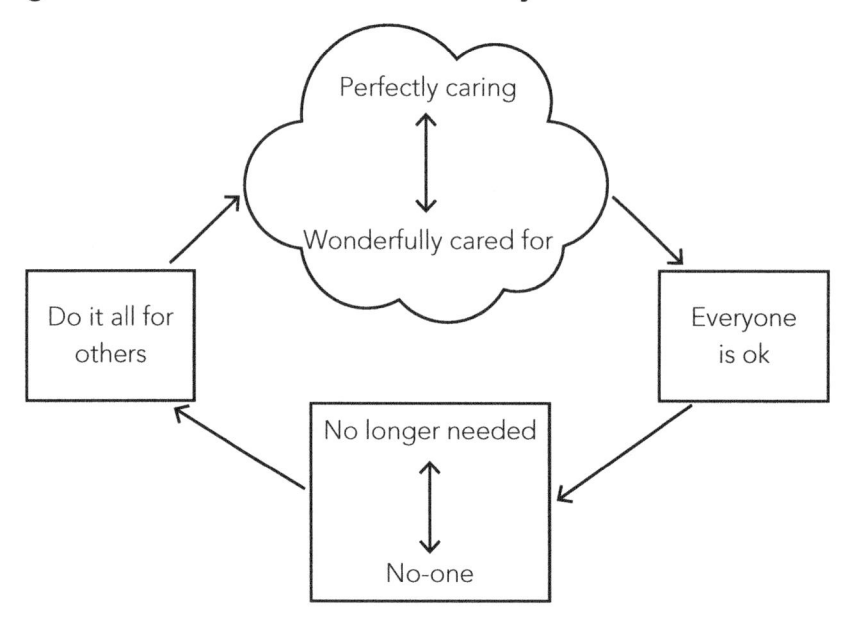

Perfectly caring ↕ Wonderfully cared for

Do it all for others

Everyone is ok

No longer needed ↕ No-one

The Wicked Stepmother and the Fairy Godmother are metaphors used to illustrate how a similar core pain of feeling dismissed and as 'no-one', can show itself in contrasting patterns and procedures. Fairy tales and fables mirror many of our desires and fears, and allow us opportunities to creatively explore them. Both parents experienced emotional neglect in their early stories, and both need to be seen and cared for unconditionally, they just had different ways, or procedures, of getting their (unmet) needs met. Many mirrors – many truths. Parent CAT working in the house of mirrors.

Reflecting on a space for Parent CAT

Psychotherapy with parents has produced real insights into the repetition of their history and the analysis of parent projections (Whitefield & Midgely, 2015). It can reflect the hidden (subconscious) self-to-self relationship with their inner child. For instance, if they have always been parented themselves to have a 'stiff upper lip', then they may be quite dismissive of their own feelings and vulnerabilities, while being similarly dismissive of their child's feelings and needs. If we are to support parents to make changes, we have to be prepared to listen, understand and hear the story of their inner child and provide space for them to see the effects on their own selves as well as their child.

CAT is sufficiently playful and creative to allow a space to explore all elements of these different relational (mirror) images and experiences. CAT is a relational model of therapy and lends itself beautifully to working alongside parents – focusing on the relational tasks of being a parent; of finding 'The Middle Way' (Jenaway, 2018). For many parents who have had strained, harmful or absent early experiences with their parents, such an approach is crucial as it allows for this to be recognised but also how it can be repeated unconsciously, and, through a better understanding, can allow to possibility of change. For parents of children whose behaviour provides clues of distress in the family or wider system, this compassionate and relational approach is vital. A compassionate and curious framework creates the foundation upon which it becomes possible to gently explore with parents the patterns that are evolving with their own children, which may be causing repeating re-enactments in the form of emotional and behavioural problems.

"It is a joy to be hidden; and a disaster not to be found." (Winnicott, 1965)

I am passionate about the role of CAT when working with parents in child-focused settings. The very name of children's services distorts the perceptions of what the service will deliver, a child intervention rather than what is *really* needed: a relationally wider focus encompassing children and their parents. So many parents, like the Wicked Stepmother and the Fairy Godmother, have unmet needs and core hidden pain, and the child becomes the recipient of this pain and these needs. Parents do not willingly place their disavowed unmet needs into their child, and they are often unaware that this has happened. Furthermore, the unmet needs of the parent can reflect the unmet needs of their own parents, and so on. Something I have so often said to the parents I've worked with is "This didn't start with you". The legacies of past relational experiences can potentially span decades of time and represent how the parent was parented themselves, alongside the social context they were in and cannot be viewed as independent of this: a rippling effect of relational evolution. In this way, when the parent speaks (and feels and acts) they are the mouthpiece of multiple voices, of many truths.

To understand the child, then, the parent *and the parent as a child* must always be held in mind. Careful listening and untangling whose voice belongs to whom can be challenging yet fascinating and vital work. To hold these multiple stories and voices in mind can be as disorienting as a house of mirrors in a fairground. All we can commit to doing in services and in ourselves, is to be willing to be curious about who you see reflected in the mirror and whether there is more to it. We must cherish the parent to truly heal the child.

Chapter 8:
Bringing CAT into the family and beyond – a systemic approach to CAT when working alongside families and their wider networks

Debbra Mortlock

Introduction

Since 2004, I have offered Cognitive Analytic Therapy (CAT) as an intervention while working as a clinical psychologist in services for children, young people and their families (CYPF). In addition, as a CYPF practitioner, I work with networks around children and young people (CYP) involving professionals as well as families. In this chapter, I will describe how:

i. I used CAT to help CYPF understand how relational patterns contribute to life challenges that brought them to seek support from services.

ii. CAT facilitates the development of helpful and coordinated responses from the young person's (YP) surrounding network, enabling them to provide good enough care for them, offering attuned and consistent responses.

Explaining my rationale for involving the network in what is predominantly an individual therapy model (Ryle & Kerr, 2002) through a more systemic approach, I shall share my experiences of using CAT in two settings: a specialist inpatient CAMHS unit and a Children's Social Care safeguarding team.

Providing an overview of these services, I will share how this more systemic approach has been helpful and demonstrate some of the processes and tools utilised in this work.

Fictitious young people's stories then illustrate how CAT can be applied in a more systemically informed approach. I have shared repeated themes from my own clinical work that have emerged through dialogue with young people and their families.

Background
My CAT story

Before diving into the specifics of the chapter, I will share experiences that led me in the direction of this way of working. As a newly trained psychologist in a CAMHS role, I worked in both specialist and generic child and adolescent mental health services (CAMHS). I was experienced in the use of cognitive behavioural therapy (CBT) and had a good understanding of attachment theory, which I drew on regularly. It quickly became evident to me that at the heart of many of the requests for help that CYPF brought to CAMHS were relational challenges. For example, challenges between a young person and their peers, parents, siblings or their wider family relationships, or even with themselves or a diagnosis they had been given.

Acknowledging my own zone of proximal development (ZPD), I embarked on CAT training, seeing a potential to build on my CBT skills and knowledge of attachment theory, being drawn to the structure, the focus on process and the flexibility of CAT. For me, CAT, through its tools such as letters and maps, offered both containment as well as space to follow the interests and respond to the developmental stages of CYP, but was mindful that CAT has not been an established therapeutic approach within the CAMHS in the UK, and therefore I was indebted to the support provided by my CAT supervisor.

In my experience, CAT in a CAMHS team offers:

- an intervention that is relational and transgenerational – complementing other commonly offered therapies such as family therapy.
- a goal-focused approach that is not dependent on CYP presenting with a specific psychiatric diagnosis in order to access the therapy.
- an approach focused on *change for the better*, which, for me, means being solution-focused rather than problem-focused, which often appeals to young people.

- a collaborative therapy that explores goals set by the client as well as allowing the therapist to contribute to the goal setting.

- a compassionate approach that endorses the idea that you do the best you can with what you have available. This avoids the enactment of blaming-blamed reciprocal role patterns that young people can often be invited into by adults.

Involving the network

Many of us working in CYPF settings are familiar with Donald Winnicott's often-referenced quote: "there is no such thing as an infant ... meaning, of course, that wherever one finds an infant one finds maternal care, and without maternal care there would be no infant" (Winnicott, 1970). When working with older children and adolescents, this quote continues to be relevant for optimal development, and even survival, as they heavily rely on care and support from the adults in their network, such as family and school. The introduction to this book describes how CAT theory emphasises how interactions with others, at interpersonal as well as societal levels, informs individuals' psychological development (Ryle & Kerr, 2002). Thus, involving important and significant others in a CYP's network offers opportunities for greater insights into the origins of their difficulties as well as exploring ways forward – in CAT jargon, 'exits' – which can be particularly important when working with younger children (those under 14 years). In my experience, the benefits of including the person's wider network include:

- Accessing the network's and community's knowledge increases our understanding of the relationships of CYP. For example, when reflecting on earlier relationships, young people may not have had the relational language to construct a narrative about such relationships, so those close to them may fill in the gaps.

- Exploring and increasing relational support from others in the network to facilitate care and change. It is extremely challenging for young people to make changes in their lives without the support of adults around them who have significant levels of power and influence over the young person.

Alongside the benefits of involving the network in aspects of a CAT framework, there can also be challenges. A young person may be experiencing abuse that one or more adults are perpetrating against them, which they may not want to disclose or may not even recognise as abuse. Therefore, it is important when moving from an individually based intervention to one that includes members of the wider network, that this is done alongside and with the consent of the young person.

Further, it is important to observe carefully how the adult responds to the CAT formulation, being mindful of any negative and positive implications for the young person's progress. If there are significant concerns raised, then sharing should be halted and a plan for moving forward made using regular service protocols, alongside suggestions from CAT supervision. It is always important to understand the motivations the young person has for requesting or agreeing for the information to be shared with family members or professionals, so that their expectations and potential outcomes are explored before sharing.

Using CAT in a specialist inpatient child and family service
Service context

There are a range of services in the UK that offer a similar approach to the model described below. Such services include CAMHS units, local authority run assessment units, therapeutic communities or specialist schools. The CAMHS unit I worked at was unusual in that it privileged a relational approach by always admitting the parent and child/young person together. CAT could be an option to support the CYPF as well as the team.

The residential service worked with children up to and around their 13th birthday. In addition to assessment and intervention with the young person, the service worked intensively with parents, creating opportunities to observe Reciprocal Roles (RRs) in action, be alongside families and work with individual family members on specific goals within the young person's care plan.

When I joined the service, its aims were to: "provide intensive assessment and treatment for children with complex emotional, behavioural and social difficulties... also offer intensive work with parents to develop their parenting skills."

This included separate activity programs for parents and CYP during school hours, education and broader learning experiences, group work for the children (social skills, art, music etc.), parenting groups as well as family time within the unit for play and creativity. Staff supported parents at 'hot spots' (i.e. challenging times for them and their children) throughout the day such as bedtimes, mealtimes and transitions, while these patterns might be explored further through therapeutic interventions offered in groups or individually, including key worker time for the children.

There was an established therapy offer from the unit that included individual psychology for children using CBT or psychodynamic psychotherapy and/or creative therapies. There was also a range of parenting groups offered that explored behaviour management as well as a parent-child relationship (e.g., Mellow Parent). All families were offered Family Therapy, and the staff on the unit were experienced in the application of systemic and attachment models as well as biopsychosocial formulation approaches.

The CYPF that attended the service were referred mostly by community CAMHS services. CYP had often received diagnoses of neurodevelopmental difficulties (autism, ADHD or Tourette's), psychiatric diagnoses (e.g. eating disorders, OCD, anxiety) or were described as school refusers. Sometimes, schools were struggling to educate and support them. A significant number of children showed high levels of violence and aggression towards their parents and others. Parents often reported that they had been fighting to get the appropriate support for their CYP, felt confused about their children's needs and felt lacking in the skills needed to support them, and repeatedly identified this service as their last hope for help.

A role for CAT

CAT found its space both as a therapy and a relational scaffold for informing wider work. There may be individual therapy for some young people, or more CAT-informed work for others, where letters or mapping felt more accessible. Parent work, including some bespoke trauma-informed practice, was supported by a sharing of CAT theory. Opportunities to observe staff and family interactions could also be mapped and reflected upon to inform further understanding and reformulation. Working with the team, through contextual reformulation (Carradice, 2004), allowed for greater clarity of the relational dynamics within the unit.

Tim's story

Tim (not the young person's real name) was a 13-year-old boy who had been admitted for assessment and intervention for an eating disorder that could not be managed in the community. He was medically stable but significantly underweight and was still struggling to eat the calories required to regain lost weight. Tim was initially resident on the unit with his father, followed by his mother, and had younger siblings who were still at primary school.

Pre-therapy assessment

Looking to explore if CAT was a good fit for Tim, alongside family therapy and the regular unit interventions, I was keen to consider whether he might be able to identify a relational goal for this work, and whether he might be able to make use of reciprocal roles and the importance of relationships. I was keen to see if he could reflect on past experiences and share these with me in our therapeutic space, but most importantly was the question, would Tim be willing to give CAT a go?

I was also keen to ensure that Tim could work alongside me, to be an active participant in his therapy, so that this would be work done *with* him, rather than for him to feel that this was something being done *to* him. Part of CAT is working 'with rather than to', including being able to say when I have got things wrong, to consider the right language to be used, and to explore what could be shared with others outside our space. Other considerations of this collaborative work are what could be shared with family, and what should be shared with the wider team, and how that sharing could happen.

Although willing to participate in therapy, young people sometimes highlight themes they do not want to explore. Tim chose not to talk with me about eating. In the end, Tim's suggested goal was a wish to be able to get on with people better, which suited the relational approach of CAT and its aims.

Given that CAT is collaborative, agreement on what can be discussed is repeatedly negotiated. Safety is always a core priority, and if someone else in the network takes responsibility for exploring certain themes with the young person, this can ensure their safety and allow CAT to maintain its collaborative stance. The beauty of CAT is that we can learn the relational patterns from any relationship the CYP is willing to explore.

Reformulation: a retelling and shared new understanding of the story

To support reformulation, and the retelling of Tim's story, a range of tools have proved helpful in supporting CYP to explore their past and present relationships, which in turn helps us to begin to hypothesise about the patterns of relating that contribute to current target problems (Ryle & Kerr, 2002). Tools that have proved helpful include the psychotherapy file (Ryle & Kerr, 2002), which I complete alongside a young person of Tim's age due to the wordiness of the document and the complexity of some of the concepts. Timelines mapped out on a piece of paper are also very helpful as school years and dates can provide good anchors. Timelines can be individualised to focus on the difficulty the young person is asking for help with or an area of their life they feel comfortable talking about. For example, relational themes can be explored through a history of friendships, or considering the toys they played with or other activities and interests that were special to them at a given age. These anchors, placed on the timeline, then allow for an exploration of what was happening around these experiences. I often draw on Solution Focused Therapy questioning strategies, such as scaling questions (Institute for Solution Focused Therapy, 2020) to understand in more depth what a young person is experiencing. For example, I may have asked about rating on a scale of 1-10, how included he felt with specific people, in different activities and even different contexts (e.g. school setting, family events). We might then explore what could have made him feel more or less included in these situations.

Reformulation, mapping and writing letters with Tim

Figure 8.1 represents some of the difficulties that Tim was experiencing and the Reciprocal Roles (RRs) that he identified as influencing his behaviour, thoughts and feelings.

Figure 8.1: Tim's map

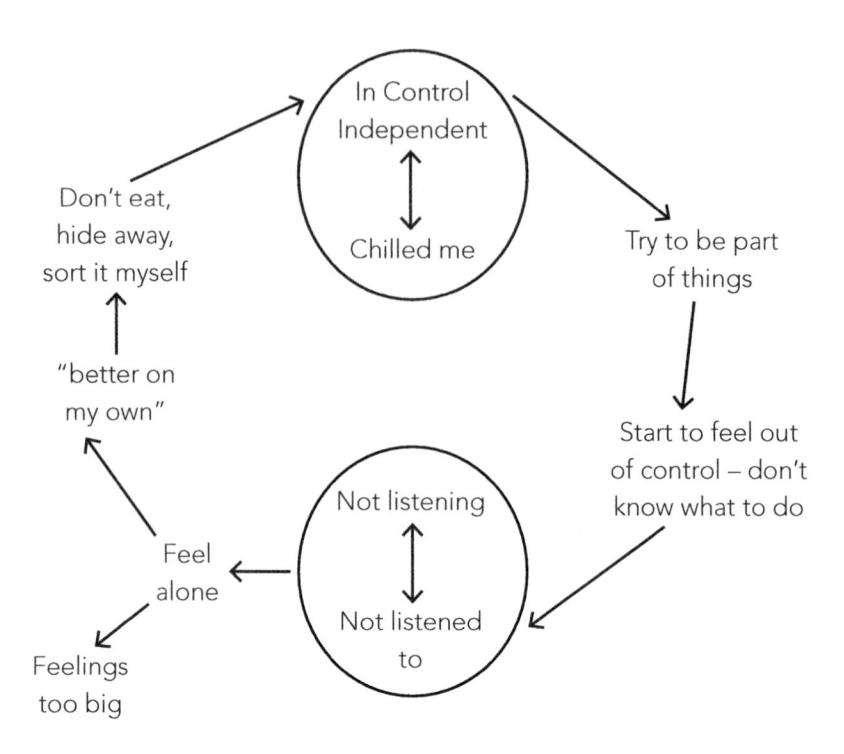

Diagram showing a cyclical map with two circles:

Top circle: In Control / Independent ↕ Chilled me

Bottom circle: Not listening ↕ Not listened to

Arrows and labels around the cycle:
- Don't eat, hide away, sort it myself
- "better on my own"
- Feel alone
- Feelings too big
- Try to be part of things
- Start to feel out of control – don't know what to do

When drawing these diagrams with young people, I have increasingly relied on the *developmental model* for CAT maps (Jenaway & Rattigan, 2011). This model, as illustrated in the map above, shows how the young person is caught in a cycle of not getting their needs met, becoming caught in a negative repertoire of RRs (as shown by "Not listening – Not listened to") and subsequently trying to get their needs met by pursuing an experience of hoped-for safety ("In Control/Independent – Chilled me"). However, this sense of safety is unsustainable, or unrealistic, and, for Tim, when looking to get to this place of safety, he places himself in harm by restricting his eating (controlling his intake), and he finds himself moving through the cycle once again.

This developmental model resonates with many CYP I work with. In many cases, more than one set of RRs (doing to – done to) is often identified but in my experience these can often be brought together into one core RRs that represent the greatest fear or level of emotional pain.

This is then the pattern to work on. "Not listening – Not Listened to" has been a common reciprocal role pattern that many young people have shared with me.

Through the narrative description in the Reformulation Letter, the cycles and traps can then be elaborated on, offering descriptions that aim to illustrate the complexity of the young person's emotional world by highlighting the breadth of feelings they experience. For Tim, this would have included how he felt not listened to by family and people at school and how this impacted him emotionally. Tim would then be unable to share this with those around him, reinforcing a sense of shame and the need for withdrawal and isolation. As a result of isolating himself, Tim then needing to take control through not eating helps him cope with these difficult feelings, thinking to himself that he will be better on his own. When feeling calmer, Tim then ventures back out to reconnect with others to avoid being alone. However, he soon feels let down and misunderstood, not listened to, and goes through the cycle once again.

Bringing the support network in

The benefit of a residential setting is being able to immediately observe the relational patterns articulated in the sessions, clarified through maps and the letter, being demonstrated live on the unit – to immediately bear witness through a systemic lens. Over time, the young person and those around them can immediately recognise the repeating patterns, and this helps provide more context to times when either positive or negative enactments take place.

Staff would have observed Tim struggling with interactions with peers more than others. Tim was reluctant to engage in physical games that the other boys were engaging in, leaving him standing on the sidelines and appearing withdrawn. In the unit's school, Tim excelled by verbally offering answers and ideas but struggled to complete written work, becoming low and withdrawn towards the end of lessons. Further observations highlighted that Tim had some specific difficulties impacting his writing ability and sporting proficiency. Tim did not share these difficulties with the adults around him. Hence, these observations helped us hypothesise that the *Not listening – Not listened* to roles have led him to believe that no one would help him or understand were he to share his difficulties, and helped us open the window for possible relationally informed exits.

Within family therapy sessions, parents shared the challenges they had as a family and their narratives about their relationships with Tim. They talked about Tim being a much-loved and wanted child, the struggles they had following the birth of younger siblings, and other relational losses that depleted their support networks. They also discussed how Tim struggled to separate from his mother when transitioning to primary school, further compounded by bullying. Experiences of loss were shared, as Tim lost a grandparent he was close to. They shared how they struggled to understand why Tim was finding it hard to attend school as teachers liked him, he had a couple of close friends he had known since primary school and things were good at home.

On the unit the parents are organised and seemed to provide good care, working together and following advice from the team, but also showing how hard it was for parents to have individual time with Tim due to the demands of his younger siblings. Disagreements with Tim usually ended with Tim isolating himself and his parents struggling to know how to react and respond.

Sharing the map with parents

Given how the map (or what is often referred to as SDR in CAT) seemed to reflect the dynamics demonstrated by the family on the unit, and that Tim's parents were keen to understand how to react and respond to Tim's distress and difficulties, it made sense, with Tim's permission, to share his map with his parents and with the wider team. A map is a simple and visual way to explore a shared formulation.

Through sharing the map, a new understanding, a retelling of Tim's story, came to light, with an acknowledgement that the "Not listening – Not listened to" had become established for Tim as his parents became busier when looking after his younger siblings, when he was struggling to settle at primary school and when his exhausted parents needed Tim to just get on and settle to take the demands off them. These roles were then being further reinforced when he could not talk about being bullied as everyone (i.e., his parents) seemed so worried about other issues.

This sharing of the map, and the unfolding of a new narrative for the whole family, helped illustrate how Tim's challenges had culminated in this current complex presentation, requiring specialist support. The parents could see and hear how much Tim had been struggling to manage these overwhelming emotions on his own.

Thinking and being together with a map

Working individually with Tim, through observing a repetition of the relational patterns for him and his family on the ward, and then sharing Tim's map with his family and the wider team, created the space for the family to experience their own reformulation. Tim's parents had been able to hear his story and, finally, Tim felt he had been listened to. The space had been created for the family to explore exits and test out a new reciprocal role:

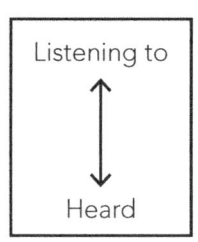

```
Listening to
    ↑
    ↓
  Heard
```

Following a session in which I share a map with parents, I would usually offer a further joint session with the young person, parent/s and the unit key workers. This session would aim to offer an opportunity for the adults close to the young person to show that they have heard what the young person has shared through the map, share their understanding of the map and perhaps share their own recognition of how they get caught up in the process. The session may also add some context that perhaps the young person did not have e.g., about their earlier life. But most importantly, the journey was no longer about repetition, and now much more about recognition and revision. A time to test out exits, not just within the family, but also through the wider network. As the original logo for ACAT stated, we are "Enabling change through understanding" (www.acat.me.uk).

Using CAT within a Children's Social Care safeguarding service

Across the UK, various safeguarding services within children's social care (CSC) have developed roles for clinical staff within their teams (Bostock & Newlands, 2020) and CAT can have a helpful role to play in such safeguarding contexts.

Service context

From a CAT perspective, CSC is a very relationally challenging landscape. Families often come into contact with safeguarding services at times of significant crisis, trauma and relational loss. Encounters with the services can be re-traumatising for often already traumatised people and there are many common RRs which can be enacted and anticipated between social workers and families:

Helpful RRs	Unhelpful RRs
Caring-Cared for	Overwhelming-Overwhelmed
Caring with limits-Cared for within limits	Blaming-Blamed
Respecting-Respected	Critical-Criticised
Generously giving-Gratefully receiving	Not listening-Not listened to
Protecting-Protected	Setting high expectations-Striving/Succeeding/Failing
Accepting-Accepted	Abusing-Abused
Connecting-Connected	Abandoning-Abandoned

Working in such a service, I was often asked to work directly with families or support social workers as they planned and completed their interventions. I found CAT helpful by being able to offer indirect work through contextual reformulation to understand the working relationships between staff and/or families, identifying some of the repeating patterns that were being enacted and were barriers to enabling change or engagement for families. Things often felt very stuck, and so understanding some of the core reciprocal roles was invaluable.

Clara's story

Clara's story reflects situations in which I was supporting a young person who didn't want to engage with me directly, and therefore I looked to work with those around her using contextual reformulation or a CAT understanding. Clara is 14 years old and lives between recently separated parents. She is the youngest of three children and her adult siblings live independently. The family experience significant financial hardship but are supported by extended family, in particular a paternal aunt. There were concerns that Clara was being groomed for sexual exploitation in her local community. Parents have been working well together and with professionals to try to safeguard and protect her.

Working alongside the service model, I would often attend child protection meetings at which the network of professionals and parents would meet together. Through these meetings, I would build up a picture of the relational traps that families, and subsequently professionals, were being caught in as they cared for their CYP. To explore this with the network, I would usually draw out an initial map of relational patterns (Potter, 2010), sitting alongside family and professionals, looking to see if the concept of RRs and mapping made sense to them. I could then offer to develop a more detailed map with them if I had captured some curiosity.

In situations like Clara's, I have often found it helpful to keep families focused on the present situation and not delve too much into their past relationships, keeping the focus on maintaining the safety of the CYP, and trying to avoid opening past relational wounds that might feel too painful to explore, and hinder possibilities for change.

For Clara's network, Figure 8.2 illustrates the RRs and relational patterns that are difficult for Clara. This includes when she feels that her needs are not being met by those who are caring for her because they appear unable to satisfy all of her demands, which leads her to feel rejected by them, assuming they do not want her. To cope, she makes plans and moves on to another family member or even to a risk-taking peer, looking for a fresh start. The family also get caught in this relational pattern with Clara. In Figure 8.2, below, we can see Clara and family enactments where P represents parents and C is for Clara:

Figure 8.2: Taking care of Clara map

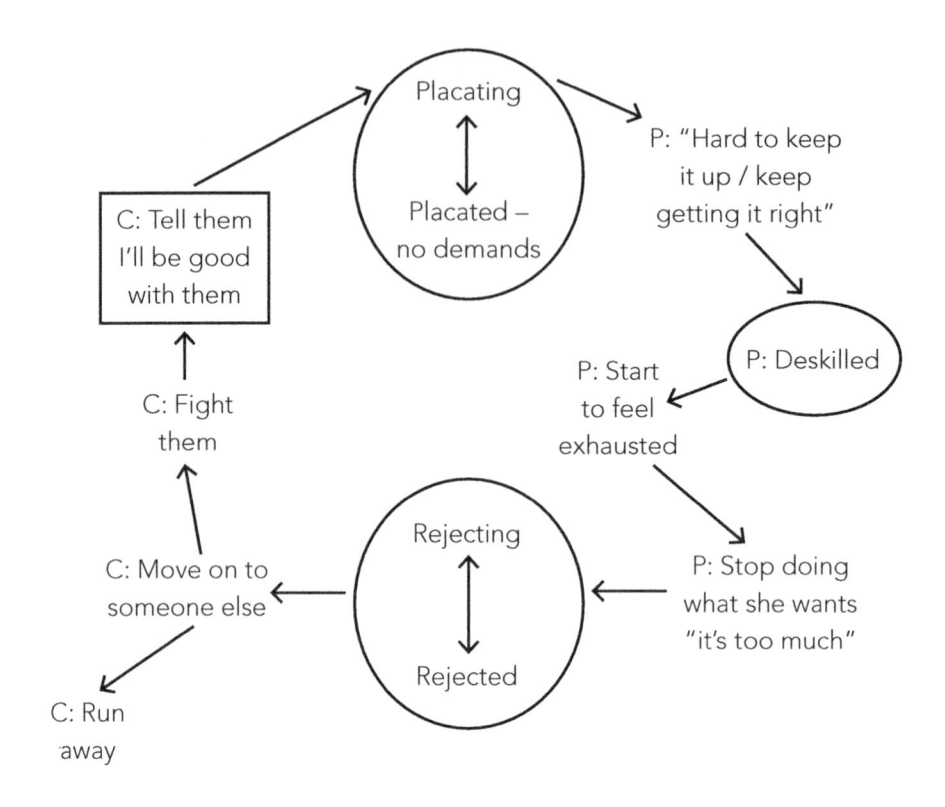

Placating ↕ **Placated – no demands**

Rejecting ↕ **Rejected**

- C: Tell them I'll be good with them
- C: Fight them
- C: Move on to someone else
- C: Run away
- P: "Hard to keep it up / keep getting it right"
- P: Deskilled
- P: Start to feel exhausted
- P: Stop doing what she wants "it's too much"

The map shows how Clara might move from one family member to another looking for support (mum, dad and paternal aunt), and shows that their approach to keeping her safe was to placate her to try to keep her with them. When they could not find the skills or energy (or the finances) to care for her in this way, she would feel rejected, and therefore reject them and move on to another family member. In the wider family context, this would then have led to conflict between those members of the family she had run to and those she had been recently rejected by, sustaining a cycle of conflicts within the family which replicated the cyclical pattern of Clara's thoughts, feelings and actions outlined on the map. This could lead them to act in further rejecting ways towards Clara and drive further conflict within the family.

As a result, Clara would look for support and care from others within her peer group or adults who were suspected of exploiting her. The map therefore helps the network understand some of the reasons why Clara may be placing herself at risk of exploitation, the potential for them to re-enact some of the relational patterns, and for those around her to reflect on how they might better work together to change their own actions and reactions, offering Clara more consistently protective relational opportunities.

Exits – finding healthier reciprocal roles

Having developed with Clara's network a map they felt reflected their experiences of trying to care for Clara, the next step involved working together to find exits from these repeating patterns and reactions to distress. In Clara's case, the network's exits would require them to be focused on goals that might include:

- Keeping her close/keep her safe enough – do the things needed to make her feel welcome.

- Keeping a watchful eye – using the time with her to try to get a better picture of what is happening for her, what keeps her there and who is she communicating with.

- Keep connected: *"We're in it together"* – keep each other up to date, offer the family member she is residing with encouragement and support and provide behind-the-scenes support when she needs to move on.

An exit that allowed for a new reciprocal role to develop, for Clara, her family and the wider network was:

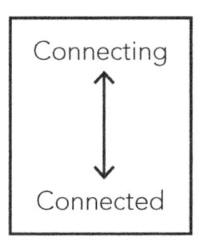

```
┌─────────────┐
│ Connecting  │
│     ↑       │
│     ↕       │
│     ↓       │
│ Connected   │
└─────────────┘
```

With Figure 8.2, the wider professional network could also see how they could support and sustain these exits for the family, and see the impact of their work, recognising that they won't get it right, all the time.

Over time, the maps can be reviewed, and developing curiosity can lead CYP and their networks to reveal new information about relational patterns that might be protective or increase vulnerability, allowing for new reciprocal roles to find their way onto the map.

149

Reflections

It is such a privilege to use CAT in the ways I have outlined above. I am forever grateful to the children, young people, families and colleagues who have allowed me to explore their relational worlds. Similarly, to have worked in services that value relationships and their power to influence change. CAT has helped me and the networks supporting young people to understand what happens in the space between them all, enabling us to use our compassion and curiosity to be relational detectives. For me, with its focus on collaboration and working in the ZPD, CAT means that the most sensitive of family experiences can be explored.

My final thoughts are to offer some guidance to those who may embark on similar journeys, sharing the wisdom offered to me by Anna Jellema and colleagues (2003) when I was "developing and promoting CAT in the NHS"; it is sound advice wherever you are working:

- Be patient.
- Establish a community to learn with and gain support from other CAT colleagues.
- Limit and tailor what you do to make a difference.
- Develop training.
- Draw and use national and strategic frameworks.
- Help develop the CAT evidence base.

Much of this advice could be rewritten as guidance or advice for parents – be patient, share the learning, be realistic, continue to learn, draw upon wider networks, focus on what works well – and all could be on the map, or in a letter. CAT, through its relational approach, has so much to offer for working with families and across wider networks of support in this systemically informed manner. After all:

"It takes a whole village to raise a child."

Chapter 9: Using CAT – a relational approach in groups with young people

Cat McKenzie

Introduction

At our core, we are social creatures, wired for connection and ill-equipped to survive and thrive alone. To belong to a group (or groups), to seek connection and safety within a tribe or community, has underpinned our survival and evolution; meaningful social bonding is a universal human need (Yalom & Leszez, 2005).

Groups can be defined as a collection of people that are placed together or considered as a unit; or a set of people who share something in common and who organise themselves to work or act together. Some groups we may choose to belong to, others are chosen for us. Just as we are shaped by the internalisation of our relationships with individual primary others, such as parents, teachers and peers, we are also moulded by the relational experience of our participation in groups (or, equally, our exclusion from them).

Adolescence and early adulthood mark a time when we are pulled to individuate and establish a self that can hold its own edges more independently from parents and carers. And yet, the innate desire to belong, to feel accepted and connected leaves us primed to seek out relationships with others. For young people, peer groups become an increasingly significant and valued source of social and emotional support and validation (Gorrese & Ruggiere, 2012). It is also in peer group settings that social injury can occur (or painful relational experiences from childhood re-enacted), such as bullying, abuse, neglect or exclusion. For young people, these experiences can forge narrow or limiting narratives about worthiness and belonging and shape expectations they have of themselves, others, and the world as an unsafe or unforgiving place. Carried unchecked into adult lives, we too often see the replaying of these hurt and hurting stories echo across people's relational lifespans and the many domains of their lives.

Providing safe, supported, relationally aware group spaces can offer reparative opportunities for us to build healing stories and integrate new ways of relating to ourselves and others. This chapter hopes to highlight the therapeutic role played by a relational approach in group settings for young people. A relational approach informed by Cognitive Analytic Therapy (CAT) can help scaffold and enrich the therapeutic group processes that assist young people to develop in their relational understanding and flexibility; allowing for healthier relationships with self and others and improved social, emotional and psychological well-being.

It is my hope that this chapter stokes excitement for the many possibilities and potential benefits of taking a relationally informed approach to group work with young people and encourages those that have yet to venture into the dynamic and enriching space of group work with young people to take the leap.

A developmental case for groups with young people

The developmental journey that carries us through adolescence into adulthood is the period of greatest psychosocial and biological change after infancy (Naar-King & Suarez, 2011). This transitional period is a time of exploration, of trying on different roles, values and attitudes, and experimenting with different ways of being in the world. The major developmental tasks as defined by Erikson (1950; 1968) are the dances of identity and role formation as well as explorations of autonomy and intimacy that develop through social interaction and are also shaped by our biology, growing up stories, family, peer groups and the cultural and political zeitgeist. I would reason that the central tasks of any process-oriented group that takes a relational approach also mirrors that of Erikson's developmental tasks for adolescence and early adulthood.

Therapeutic group settings can offer a safe and containing place for young people to explore and experiment with roles and responsibilities, as well as intimacy and belonging, in a supported and supportive group context.

They offer human experiences that can contribute to young people internalising a range of protective and flexible relational roles including the freedom to step into both poles of relationships i.e. offering care to others while also being cared for, witnessing others while simultaneously being seen. These experiences of duality can assist in shaping a positive sense of self and a greater capacity to be with self and others in a caring, flexible and skilled way. In CAT, we are seen as more interpersonal when we can move more flexibly from one pole of a relationship to another (Ryle & Kerr, 2020). This makes sense as, to be in a loving relationship, we need not only to be in the state of 'loved' but in the more active state of 'loving'. A group can offer a safe space to play around and experiment with being in different poles of relationships, not just different relationships. This peer-to-peer group dynamic is a helpful adjunct to individual therapy where opportunities to step into more active caring roles are more limited.

Our aims as facilitators are to support the group to work together to co-create a collective identity for the group around shared values in which each person is a stakeholder and has responsibility for maintaining. Intimacy and autonomy in a group context can be seen when a group shifts from being facilitator-led to being peer-led. This can be achieved by building in invitation and opportunity for the group to make decisions, facilitate activities, set agendas, share wisdom and demonstrate care towards each other, all the while developing in their skills and confidence for shared ownership and leadership. If you do a good enough job at this as a facilitator, you will need to tolerate no longer being needed but the opportunity to bear witness to connection, community care and interdependence originating from group members back to the group is the ultimate redundancy package.

Evidence base

Therapeutic group interventions with children and young people have been practised since the turn of the nineteenth century (Shechtman, 2007). The bulk of research has focused predominantly on cognitive behavioural approaches to group work, which typically focus on skills training and addressing individual presenting problems within group work settings (Martin *et al*, 2020). There is solid evidence for skills-based groups in symptom reduction and I acknowledge the place for such groups (Martin *et al*, 2020). It is my experience, however, that groups that take an integrative process-oriented approach through considering the relational experience of the individuals and how they may notice themselves in the context of a collective, offer rich insights. These groups not only build skills, particularly the skill of noticing themselves in relationship with others but can also be a space for deep interpersonal growth and transformation as they are noticed by others in different and (hopefully) more empowering, strengths-based ways. For instance, a young person who is often bullied at school can have a different experience in a group as they take on a leadership or spokesperson position. Equally, a young person in the role of a young carer for a family member may have the opportunity to step into the experience of being the one that receives care in a nurturing peer group space.

It has been argued that behaviour and skills acquisition might be most efficiently achieved through process-oriented groups where re-experiencing positive relationships can be internalised, rather than through purely skills-focused groups that could overlook the relational context of the group (Shechtman, 2007). For it is the intricate interplay of human experiences in a group process that contributes to the therapeutic properties that help individuals in their process of change (Yalom & Leszez, 2005). Aside from psychoeducation and skill building, Yalom highlights a number of therapeutic factors that relational process-oriented groups offer including: the installation of hope, universality of experience, opportunities for altruism (the opportunity to sit in both a caring and cared for relational roles), the corrective recapitulation of the primary family group, imitative behaviour, interpersonal learning, group cohesiveness, catharsis and existential factors (Yalom & Leszez, 2005).

The bulk of research into therapeutic group work has predominately focused on adult populations and the evidence base for therapeutic group work with young people specifically is relatively underdeveloped (Martin *et al*, 2020). CAT has been used in group settings successfully in the UK and other countries, however it is still building its evidence base and the pool of evidence for CAT and group work with young people remains shallow, although what has been shared so far is very promising (Martin *et al*, 2020; Mulhall, 2013).

CAT and group therapy with young people

CAT as a relational model of therapy lends itself organically to process-oriented group work by offering tools and language that make the shared relational space between people more tangible and accessible. CAT aims to support people to build awareness (and therefore choice) around their relational ways of being in a compassionate and non-blaming way, bringing into focus patterns of thinking, feeling and behaving that play out relationally and either serve us or maintain difficulties, at an intrapsychic and interpersonal level (Martin *et al*, 2021). As a model, it encourages individuals and groups to reflect upon what they are bringing to the group dynamic from their previous relational experiences as well as what is being played out in vivo within the group context. This relational stance invites a rich dialogic narrative and opportunities for supporting one another's awareness and growth; shifting the focus from individuals to examine and 'fix' their difficulties in isolation or solely in an individual therapy room to a multi-perspective group where one can move in and out of different relationships, reflecting on what best suits and fits with themselves and the relationships they want to build on.

The group space is influenced by a number of factors including the individual and shared capacities of the group to engage in learning relationships, the relational stance of group facilitators, the participants' own ways of engaging, their developmental stage and relationship history, the physical space and mediums and the task. I will discuss some of these concepts and how they can be used to create a group that both supports and challenges young people to be both interpersonally and intrapersonally more aware and relationally flexible.

Introducing CORE Group

In 2019, my colleague Lee Crothers and I developed and facilitated an integrated CAT and Art Therapy group for young people aged 18 to 25 that ran once a week for six weeks. CORE group set out to foster a safe and supportive environment for young people to explore their patterned ways of being and increase their relational flexibility using CAT and creative expression. The group focused on building a shared narrative of a presenting problem (they identified their shared target problem of feeling 'alien' and not belonging) while holding space in tandem for the unique individual stories and experiences of members. Recognition of patterns was practised through mapping and reflection as a group and the group came to explore shared exits and a co-authored goodbye. The group took a creative and experiential approach to introducing CAT concepts and tools, integrating art and music therapy modalities.

Participants had varying degrees of exposure to CAT, with the majority having little to no experience with the model. The ten participants were aged between 18 and 25 years with a mixture of genders and gender identities. There was some diversity in cultural background with the majority of participants being white Anglo-Australian. A diagnosis of mental illness was not a pre-requisite for participation in the group, however there was a broad range of mental health presentations within the group including mixed depression and anxiety disorders, eating disorders, personality disorders and histories of psychosis.

I have made reference to CORE group throughout this chapter to illustrate the application of ideas, concepts and learnings.

A relational understanding of group learning: The Zone of Proximal Development

The zone of proximal development (ZPD) is a relational concept that helps us to consider how we, as group facilitators, can optimise individual and group development and learning (Ryle & Kerr, 2002). Lev Vygotsky, a Russian philosopher and psychologist, used the term to describe the 'zone', gap or space between being dependent on another , more-skilled person to help, and being competent to perform that skill independently. When the pupil is met by the teacher (one being more skilled in one area than the other) within the ZPD they are relating to each other and the task in a way that is conducive to the pupil learning the skill and access it independently (Ryle & Kerr, 2002).

The ZPD can be overshot or undershot but there is a 'sweet spot' or window where the teacher and pupil are mutually understanding of each other and able to challenge and be challenged enough so that learning occurs. The ZPD can fluctuate depending on each of the individual's state (e.g., if we are very hungry our ZPD typically shrinks as we tend to shift our focus towards finding a meal rather than learning or teaching a new skill), but it can also depend on how one generally relates to others or whether we can be socially flexible and tolerate being in teaching and learning relationships. Vygotsky was fascinated by how some individuals could learn more rapidly than others even if they had the same IQ and education history, and put this down to how they could better relate, self-regulate, and be in a learning relationship (Ryle & Kerr, 2002).

This social and relational concept of learning – that we can only learn through others – is useful in considering group facilitation with young people. In a group context, the ZPD is held not just between an individual and teacher (or in this case, facilitator) but is also shaped and held by the group. So there exists both individual ZPDs and a shared group ZPD. In a group context, we are influenced by our peers and the spectrum of experiences and skills the group bring can help to stretch and extend the shared ZPD of the group as young people learn not just from the facilitator but also from each other. Given the developmentally weighted importance of peer group acceptance, it can also enhance and push the group's learning edge as young people in the group lead by example. I can think of many occasions when I have witnessed young people who have felt stuck in their individual therapy sessions make gigantic leaps when they find connection, comradeship, leadership and learning opportunities from their peers in group spaces. The challenge for the facilitator is learning to hold and accommodate both spectrums of the group ZPD. A relational approach helps with understanding a group's stage or ZPD, alongside the individual's ZPD and what it may take from both to further develop.

Scaffolding the ZPD of the group

Meeting the group in its ZPD in the initial sessions of therapy requires thoughtfulness in scaffolding an environment that establishes a sense of safety, as well as shared control and ownership. For CORE group, we approached meeting the broad ZPD of the group by scaffolding an opportunity for participants to engage in different ways so that they could make choices about the level of vulnerability they shared based on their readiness and regulation. Group members were given the opportunity to contribute verbally in large groups, small groups, or non-verbally through other means of creative expression, or opt out of sharing but encouraged to remain present with each other in the room. Taking the pressure off, while maintaining an open invitation, allows enough room for participants to move between a desire to be seen and a need to hide.

To scaffold a sense of safety (a core element for connection and learning and stretching the ZPD) we invited the group to participate in building a group art installation; identifying values important to them in order to cultivate a culture of care and inclusiveness. This bridged conversation that helped individuals connect in their co-creation of the space and the installation remained present in the group room each week as a representation and reminder of the values they aspired to maintain.

The relational stance of group facilitators as a way to scaffold the group

How we position ourselves as facilitators and the relational stance we consciously or unconsciously step into has a powerful influence on the group dynamics we cocreate and the ZPD of the group. A group that uses the relational understanding that we all have a learned way of interacting (which helped us get our emotional needs met or seemed to be the better way of protecting ourselves as children) offers group members and facilitators flexibility in the way they understand and meet each other in a compassionate and non-blaming way. In CORE group, we had a number of young people who had experienced bullying by parents, peers and teachers, and entered the group with a fear of this experience being repeated. In bracing for this, they positioned themselves, accordingly, to being silent and wary as a way to test out the safety of the group but in doing so could have elicited suspicion and wariness from group members. A purely skills-focused group may have unwittingly overlooked this enactment and set the group up to re-enact the bullying-to-bullied relationship in the group by the group. In taking a relationally informed approach, we chose to be explicit in educating the group members about our tendency to position ourselves (largely unconsciously) to repeat relationship patterns because of our history and learnt ways of relating, which invited participants to move from a judging or scrutinising stance into a more curious, empathising and connecting position.

This approach to group work also provided us, as group facilitators with this understanding so that we could be mindful of not being drawn into repetitions of unhelpful patterns as easily, and thus model to the group a different way of relating. CAT offers a language and multiple perspectives that can help group facilitators (and participants, once they have been introduced to the model) to notice and reflect on the relational pushes and pulls and use this awareness to make more empowered decisions about how they position themselves and participate. This is often referred to as the relational 'dance'. As Steve Potter (2020) references, "we can easily be so entangled in one style of helping that we neglect, or don't see, the need to talk about the process of helping, in particular the changing quality of the helping relationship between us". A group facilitator, in response to the withdrawn and wary young person (who is worried about not fitting in or being bullied), may unconsciously try and draw that person 'out of their shell' so the group can include them, but this could lead to the young person feeling pressured, leaving them to rely on their protective way of shrinking and consequently elicit more coldness from them. The other response many facilitators get into is to notice this person is wary and so not push at all, overlooking the person in the group to not repeat the bullying experience. This approach also has good intentions but leaves the young person with an experience of not being seen and remaining on the outside.

CAT invites group facilitators to adopt an open, humanistic, 'doing with/alongside' stance (Hepple, 2012). This is supported by the tools that can be used throughout the process, such as group letter writing and maps that invite participants and facilitators to collaborate, explore and make meaning together. It can also be supported by the relational stances a facilitator takes, often moving flexibly in order to help the group as a whole move forward in a task and then zeroing in to help individuals in their personal development and out again, thinking of the whole group. In the spirit of the Helpers Dance list by Steve Potter (2020), I have identified a handful of common relational stances that group facilitators might feel drawn to in a group setting. These examples are not intended to be a binary of 'right or wrong' ways of approaching group work, as it's been my experience that this can lead us to overly scrutinise ourselves for fear of 'doing it wrong' and stifle the way we approach group work (which flows on to limit the experience of the group). This is simply a list of a few ideas intended to support group facilitators to reflect on the relational position they are taking up and whether it may be useful in developing the group ZPD or not.

Group helpers checklist

The Host with the Most

The Host with the Most feels pulled to perfectly curate a space and a session plan with the hopes that people will feel valued, celebrated and special. This can be helpful in the first session or two and might be experienced as containing and caring, but if we always curate sessions this way it can send the message that 'everything has been done for you' or 'this space does not belong to you', leaving young people feeling stifled and limited in their freedom to cocreate the space or make a mess. It can also fail to overlook the creative capacity of young people to define their own spaces. It connects with the helper's dance of: *I can lose perspective: I get so involved in the detail I forget the big picture.*

The Mate

The Mate wants to create an experience where young people feel comfortable and related to. In this dance, we seek to be friendly and emphasise the things we have in common which can aid engagement and rapport building. An over emphasis, however, on being accommodating and accepted by the group can leave The Mate reluctant to step into other roles required to hold the space or model appropriate vulnerability for fear of being judged or unliked. In turn, participants may be reluctant to give critical feedback for fear of 'upsetting', may feel insufficiently held or safe, or similarly be reluctant to open up and try new things for fear of being seen as 'silly' or not accepted. It connects with the helper's dances of: *Mostly a hero, rarely a villain and; Not here, not now: I see the need to talk about what is happening between us but find it unpredictable or embarrassing and tend to wait and miss the moment to name it.*

The Helicopter Parent

The Helicopter parent wants to protect and nurture. Here, we try and anticipate others' needs before they have an opportunity to identify or express them themselves in the hope of shielding people from feeling discomfort. Consequently, we minimise necessary risk-taking, holding so tightly to the reins and keeping the parameters of the group restricted. We find ourselves in a perfectly caring and protecting dance which can leave people feeling both perfectly cared for but coddled and controlled. This limits young people's opportunities to practice →

articulating their needs, demonstrating their independence, modelling their capacity to take care of themselves and be caring towards each other as well as their ability to tolerate and sit with uncomfortable feelings. In this dance, we undershoot the group ZPD and overlook the resilience of young people, giving the impression that 'I cannot bear or think you cannot bear any discomfort'. It connects with the helper's dance of: *If I don't help no one will: Other people won't see the need or have the know-how to help so it is left up to me to provide the care that someone needs.*

The Lecturer

The Lecturer wants to impart and teach or 'upskill'. They feel safest with participants in the role of student. The role of facilitator will often include that of teacher, particularly when introducing concepts, but when we lean too heavily into this dance we risk overlooking the suite of competencies the group already has. This dance can lean towards didactic models of group work that feel safe and controlled but limiting and can stifle more robust conversation, learning and opportunities for participants to also be teachers. To young people, this dance might be experienced as patronising, infantilising, distant and stoic. It connects with the helper's dance of: *Safe but less real: I safely hide feelings, appear professional but less the real me.*

Hands off

As a group matures, our aim is to hand over power to the group. However, when we adopt a 'hands off' approach before the group has a handle of itself and the culture and skills to hold itself, it can communicate a lack of care and lead to harmful experiences that can be re-traumatising for group members who have too often felt neglected, overlooked, or unsafe in social spaces. It is my experience that a laissez-faire or 'hands-off' approach to group work rarely reflects a lack of care on the part of the group facilitator but a lack of time and resources to adequately prepare for a group, or the confidence and support to step into the role in a 'hands on', relationally informed way. Examples of this may be little or no scaffolding of group values and norms, insufficient session planning, poorly defined group aims, hesitancy to intervene when indicated, or an inadequately set up space. It connects with the helper's dance of: *Let it be and wait and see: I am not sure what to do so I tend to let it be and wait and see.*

The beauty of a relationally informed approach to group work is that the dance is fluid and changeable. Inviting 'noticing' helps us to consider the many different ways we can show up as facilitators and support the unfolding needs of a group. It is also a parallel process for participants who are developing their own capacity to observe without judgement, practice flexibility, and make more empowered choices in their relationships. In this way, there is no wrong dance if we show up with curiosity, authenticity and a willingness to participate in the process.

The task, the space and the mediums

As mentioned, a central task in a relationally informed group is for the group to become increasingly peer led. It is the role of the facilitator to "allow the group to evolve its own identity" and for the facilitator to transfer the role of leader to the group (Hepple, 2012). So, while the destination or task of the group is to form its own identity, culture of care, and shared ownership, the activities or mediums you build the group around and the space you create for the group help to facilitate the journey.

I consider the space and the mediums or activities we offer to a group to be co-facilitators in that they carry a relational dialogue and can be used to help establish safety and containment for a group while simultaneously creating an opportunity for the group to express, evolve, challenge and mould itself. This aligns with the Vygotskian viewpoint that signs, such as gestures, rhythms, sounds and jointly created rituals and symbols (and I would extend this to spaces and places), communicate wishes, intentions and meanings (Ryle & Kerr, 2002). In this way, the space and activities can be used to hold the spectrum of a group's ZPD and be adapted across the scope of a group to meet the group's learning needs.

In setting up the space for CORE group, we used colourful rugs to demarcate different zones in the room with a central gathering place in the middle. Cosy nooks were created around the edges with cushions that invited people to take small group chats or time out alone. Food and refreshments were readily available to people throughout the group, and art materials, instruments and sensory aids were easily accessible, encouraging self-care, exploration and play, as well as self-regulation. Music was also played in the background of the group, which was adapted to meet the needs of the group and, over time, it was curated by the group as they created their own playlists.

In CORE group, integrating art therapy with CAT provided an opportunity for participants to engage in creative exploration and experiential activities with a range of mediums which helped to scaffold and support reflections and integrate CAT theory and tools in a less prescriptive and non-traditional way. This made the group more accessible as it created a broader range of ways that young people could explore and express themselves, and was particularly helpful for young people who found purely talking-based approaches inaccessible. While art-making lent itself well to the cohort of young people we were seeking to engage, the beauty of a relationally informed group is that it could just as easily integrate different therapeutic modalities or activities to support inquiry such as team sport, Dungeons and Dragons, cooking, social action groups, or nature-based activities.

Conclusion

Group work is developmentally indicated for young people whose relationships with their peers are a priority. A relationally informed, process-oriented approach to group work with young people can help us as facilitators consider the individual and collective needs of the group and meet the group in their ZPD. A relational approach helps with scaffolding to maximise opportunities for learning and growth, including how we position ourselves relationally and how we code and imbue the spaces we set up with relational meaning. A relational approach can also give us insight into the counter positions we might take on to reassure people or even rescue them, and how this can be counter-productive at times and leave little for the group to help out with. CAT, as a relational model for group therapy, offers tools and language that can help the group to increase relational awareness and flexibility, and in doing so, can support young people to internalise new ways of being with themselves and with others.

Case Study 2: 'A Game of Two Halves' – CAT in the world of football

Nick Barnes

Love it or hate it, we all have a relationship with football. For some, it is the beautiful game, with a global reach that transcends division and dispute, even when the FIFA president states, "Today I feel gay, I feel disabled, I feel a migrant worker" (Infantino, 2022). For others, it typifies a legitimisation of aggression, most easily demonstrated by the rise in recorded domestic violence following each England international fixture (Oppenheim, 2022). As either a participant or a spectator, the world of football can divide and polarise us, but for some young people, it is a world that enables a sense of belonging, an experience of connection, and a possibility of dialogue.

'A Game of Two Halves' is a CAT-informed, group-based programme that looks to take a radical departure from more formalised therapeutic experiences and settings, delivered through the language and social meaning of football. It evolved out of a sense of frustration at a model of working in children and young people's mental health services that felt inappropriate and meaningless to the young person sitting in front of me. On many occasions, I had been asked to meet with a young person who was at risk of being excluded from school because of concerns about their 'behaviour', and that a mental health opinion was needed to make sense of what might be going on for the young person. The young person would feel embarrassed and humiliated for being referred to a mental health service, the parents often felt ashamed, while the referring school were anticipating that something magical might happen to ward off the possibility of exclusion.

While I fully accept that an exploration of a young person's mental health needs can be pivotal in preventing the possibility of exclusion, and particularly when thinking about any underlying neurodevelopmental needs that may have been missed in earlier years, there is often a need for timing and pacing of such interventions and assessments. Otherwise, they arrive at the point when the child is on their way out of the education system, and the prospect of a meeting with a mental health practitioner can feel intimidating and negating of the social or cultural context. Hence, the possibility of meaningful engagement and any collaborative working can feel far away from this clinical space. Certainly not a space that feels conducive to conversation and dialogue.

However, working in North London, under the shadow of White Hart Lane stadium, I was very aware that football had a currency and emotional capital that was far more accessible for some young people, and certainly offered a more meaningful space for dialogue. I reached out to Tottenham Hotspur FC community foundation, and from these conversations emerged 'A Game of Two Halves'. Over the last twelve years, 'A Game of Two Halves' has been in constant evolution, but the original model developed with Tottenham has informed all other iterations.

The key aim was to develop a group experience for young people who might be reluctant to engage with anything 'therapeutic' or based within a clinical mental-health setting – but who might be willing to explore how they connect with themselves, with each other and with the world of football around them, through a programme facilitated by the local Premier League club.

Our initial programmes were aimed at young people who were at risk of exclusion from secondary education for a multitude of reasons, it being important to stress to schools that asking us to work with a group of young people who were all seen as highly disruptive, would simply provide a setting for a group that would reinforce the challenges, not offer a space for testing out new ways of being with others. We also sought to recruit young people from different schools, so that there could be a coming together and team building that felt new and different for those involved, although we needed to be constantly vigilant to the possibility of postcode disputes.

The programme would run for up to twelve weeks, with sessions taking a morning of school curriculum time, one day a week. The key focus was to create an awareness and insight into how emotions might impact how we manage and relate to others, and hence on our actions, but initial conversations were kept at a safe distance from anything that might feel too exposing or humiliating – as it was this fear of humiliation that then informed how they might act and react within the world around them.

Each session ran with a similar scaffold – a minibus would collect the young people, and a member of staff from each school and the team would be brought to the training venue. An indoor team talk would take place, followed by everyone getting changed and heading out on the MUGA (multi-use games area) to do some skills training with the coach, followed by a match. A session debrief would happen on the MUGA before everyone would get changed and be taken back to school in the minibus. Throughout the programme, the emphasis was on developing and belonging to a team.

Team talks offered spaces for conversations that might explore what had happened in the Premier League the week before – so often fertile ground for dispute and disagreement. They might reflect on their 'idealised' (Premiership) clubs – on times of joy and times of despair, on times of success or failure. Teams could be idealised, favourite players could be admired, and yet, within a short space of time, they can just as easily be denigrated or dismissed. Think of the views of David Beckham after the World Cup against Argentina (1998), vilified across the nation for kicking out at an Argentinian player and getting himself sent off and being seen as contributing to England's exit, and then think of him as the 'role model' and the ambassadorial role that he holds today.

Working with a club like Tottenham Hotspur allowed for an exaggeration of these positions (or states) – admiring or dismissive, idealised or denigrated – with the brand of the football club being an important draw for the young people to take part. By reflecting on how we find ourselves in different places in relation to the club (and to others), we could then articulate the reciprocal roles being enacted, but still keep well within the language of football. Through role-playing incidents from Match of the Day, or speculating about ways of managing others, such as the Fergusson 'Hair Dryer' technique, the team began to reflect on how they might deal with such pressures.

This emerging awareness and understanding could then be taken onto the pitch – in both the training session and in the match. After all, football is about learning, working on, developing and implementing skills both as an individual and as a team, and then applying that learning in a way that it can be tested and revised – not too dissimilar to CAT. Skills can be about ball control or dribbling, passing or positioning, or even trying out set pieces. At the same time, CAT can be about learning skills, developing an awareness of a need for skills, and then implementing those skills to keep you on the field of play. Or, alternatively, to keep you in school.

The coaching was delivered by a Tottenham Hotspur coach who would use the sessions to work on specific drills and skills, informed by being part of the team talk previously. Any difficulties that may arise on the pitch, and there were many, could then be dealt with within the context of a different understanding. Sometimes players needed timeout or a yellow card, but the space always existed for the player to be able to gain some insight as to what had happened. The chance to move on from "it's not fair ref", or getting another red card.

At the end of each programme, the young people would go to a celebratory event at White Hart Lane stadium, and parents/carers would be invited to see them receive their medals and certificates to acknowledge what they had achieved. They would also be invited to train as peer coaches for the next cohort of young people coming on the programme.

This way of working perhaps best articulates the flexibility and creativity of CAT, building on the scaffold provided by Vygotsky's Zone of Proximal Development and looking to test out where we provide a necessary space, or gap between what a child is able to do along and what he/she could do with the provision of a more competent other – teacher, parent, peer, coach. But we are also providing an opportunity to reflect on self, and our relationships with others, as well as the world around us, that feels accessible and meaningful. Football offers these young people a tool for dialogue that has the credibility of being linked with coach and club, and is reinforced by working alongside peers – sideways support.

The project has evolved to work with those who have been excluded through working within a pupil referral unit. It was also adapted into a more individualised relational mentoring approach (advantage mentoring) that focused on young people who had been profoundly impacted by the COVID-19 pandemic with a genuine impact on experiences of exclusion and isolation. But one of the most significant results came through Strengths and Difficulties Questionnaires completed by the teachers, showing an improvement in prosocial behaviour. These young people were being seen, understood and connected with differently after A Game of Two Halves. Football had enabled, for some, a sense of awareness and connection, and an opportunity to prevent exclusion.

For more information about A Game of Two Halves, see: https://rsquaredservices.com/projects/a-game-of-2-halves.html

Advantage Mentoring: www.advantagementoring.co.uk/

PART 3: Relational approaches to service provision and the workplace

Chapter 10: Relationships matter – a case for CAT in an Early Intervention Service

Wendy Giovanelli and Kiara Wickremasinghe

"Inside the Sack"

White sheets piled high
Lying under dreams
Breaking glass under feet
Boxed in lines
Four eyes
Palms meet streams
We were once those trees
Now symbols
Revealing symmetrical pasts
Unknown futures
Question "safe"
Borderline hope
When you're ready
I'm here.

(Produced with permission from Celia Bax[8] 2023)

Introduction

A key component of any relational therapy is creating a safe and supportive environment in which to share and explore what has felt difficult. We consider this book a safe space for us to reflect on our meeting within an Early Intervention Service (EIS) as a care coordinator

---

8   Celia Bax is a London-based poet and creative who speaks with the voice of lived experience.

and a service user who had experienced a first episode of psychosis (FEP), and how our relationship led to this collaboration. We hope that by sharing our narrative, we can help support the recognition of Cognitive Analytic Therapy (CAT) as a useful relational addition to what is already on offer within this type of service.

Like a CAT reformulation letter, this chapter will not include all that could be spoken about in relation to us, CAT, EIS, young people, or what is understood as psychosis, but will support dialogue and give a sense of what allowed a meaningful connection between us as people, then and now. We have written this chapter as a way to demonstrate the dialogue between us and the social context in which we met: it moves between conversation, service-based information, personal reflection and poetry as a way to articulate a commentary on the importance of working relationally within this setting.

Magenta Café London, January 2023

Trust, tea, and the odd sushi roll offered us a place and time to meander in conversation, and to reminisce about our relationship and the path it had taken us. A way of speaking that allowed us to reconnect and consider the dialogic possibility of CAT and how it could imbue this chapter.

Kiara: Wendy, do you remember that time we sat here the day before my singing exam helping me write programme notes?

Wendy: Of course, I even included it in your CAT goodbye letter: "Kiara, I will miss our conversations, especially since we discovered the Magenta Café! Also, who else is going to give me the chance to analyse classical verse?"

Kiara: Yes, I'd come off my medication and had a limited sense of urgency and focus, and sitting here together was really helpful…

Wendy: Yeah… it's nice to be back.

Kiara: When you were invited to contribute to this book Wendy, what were your thoughts?

Wendy: Initially, I wondered if I was right for the job, then took a breath and considered what felt possible to share, including how it was offered to the reader. I felt a need to emphasise a way of being as a clinician, that holds and gives hope around healing and recovery for any young person experiencing what is understood as psychosis. Also, to convey respect for authentic collaboration with young people (and their networks), to make sense of, give agency, and move beyond what led to their referral to secondary mental health services, a system that has the potential to harm as well as heal. I wanted to offer a perspective around mental distress in which the impact of trauma, discrimination, poverty and loss is acknowledged, and every young person is understood within their social context. This is a position that advocates for relational work within EIS/psychosis-service lines and that CAT therapy is a good addition to what is already on offer. I also knew I didn't want to be writing about others, but writing with them, and so asked you to join me.

Wendy: So, Kiara, what were your thoughts when I approached you about this?

Kiara: Well, I was excited by the prospect of working with you again, following meaningful past collaborations – most memorably co-producing music for recovery workshops in EIS back when I was a service user. Butterflying into an anthropologist and practising and researching peer-supported Open Dialogue in mental health services, I enjoy experiencing and writing analytically about things from a 'peer' perspective. However, this chapter marks the first occasion that I'm sharing personal insights in published form, but also embarking on a dialogical writing process that feels different from what I'm used to. The challenging aspect of this collaboration, then, has been reflecting on vulnerability with respect to disclosure. But, equally, I want to convey how a label or diagnosis can still be a ghost towering over you and so finding my own relationship with this experience is important. Accordingly, I find the CAT-informed relational work we began together still informs and comforts me. Overall, my experience of recovery from psychosis has led me to a place of understanding, meaning, purpose and happiness around who I am and how I got here – both personally and professionally.

Understanding Early Intervention Services

Within the UK, an Early Intervention Service (EIS) team will work with any person aged between eighteen and sixty-five who experiences a first episode of psychosis, ensuring they receive a diagnostic assessment and, if accepted, an evidence-based, NICE-approved (2016) care package of support. A NICE-approved care plan includes the allocation of a care coordinator, an offer of cognitive behavioural therapy for psychosis (CBTp), family work, psychiatric medication and psychosocial interventions. As CAT is not NICE-approved within EIS, it fails to register in the data collection. However, there is increasing evidence that meaningful therapy with a relational focus offers better therapy outcomes for people experiencing FEP, and that the strength of the therapeutic alliance is a key indicator of positive or negative therapy outcomes across any psychosis pathway (Goldsmith *et al*, 2015). Growing evidence suggests that CAT, when used flexibly in a needs-led way, is a safe, relational, cognitively informed therapy that brings positive choice to the current treatment pathway (Taylor, 2017). CAT also equips the therapist with a theoretical frame and tools to scaffold work with this client group. However, as with CBTp, helpful, safe and meaningful therapy requires the therapist to hold certain key values and principles around psychosis and recovery (Morrison, 2017; Brabban *et al*, 2016).

Psychosis and other

"Voice-hearing is a complex, multi-faceted phenomenon that takes many different forms and resists reductive explanations." (Woods *et al*, 2022, p7)

Fortunately, a dialogic model like CAT has the potential to hold and listen to multiple perspectives; a helpful stance when there remains much uncertainty around the origins of 'psychosis' and how to define and refer to an experience that can involve unusual beliefs, paranoid thoughts, dissociation, bodily sensations, voices, noises and visions not experienced by another. Despite being intrinsically human, the othering of 'psychosis' continues to foster stigma and shame. Fortunately, increased representation from the voices of those with lived experience is effecting positive change in how we understand and relate to this phenomenon. Ted Talks (Longden, 2013), Healthtalk.org (2019), Hearing the Voice Project (2019), as well as Alex Bretherton and Kiara Wickremasinghe (contributors to this book), are all helping create greater awareness. Hopefully, having these more accessible narratives can aid young people and their families to better identify and seek support for an experience that can be hard to comprehend and distinguish from more expected responses to social stress and pressure (Boydell *et al*, 2012).

For many reasons, not everyone who experiences 'voices' has contact with mental health services. Romme and Escher (2000), founders of the Hearing Voices Network, draw attention to the importance of the relationship between voice hearers and their voices. They compared patients with non-patients and found the key difference between these two groups was that the non-patients' ratio of good to bad voices was higher than the patients', so they were unsurprisingly less fearful of their voices. Cultural and religious norms can also influence how an experience that is perceived by Western psychiatry as unusual or as an illness is understood and acted upon by that individual or community, while other cultural backgrounds may lead a person to perceive the experience along more spiritual lines, for example. This highlights the need to consider the role of spiritual care if we are to respectfully address the whole person within their socio-cultural context (Ryle & Kerr, 2020).

Although there may be multiple labels associated with psychosis and many diagnostically driven pathways for people who experience mental distress, in EIS there remains a reluctance to formally diagnose beyond the label of psychosis, and for some people, the offer of a diagnostic understanding may feel helpful. However, many highlight the poor fit between psychological difficulties (DSM-5, 2013) and the use of diagnostic categories including Johnston (2018) through the Power Threat Meaning Framework: a trauma-informed social perspective on mental distress. Indeed, alone or in combination, any traumatic event, acute stress, sleep deprivation, drug use, alcohol withdrawal, poverty or discrimination, can trigger a psychotic response. Thus, the British Psychology Society (Cooke, A 2017) advocates a cognitively informed continuum approach to psychosis, where we are asked to consider this experience as a meaningful response to adverse and painful life conditions. Seeing psychosis as lying on a continuum of normal human experience challenges the notion of psychosis as a symptom of underlying mental illness. It can therefore be responded to like other types of psychological distress. By building a 'meaning bridge' to an utterance or concept that has been othered, there can be integration into the collective conversation where the previously unsaid is articulated and validated, allowing for the joint creation of fresh meaning between those involved (Stiles, 1999).

CAT thinking and theory

"Playing the inscrutable withholding therapist, aloof consultant or 'scientist-practitioner expert' has no role, especially with this [group of people]" (Ryle & Kerr, 2020, p198)[9]

Therapy in EIS should feel safe and welcoming, a kind and flexible space that values uncertainty and the creativity that not-knowing affords; a way of being together that frees up possibilities and encourages collaboration (Peebles, 2022). Necessary flexibility within the CAT scaffold is afforded by Vygotsky's concept of ZPD, in which session number, use of tools, pace, depth and content of therapy is informed by client-need (Taylor *et al*, 2017).

The same relational understanding is used to make sense of distressing 'psychosis' as it is for other psychological difficulties (Taylor *et al*, 2018) and involves the concept of the 'dialogic self': we learn and evolve as beings in relation to others and our wider social context (Ryle & Kerr, 2020). This is an inter- to intra-personal understanding that involves the internalisation of dialogic voices, including the voice of the world we inhabit. Once internalised, communication with these 'voices' informs how we treat and view ourselves and connect with others, understanding which supports the well-documented connection between childhood adversity and voice hearing (Varese, 2012).

CAT views distressing psychosis as represented by "muddled, amplified or distorted enactments of RRPS as well as their associated dialogic voices" (Kerr *et al*, 2003, p517), which can then be mis-attributed as coming from a critical or threatening external other. Most voice content, if upsetting, appears linked to a threat from a more powerful other, eliciting shame and self-criticism (Heriot-Maitland *et al*, 2019).

The overall impact of FEP, including current treatment, may leave some young people feeling pressured, less confident and uncertain about what previously felt straightforward, including who to trust and how to disclose associated feelings. Authenticity as a therapist informs trust, is non-judgemental (this involves seeing the young person as a real person), wants to connect, and can provide safety around what is shared; a kinder reflective way of being together that, if internalised, can sow the seeds of a more compassionate internal and integrated dialogue. I have been told several times by young people that they have heard my voice reminding

---

9   Alteration from original text – agreed with author

them of things we had discussed when together. What is said may not always be verbatim but offers support through a sense of our relationship.

Steele (2013) connects a therapist's knowledge of their own 'CAT Map' through their own personal therapy and ability to collaborate in a genuine way. I recognise being curious about what I 'bring' as a clinician, or why certain words or phrases are included in maps or letters. This supports in me a sense of 'being with' as opposed to 'doing to' for young people, particularly those who may also struggle interpersonally or who are not yet ready for formal therapy.

The Trees

*Spiders have eight legs
because… therefore…
Silk slips like water
and we exist in a constant womb
Spiders have many eyes
Like my family
Loosely connected like verbs or
roots or boats
I am the constant lighthouse
I drew a mirror today, atop a tree
below a web
Balanced "I" the dot between
(I am, I am, I am.)*

(Produced with permission from Celia Bax, 2022)

Being in an EIS

Working relationally benefits a whole team. Making space for respectful conversation between colleagues is invaluable, particularly in a beleaguered mental health system that exists in a constant state of flux. Unconscious bias is relevant to how a young person enters and is viewed within the mental health system, and their ability to trust and use the support on offer will be informed by this first contact. A community referral via a GP is different to a referral via a police station followed by psychiatric detention. Resulting distress is universal, however there continues to be a greater likelihood of black Caribbean people entering services through an aversive route that involves arrest and detention

(Degnan *et al*, 2020) which confirms there is still work to be done to address the barriers to early engagement for African and Black communities described within the Breaking the Circles of Fear report (The Sainsburys Centre for Mental Health, 2002).

Brown (2019) rightly questions the ability of a white clinician to validate the real-life causation of mental distress for people from black and other minority ethnic backgrounds, without accepting their own relationship with privilege and power. I personally strive to hold an open stance that acknowledges the complex interplay between class, race, gender, sexual orientation, disability, religion and age, and the multiple factors associated with the creation and maintenance of systems that discriminate and oppress (Turner, 2021). CAT's social perspective can explore the relationship between power and disadvantage including within the mental health system. All trauma inflicted through a loss of liberty, including medication administered by force and detention in out-of-area beds with no connection to family and support networks, needs validation before meaningful exploration around initial referral can begin.

Before starting therapy, I invite the young person and their care coordinator to an introductory session to reinforce the sense of collaboration, continuity and connection within the team. As CAT is client-led, no therapeutic encounter is the same and, despite being on a psychosis pathway, this phenomenon may not be what a young person wishes to discuss. However, if a young person does want to explore 'psychosis', CAT tools support creative ways to facilitate dialogue. During one therapy, the word 'psychosis' was concealed under a Post-it note on the map until the young person felt secure enough to address it. In another scenario, persecutory voices were present on the map from the start, but only after a narrative around assault was discussed and the resulting distress validated, did the map come to life. It involved the perpetrator's name being written next to the symbol used to identify an unknown 'voice' who took responsibility for the attack. Once the name and symbol were integrated on the page, a different view was offered in which the young person was not to blame 'as they had done all they could'. Our work resulted in the relationship with the persecutory voice changing, its power weakening and the young person connecting with empathy in relation to their experience. Perry (2012, pp16-21) discusses how CAT has the potential to support negotiation with voices to free up alternative explanations and alter perspective in relation to power without "getting caught up in whether voices are 'real' or 'not real'".

For those young people who are not ready 'to talk', shared group activities such as a bike project, gardening, creative writing, fitness, social outings and the peer-led gaming group (see Chapter 15) are all relational examples of what can support healing. The power of having respected peer colleagues in a service is immeasurable and can be recognised as being an organic relationship with hope and recovery.

There is a lot of talk in CAT around ownership of letters and maps, including how and with whom they are shared. The map and the letters clearly belong to the young person as opposed to the service, and any 'letters' I receive – like the beautiful end-of-therapy poems shared in this chapter – are held by me. Decision-making around how documents and insights from therapy are shared with the wider team, family or beyond, is granted through collaboration and respect for agency. A compassionate CAT letter offers something different from a medically informed discharge summary, and a co-created map has depth beyond any psychologically informed template, so the meaning of CAT documents post-therapy is open to future possibilities, as evidenced by the poems and the conversation below.

"The Map that Travelled"

"I'd never linked my psychosis with leaving my home country, identity, place of belonging, community, support, all of these things. I didn't make that connection earlier because you think that was 2-3 years ago, so why is it relevant to what I'm facing now? It opens the possibility to really process or start to process that move. I'm still processing that." – Kiara

My family immigrated from Sri Lanka to the UK when I was a teenager, and for years I had bottled up the struggles of losing my home, identity, social support networks and sense of belonging. I now believe my mental distress stemmed from 'leaving' my home, a view corroborated by research (McKenzie & Shah, 2015). Indeed, I'm still fighting to belong on British soil; the difference being that I now see it as having two homes, both of which I can put down roots in. The map below, co-created with Wendy many years ago, is a 'sign' between us, and with the letter, has helped me better navigate elements of life going forward.

> **Wendy: Thinking about our relationship, what mattered and what helped you connect with EIS during your recovery?**

Kiara: Definitely a sense of warmth from you and others in the team who were involved in my care. And also just this feeling that I could slowly become myself or even understand who I was – because I didn't have that self-awareness before and that took time to cultivate. So just having that inclusive and non-judgemental space where I could be free of the critical voices that I maybe had in my life (I was very self-critical as a person but also family, culture, society – the voices of pressure). I think I always remember you recognising that I had a sense of humour, which nobody else had really told me since moving to the UK. But obviously, when I was young, I did have that sense of humour that was recognised by my grandma and friends, and people would say I was very witty. But I had lost that, or not lost entirely, but it had kind of disappeared. But you recognising my humour and wit told me that you really got me, and I saw it as a really nice compliment.

Wendy: Yeah, I noticed, and humour definitely played a part in how we connected.

Kiara: It helped me feel more like myself, more confident. I think even though we're different personalities, there's something about us that clicked really well from the start and that's why our relationship has lasted as collaborators and colleagues.

Wendy: You were planning on returning to university and I wasn't too sure if I would see you again after our first meeting, but there was a change of plan?

Kiara: It's the part I avoid in my broader narrative of recovery. If people ask me, I say I took a year out for health reasons, but I forget that actually I did have my psychosis in the summer after the first year of university and still thought I'd make it to the second year. Because, throughout my life, I'm just someone who's always had a plan with the next thing on my mind. I'd never had a break in life up till that point. I felt I needed to just keep going – until I got to my university accommodation and realised I was overwhelmed. But making that decision to stop was hard as I worried that taking time out would be like a year of life lost. But, actually, taking that time out was the best thing I did for myself.

Wendy: Yes, taking a pause and finding space to work through your experience is so important...

Kiara: Tolerating uncertainty is hard. I thought I'd go back and finish my degree but my GP didn't think I'd ever be able to go back. Not everyone has the best experience of initial referral pathways like GPs and home treatment teams. But ending up in EIS, I had a named care coordinator and continuity in care which I didn't have until then. You and the EIS team more broadly allowed me to build trusting relationships and maintain the belief that I could return to university.

Wendy: Is there anything else you'd like to share regarding your experience?

Kiara: Alongside the usual EIS family work, I really appreciated the one-to-ones with you as they helped me work out who I was and what I wanted. Another thing that helped my recovery was feeling integrated into the EIS team and being invited to sit on recruitment panels. Knowing that my opinions were being heard made me feel valued. Similarly, our collaborations, like co-producing those music workshops. And you encouraged me to pursue singing as a means of self-expression. I joined a church choir which was a pivotal moment in my recovery as it offered me a community to feel grounded through collective commitment to faith and music-making. But recently, I've also been thinking about the necessity of a spiritual community that's inclusive and makes room for people like me who don't fit the mould.

Wendy: Shall we talk a bit more about the map and how CAT-informed work came into our relationship?

Kiara: I think all these feelings like 'judged', 'criticised', 'stigmatised', 'shame' – I just never even thought about these words before. Isn't that weird? Hitting 19-20 and you've never conceptualised things in this way? You've bottled things up and don't have a language: 'can't express myself'. Because my degree was in geography, I obviously did have some affinity towards maps and diagrams. I love that CAT maps were a way I could digest things but also take them away with me. Because when you're recovering and medicated still, you're not going to retain all this. As I told you before, there's a lot about this map that I benefit from now and I can still see some of these patterns in my life, because this is kind of who

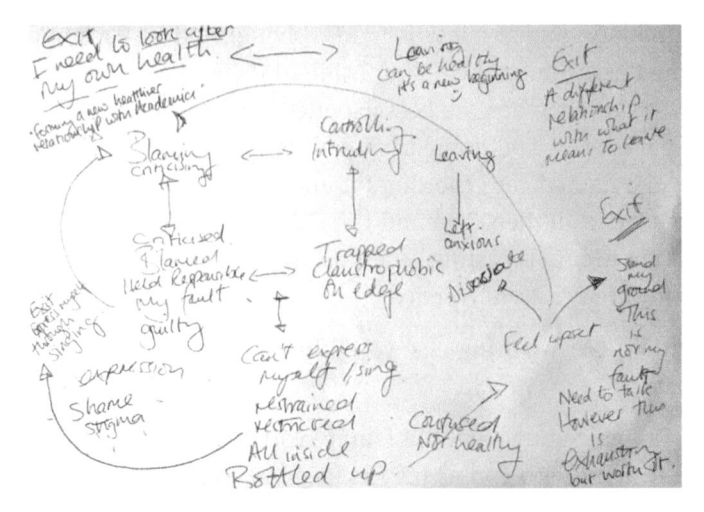

[Handwritten diagram of a CAT map showing exits, traps and reciprocal roles]

I am. I think, for the first time ever, I realised that 'leaving' or 'being left' was my vulnerability. So now I can actually have more self-compassion when it comes to the point of having to exit something unhelpful. I can find a healthier way of dealing with that and it doesn't have to be a negative thing. For example, in co-creating the map, you helped me see that leaving services was a needed exit and that I couldn't have thrived otherwise.

Wendy: Ultimately, this is its beauty, connecting with what works well and reflecting on how that can offer support or help in managing what's difficult.

Kiara: But also, see this word 'dissociate'. When someone dissociates, they can feel really anxious that it's a symptom but when it's put down on a map it's somehow connected, it doesn't have to be pathological – it's a natural, protective response. It's really alright to have a diagnosis if you find it comforting but setting things out in a social context on a page where you can see all the difficult things going on was helpful for me to make sense of the situation.

Wendy: Seeing it on a page, you step back and gain a fresh perspective.

Kiara: And that's why the map is a very living thing because you keep coming back to it with a new take on it. I keep it and the letter in my desk drawer and, when I feel a bit challenged, I pick them up and read them.

Wendy: Shall we talk about the letter and how it might mirror the map?

"As we come to our ending, I am aware the concept of leaving and or being left can bring up much for you – however I am glad we took time to focus on this and begin the process of understanding that leaving or being left is not always a bad thing. This is, as every ending introduces a new beginning, with the opportunity to try out ways of being or feeling that needed a fresh environment in which to thrive…" (Excerpt from Wendy's goodbye letter)

Kiara: The letter made me feel that a genuine connection was there throughout with you, and I realised how much care you had shown me. The thing about an EIS service is that you build a close therapeutic relationship with someone but it has an ending. But having your letter felt like you were still in my life in a deeply influential and healing way. And it's something tangible isn't it, with your name signed at the end – hand-signed, not typed.

Wendy: Yeah, working with the feelings connected to ending is a real strength of CAT and I still have your beautiful goodbye letter to me kept safely.

Kiara: But, ultimately, our relationship didn't just end with me being discharged. We've collaborated in various ways over the years and you've continued to hold me in mind. Even with the PhD I'm now doing, you heard about the role and connected me with the professor running the project.

Wendy: Well, I'm really proud of you and fully trust your ability to keep growing. To be honest, it's about recognising someone's potential whatever it is – be it academia, music, sport, dance or just the ability to have a calmer life. It's important to 'see' people.

Wendy: Lastly, I was so happy to learn you'd been using your CAT map as a training tool for clinicians.

Kiara: I was collaborating with a psychologist and we were running workshops on recovery-oriented care, so I spoke a lot about our therapeutic relationship and how healing that was. And that's how your maps came in.

Wendy: But maybe they're more 'your maps', than 'my maps'.

Kiara: Ok, they're our maps.

Wendy: Yeah, our maps [laughs].

Kiara: We'll have to have a debate on ownership of the maps! [laughs] Interestingly, I wasn't using them to demonstrate anything about CAT specifically.

Wendy: I love the idea of you taking a CAT map with you to a different place, and then you used it in a new way and it meant something different, evolving, very dialogic, very Bakhtin… [laughs]

Kiara: The 'map that travelled' has had a variety of functions and meanings in my life. It has been recycled in public settings like the training, but also in terms of personal growth. I still struggle with leaving unhealthy situations, but looking at this map gives me the courage to weigh up whether situations are worth sticking out or walking away from.

"The Ending Map"

"Creating a new map felt like a meaningful way to acknowledge and celebrate our collaboration on this chapter." (Kiara and Wendy)

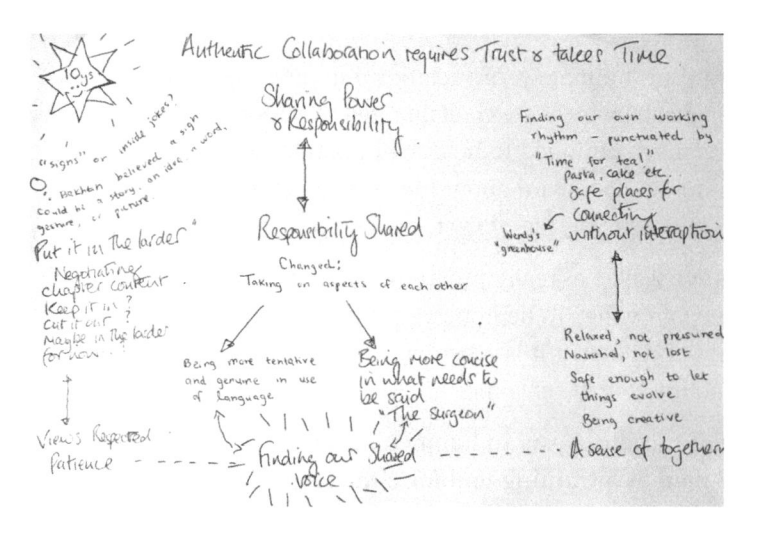

We hope that the story of our relationship and our reflection on it can show how value for reciprocity offered a way of communicating that was flexible, held uncertainty and met the concept of psychosis with kindness, interest and respect. As such, we are making the case to offer CAT and relational working within EIS services for the benefit of young people and staff. We ended this process convinced that working relationally is tantamount to healing.

Chapter 11: Creating 'just enough' space – setting up a new psychotherapy service in Chennai

Sivakami Suresh Prabalkumari

Introduction

In this chapter, I look to offer a window into my clinical practice and experiences in setting up a new psychotherapy service in Chennai. When invited to write this chapter, I was asked to consider whether there were specific societal and cultural contexts that needed to be considered when establishing this new practice, being mindful that I was applying a model of psychotherapy – Cognitive Analytic Therapy (CAT) – that I had learned about and trained in, within the UK. These initial questions have enabled fruitful conversations and dialogue that have allowed me the space to consider how culture is discussed and considered within our work.

I have always struggled with the binary position or stereotypical assumptions that can be made when exploring issues of culture. While some assumptions may be needed initially, I believe a therapeutic space needs to be safe for an individual and family to explore such issues without becoming a place influenced and informed by prior notions of who they are. When I came across CAT as a psychiatry trainee in the UK, I was struck by how it includes context and culture without making generalisations. I value the flexibility and creativity that CAT allows, enabling me to think about the needs of the individual, as well as the wider context of family and their surroundings – being able to consider the within, the between, and the around.

I start this chapter by offering an understanding of the context of setting up a new psychotherapy service in Chennai, followed by an account of seven stories of young people that reflect my practice of CAT, and the push and pull of working with a young person alongside their family. The stories have been chosen to reflect the diversity of care and support, but I am hopeful that readers may see aspects of their own approaches and ways of working reflected in this case material: case working that reflects and holds the diversity and plurality of our societies.

The wider context: Chennai

Chennai is one of the four metropolitan cities in India with a population of ten million. It is a sprawling city that is constantly expanding. It has a long history from its days as the state of Madras in pre-independent India. Home to the 228-year-old, government-run Institute of Mental Health, Chennai has one of the largest psychiatry hospitals in India. Mental health care is delivered in a variety of other settings, such as community-based clinics, general hospitals, psychiatric hospitals, in the private and public sectors. Out-of-pocket spending by individuals and families supporting them covers a large proportion (50.59%) of health care expenditure (World Health Organization database, 2023).

In the community at large, there are a multitude of voices speaking about mental health and many innovations are being made to make services more available. In recent years, there has been a wider recognition of the existing need and a call to strengthen governance, health systems and build care models relevant to the local context (Cuijpers *et al*, 2023).

In most parts of India, in the current mental health service context, the treatment of severe mental illness like schizophrenia, particularly in the acute phase, gains a far greater emphasis (Gururaj *et al*, 2016). The provision of psychotherapy or rehabilitation services compete with the same for resources. In such a competition, it is not surprising that the need to develop psychotherapy services gets overlooked by different stakeholders, including mental health professionals, administrators, patients and their families. There are few specialist psychotherapy services.

India is among the most unequal societies in the world (World Bank database, 2019). Currently, it is also the most populous country in the world. The inequality is stark in access to good quality healthcare and the use of available services (World Health Organization, 2021). There is also evidence to suggest that health professionals' communication and decision making with regard to treatment plans are influenced by their own social biases, resulting in the exclusion of certain groups in the community from receiving certain treatments (Gopal *et al*, 2021). This is compounded by other assumptions such as the need for *psychological mindedness* to engage in treatments like psychotherapy and, in turn, excluding groups who are deemed to lack the same (Thara *et al*, 2001). Inadvertently, this tends to discount the responsibility of services to evolve with sufficient complexity and nuance, leaving access to psychological treatments to a privileged few.

Trying to keep an even focus on the health needs across different sections of the society reminds me of the Tamil adage "So, is it blood when it flows from your body and tomato chutney when it flows from mine?". For conditions with complex needs like personality disorder, medically unexplained symptoms, substance dependence and 'treatment resistant depression', psychotherapeutic work is an established key component of a care plan, highlighting the need for innovative psychotherapy models and service delivery systems that are sensitive to the different socioeconomic pressures and contexts.

Against this background, I started a psychotherapy service in Chennai in 2019 in two locations. One alongside an existing community psychiatry clinic, and another in a children's hospital. Without any other psychotherapy service provision, the service attends to individuals aged twelve and above. Patients can be referred by other doctors or psychiatrists, or can seek help independently. The CAT model, benefiting from being transdiagnostic and time-limited, is used as the main model and offered in a stepped care approach (between six and twenty-four sessions) to match the presentation of the patient.

Common themes in creating 'just enough' space within this context

There have been considerable challenges in the setting up of a service offering this type of help. Challenging aspects within the wider healthcare system are outlined above. Some other factors occur at the level of family and culture. Some of the themes described below can appear to occur in families elsewhere in the world, too. The anxiety of talking about one's family to a third person around the reformulation process with adolescents has been expressed by Mulhall in his writing about using CAT with adolescents (2010).

With such caution, it is now safer to consider some common themes that are prevalent in a context like Chennai. One is a powerful and established hierarchy within the parent-child dyad. At its extreme, parents are framed as gods, with young people being required to honour and revere them. This is expected to manifest to varying degrees across individual families and needs exploration at that level. It could be held with varying degrees of flexibility. Families are also sources of strength and support. Healthcare systems (public and private) are designed with the expectation that families will take an active part in the individual's care, including meeting practical demands like organising care and funding the same.

Within this psychotherapy service, I have observed some general themes emerging at the time of seeking help and engaging with an activity like psychotherapy using the CAT model. One of these is the tug-of-war between the young person's interests and the wider family's interests. Another challenge is the invitation extended to the young person to discuss their experiences in the family environment. This can be traced as a CAT dilemma:

> "I express what is difficult for me, feel heard and understood" or
>
> "I am not allowed to speak my mind and I can never feel seen or understood".

The nature and level of involvement from parents vary with every family. Different degrees of separation seem to be available and the negotiation for 'just enough' space for a person to consider their own mind and their own needs is ongoing.

In this, I find that the CAT model offers the therapist ways to reflect on these issues. There is a need to meet every patient in their Zone of Proximal Development (ZPD). This offers flexibility in choosing what is done in every therapy. The time-limited aspect supports aspects around spending and other indirect costs.

Importantly, CAT encourages every therapist to have an active interest in the person's wider context, their experience of it, and their attitudes towards the same. This includes the therapist needing to have an awareness of their own assumptions and relationship with wider societal norms (Rafi & Prabalkumari, 2019). This opens a lot of space to address and attend to them at the level of the individual in a collaborative way.

In my work, staying in the here and now was valuable, and being attentive to the developmental stage was key. Engaging with young people and meeting them "where they are at" at different points in time becomes central. A more tentative approach in naming and using reciprocal roles can help them work their way through experiences in the family and explore more middle ways of relating. The words become handles to grasp and not rigid conclusions about the emerging self. An invitation to play can be packed into the process of mapping, by the use of metaphors or drawings, and helps the therapist occupy this stance.

Young people's stories and experiences of CAT

In the following section, I will share excerpts from the work done with young people (aged eleven to twenty-one years) who have attended the service, to illustrate the issues raised above and to reflect on other experiences of using the CAT model in this context.

Meeting complex needs: Abhinav's story

Abhinav was nineteen years old at the time of his referral from his consultant psychiatrist. His presenting difficulties included obsessional thoughts followed by compulsions that spanned multiple themes including fear of harm from others, recurrent doubt and guilt. He experienced his obsessions with a high level of conviction and was unable to question them. The symptoms involved his mother, and she often responded to his obsessions by accommodating and reinforcing, and hence, sustaining them. He spent multiple hours a day engaged with this and was unable to function in his daily life. Additionally, he was identified to have features of Autism Spectrum Disorder. This opened a need to engage with him using a flexible framework. He experienced his prior engagement with a different course of psychotherapy sessions as very demanding and unhelpful, as if he was being asked to do something that he could not.

During the therapeutic assessment, he expressed having ideas of being watched or heard by others. He was unable to explain this further. He needed to be quiet in his conversation as a response to this. The extent to which he believed this and its effect on him seemed to vary across time. He shared his experiences of rejection within his peer group from the start of his years at college. He experienced abrupt shifts in his mood characterised by intense feelings of loneliness, anger and hurt. He was found to act on these feelings by taking extreme measures such as, on one occasion, trying to jump from a height.

We engaged in a course of sessions with a view to addressing the severe obsessive-compulsive symptoms, emotional dysregulation and his wider interpersonal difficulties. The CAT model seemed to open multiple opportunities within the therapeutic space. We were able to map the reciprocal roles from his different relationships within his family, with peers and in the therapeutic relationship. Locating it in a third space as something that can be looked at, helped him gain a distance from the intense emotional states (Potter, 2010).

Following the reformulation stage, we engaged in jointly recognising the emotional states that he entered during the session and outside sessions. By then it became possible to design and implement Exposure Response Prevention (ERP) exercises to address the obsessive-compulsive symptoms more directly. Joint sessions were organised inviting his mother to participate and develop ways of stepping back from accommodating his symptoms. There was room to notice other aspects in their relationship and facilitate the move towards more independence for the young person. In the recognition stage, a shared humour emerged in the therapeutic relationship, supported using memes.

The end of therapy gave us an opportunity to face the disappointment of what did not change and the loss of the therapeutic relationship. We were able to recognise the feelings of rejection that he felt. He viewed them as inevitable and joked about how he was warned about therapy ending even in the beginning.

Blinded by prejudice: Sriram's story

Sriram was twenty years old at the time of his referral, living with his parents and sister, and experiencing recurrent outbursts of intense feelings of loneliness, anger, mistrust and fear of rejection, both at home and work. In the weeks leading up to his referral, he lost his employment as an office aide in a small firm.

These unmanageable states appeared and continued through his adolescent years and were associated with compelling thoughts of suicide, at times acting on them. Typically met with physical punishment within the family environment, the helplessness and mistrust gained further strength. He struggled to cope with friendships, with frequent conflict and ruptures that seemed irreparable. These years were also marked by a premature dropout from education and, later, from an opportunity at vocational skills training. Engaging with street drugs and entering street fights became his way of coping and further alienated him from his family.

He participated with interest in the therapeutic assessment. It soon became apparent that the loss of employment resulted in severe financial strain on him and his family's already fragile economic situation.

The language used was important to our work, using his own words to name his experiences extended a sense of ownership as we progressed through the stages in therapy.

In the therapeutic relationship, I experienced the divide and differences in our socioeconomic background in a variety of ways. My general assumptions about his lived reality interfered with witnessing and exploring "what it was like for him". The CAT model supported me in recognising my own prejudice and to suspend the same. Furthermore, we were able to recognise and name the asymmetry in the relationship. I was able to challenge my automatic response to 'normalise' violence as an inevitable part of life in some sections of society. Taken to its extreme, such a notion can disallow attending to certain needs in parts of a community. It was as if I was in a dilemma, in turn condoning violence or entirely overlooking its existence. The CAT model explicitly invites the therapist to engage with the person in the room, while being aware of their prejudice (Ryle & Kerr, 2017). It also extends the same invitation to the patient, affording a space to wonder about rigid, prior norms. For example, we were able to wonder about and question some 'givens' that he held. "On the streets, saying no to an invitation to fight is cowardice", was one such given.

Gradually, he started experiencing the therapy sessions as a more comfortable and secure place. This was a shift for him. He described moving away from the experience of having to rise up to a powerful other. The power can be attributed to a mix of aspects like age, social status, economic and educational background. We were also able to attend to experiences within the close family environment that helped us have a shared understanding of his sense of self and usual responses in relationships.

In the recognition and revision stage, we saw the spontaneous emergence of exits that supported tolerating extreme emotional states and these supported connections with his peers. Playing games of carrom in common spaces was a typical way of relaxing in the evenings, among his peers in his community. He started participating in this and experienced a growing confidence with them.

"Watching out for what is allowed": Brinda's story

Brinda was sixteen years old when she attended the service for her first assessment along with her parents. This initial assessment aimed to explore her presenting difficulties and reflect on other aspects such as the experience of being with the therapist and responses to the observations being made. Typically, parents or other caregivers are involved and are invited to share their concerns.

In our assessment, she terminated the meeting after a brief period (ten to fifteen minutes). She expressed a strong sense of mistrust towards me and politely asked to leave.

Some of her presenting difficulties included significant difficulties in coping with intense emotional states, with frequent feelings of suspicion towards others. This had evolved over the preceding two years. She described a strong sense of isolation from others. Occasionally, during times of increased stress, she heard voices being abusive towards her. She also described experiencing herself as a 'machine', devoid of feeling. She noted withdrawing from people around her as she could not possibly reveal her thoughts or feelings to others. We agreed to end the assessment at the point at which she requested the same. I shared with her that she could access the service again when she felt more able to, and perhaps she should continue to discuss this with her doctor, who made the referral. We also agreed that I would give feedback to the consultant psychiatrist who was involved in her care. The meeting ended with her parents feeling perplexed and disappointed.

Within a few weeks, she attended the service again and wanted to complete the assessment. We were able to proceed with this and gain some more clarity regarding what she perceived as her difficulties. Among other things, the possibility of naming her sense of suffocation, particularly in her relationship with her parents, without being judged for the same seemed to surprise her. She was intrigued by the experience of being able to speak about how revealing her true thoughts or feelings always came with a cost.

In the course of her sessions, we identified a frequent expectation of rejection from the therapist and caution, as if being watchful of doing or saying the forbidden. She proceeded to share the experience of high levels of unpredictability within the family environment, with intense hostility between her parents and excessive control in their relationship with her. We identified alternating feelings of relief and guilt as we proceeded through the initial stage of therapy.

Within the sessions, we experienced the process of mapping as an anchor that enabled us to stay with emotions that seemed otherwise forbidden. It appeared to offer a holding space to negotiate contrasting experiences in her relationship with her parents. The space extended to considering wider social norms like gender and sexuality as experienced by her. She was able to voice the experience of having romantic feelings towards a young man and to explore having healthy boundaries in new relationships.

The individual therapy sessions were combined with family work that involved independent sessions with her parents, mapping their reciprocal roles in their relationship with her. Within the family, this allowed naming of her father's difficulties in managing his own emotions and the need for help-seeking.

"I don't need to be perfect": Sandeep's story

Sandeep was thirteen years old when he attended the clinic. He was experiencing recurrent dissociative episodes during which time he was found to wander away from his home for short distances. At other times, he was found to enter a completely non-responsive state that lasted between minutes and hours. He experienced repeated episodes of vomiting that were not medically explained. He was unable to engage with any schoolwork and noted episodes of 'going blank' when he tried to. He also described hearing voices of multiple persons being very critical of him.

He was described as a very bright boy who took pride in his schoolwork. His mother was puzzled by his inability to cope at school. She also described a change in his way of relating towards her, as if becoming very hostile and argumentative with her. He experienced mood fluctuations, switching between states of intense fear, sadness and anger. This occurred against a background of intense, recurrent conflicts in the family with parents being separated. Living with his mother, he continued to feel abandoned by his father and as if he was seeking to be accepted. His mother experienced these feelings as a betrayal of loyalty and perfect goodness that she needed from him.

He engaged with interest in therapy. We identified and named a 'Super detective' state, in which he required himself to be perfect, all-knowing and all-powerful. This place was very severe and devoid of anything childlike. When he engaged with the therapist in this state, we recognised him becoming overbearing and shut off in the interaction. Gradually, we understood that he needed this state to have a sense of control over what was otherwise confusing and chaotic.

This alternated with the 'helpless child' who was repeatedly overwhelmed and lost. We also started mapping out the more harsh reciprocal roles using his words and viewing them as different characters from the movie 'Transformers'. These attempts led to more humour and play in the sessions, which otherwise resembled a very adult-like conversation where he discussed his difficulties using complex medical terminology. We started naming feelings in the here and now and exploring ways like journaling to continue this between sessions. More immediate exits such as grounding were introduced and rehearsed. He started feeling more connected with himself and able to communicate how he felt with his mother. Family work was offered. A challenging and yet rewarding joint session with his mother allowed the sharing of the understanding that emerged in therapy.

"I don't want to lose my sides": Amrita's story

Amrita is a fifteen-year-old girl. After recognising her intense and impairing mood changes, she decided to seek help and encouraged her parents to consider this. In her presentation, the CAT model started supporting the identification of different states of mind that she finds herself in. She experienced these as separate characters and referred to them as such. She described how every state becomes consuming and disconnected from others.

Through mapping, we recognised and engaged with the different states in turn, enabling us to hold them together. This seemed to become an entry into talking about difficult feelings, when the dominant state was one of being 'cut off'. In such a state, becoming vulnerable was viewed with disdain and nearly prohibited. Towards the end of the initial stage in therapy, she shared a sense of clarity and increased coherence in herself.

Figure 11.1: Amrita's Map

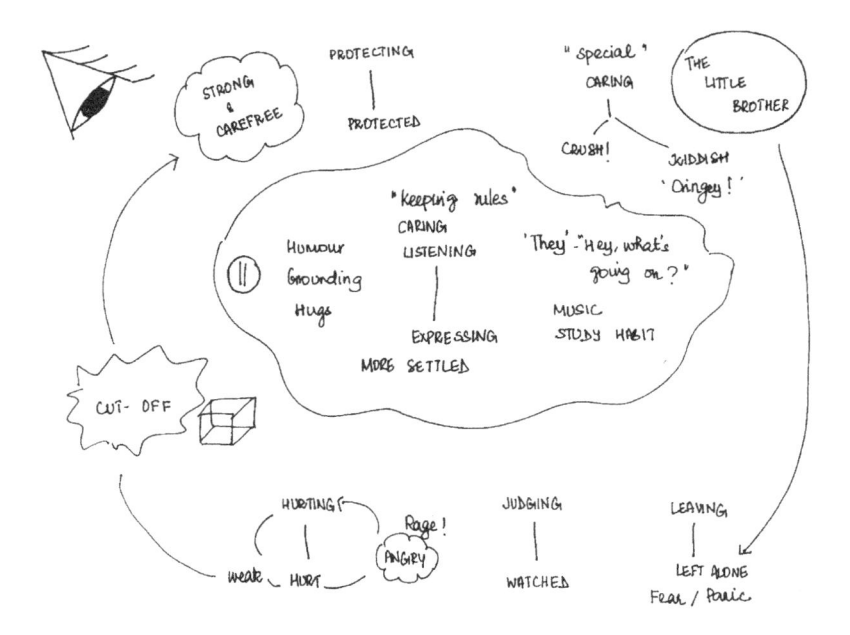

The latter part of the therapy opened up spaces to explore the distress in her female body and her identification with the male gender. Her choice of a more masculine way of dressing allowed her to be more comfortable in herself. She was unable to disclose this within her family. She anticipated a lack of acceptance and this appeared to be based on the strong disapproval she faced with regards to her masculine way of dressing. We identified this as another focus in therapy. The map (See Figure 11.1) continued to support this exploration, as we wondered about how she viewed the gender of her different states. She experienced some of the states as male and others as more female. The CAT model creates enough space to bring in complex and at times competing needs. Each may require varying levels of attention and priority. It enables one to have a clear goal without ignoring other important aspects. It invites us to recognise our multiple selves, rather than feeling constrained by a binary position – e.g., we are either male or female.

"Father and son": Kiran's story

Kiran, eleven years of age, attended his appointments with his father. For two years he had been experiencing increasing levels of anxiety interfering with school attendance and other activities like play. He started isolating himself in his room. He described entering a "daydream" repeatedly and remained preoccupied with very challenging ideas that revolved around harm from others without clear evidence of the same. He felt threatened by minor physical symptoms and sought reassurance by multiple hospital visits. Most importantly, he felt alienated from his parents, with whom there were frequent and intense arguments. He entered unmanageable states of anger hitting out at them and breaking objects in the house.

He was referred for an assessment regarding suitability for psychotherapeutic work while also awaiting assessment for Autism Spectrum Disorder.

During the initial assessment, he spoke with interest and wanted help. He was bewildered by his experiences and certain that a doctor was needed. His father moved between reassuring him and falling into a state of helplessness, as if overpowered by Kiran's thoughts. We explored other relational experiences in the family environment. We identified how his father tried to keep up with lengthy, seemingly intellectual conversations, trying to reassure him. I suggested that we invite his father to join the sessions; Kiran preferred this, and so they entered therapy together.

We started by identifying and naming feelings that Kiran experienced. In the weekly sessions, he brought experiences that he found overwhelming. We started putting down words that matched his different emotional states. Across the sessions, we started going back to them and using them to stay with difficult experiences. He started experiencing a reduction in being disconnected from his surroundings and more available to the present. He welcomed this.

We also named the reciprocal roles that recurred across situations in his relationship with his parents. His father found this helpful and joined in by reflecting on his own responses to Kiran. He observed that he was trying to provide him with a high level of certainty, as if working hard to answer all his questions. He started seeing how this left little space to notice and talk about how Kiran was feeling. Father also recognised his own helplessness when Kiran was losing control and entering very intense states of anger. We introduced some ways to self-soothe and his father was able to help Kiran access these during times of distress.

We invited his mother, who participated in one of the sessions, and the map allowed recognition of the recurrent enactments within the family. The relational approach seemed to naturally invite parents to consider their own upbringing and the roles that seemed to have emerged there.

Such an engagement may not be possible with families who have higher and more complex needs, with parents experiencing significant mental health difficulties or in the presence of significant harm within the parent-child relationship. However, CAT appears to offer a lot in engaging the parent-child dyad directly.

"A different experience of speaking openly to someone older and more mature" – Saroja's story

Saroja made a decision to seek help at twenty-one years of age, when she had the means to support herself. After being unable to convince her mother and grandmother, she decided to attend the clinic on her own. They did not perceive her difficulties as something that required professional help. She was experiencing episodes of intense sadness and fear alternating with 'blanking out', combined with a persistent sense of guilt. At times, she coped by cutting herself with a blade and at others, she experienced compulsive thoughts of ending her life. She was unable to engage in social interactions and had thoughts of being watched and judged by others. These worsened after she failed a professional exam, which prompted her visit to the clinic.

In our relationship, I found myself balancing the urge to compensate in sessions by speaking, with a need to wait and allow space for her voice. In our sessions, I was also able to recognise a strong pressure from my own relational experiences growing up in the same orthodox community as her. She shared her experience of feeling crushed by the demands to live up to certain expectations held by the elders in the family. This occurred at the cost of not having herself heard. Spoken in a language very familiar to me, I experienced a strong pull to view the conditional acceptance prevalent in that family as 'typical' or 'innocuous'. This had the potential to overlook her individual experience. Within the CAT model, I was able to recognise my response and bring in a more curious stance.

Towards the latter part of the therapy, we became more comfortable in recognising the role of enactments and she noticed a sense of safety in speaking her mind. She remarked how the experience of speaking openly to an elder without the fear of making mistakes was new. Over the course of therapy, she developed a more caring approach to herself, especially her failings. She also worked through her experience of her parents separating at a very young age and the compelling need to be the 'good one' for her mother.

Closing comments and reflections

The setting up of a new psychotherapy service in Chennai has been a challenging experience. Reflecting on the initial experience within this service, the CAT model appears to offer some unique advantages with regard to working with young people in this context. The relational approach used within this service is not yet part of mainstream practice in mental health services. Drawing from the experience within this service, it appears to be an approach that young people and families value.

I have chosen seven stories that offer very different levels of need, and arise within markedly different contexts. Abhinav's story shows how CAT can allow us to embrace the complexity of a person's presenting needs, while Sriram's presentation reminds us that we need to be careful and mindful of our own prejudices and assumptions. Brinda speaks to our need to work within the ZPD and "meet young people where they are at", while Sandeep exemplifies how naming and mapping perfectionism might allow for more humour and play to come into the sessions. Amrita demands the need for us to embrace the plurality of our young people, and engage with "How to be Both". Kiran's story offers an account of being flexible and adaptive, allowing the father to join in and to be part of the conversation, while Saroja's story really exemplifies how we need to ensure we are seeking and listening to the individual's voice. Seven stories, all connected by my practice of CAT, and all speaking to how we prioritise relationships in our practice.

CAT speaks to a possibility of meeting people where they are at and joining in with how they already feel, think and talk about their difficulties and experiences. In a setting with very few specialist psychotherapy services, such a model can offer a lot in regard to issues that can be attended to. Complex difficulties can be addressed and the wider system surrounding the young person can be engaged directly or indirectly. One can choose to stay in the past or in the present, depending on what seems more relevant at different times. The therapist is well supported by the safety of working within an established therapeutic framework with a degree of autonomy and flexibility. This flexibility is invaluable when working with young people in this context.

Some of these advantages have been valued and widely discussed in other contexts across the world. Within the limits of a community-based psychotherapy service in Chennai, the model appears to enable both the therapist and the young person to co-create 'just enough' space to address presentations at varying levels of need, context and complexity.

Chapter 12:
Can you even relate? Invitations to think and work relationally in Out of Home Care

Katherine Monson and Kiera Kauler

Introduction

Central to this book is the idea that we are shaped by our experiences of relating to others. When we enter into working relationships with young people in statutory Out of Home Care (OoHC) (what readers from the UK will refer to as Looked After Children (LAC)), we are typically all too aware of the kinds of relational experiences that have impacted them. Our alertness to the possibilities of young people's distrust, fear, pain and lack of control might lead to a lack of attention to how we bring our own relational experiences into our work with them. Maintaining attention on our own ways of relating is not only ethical but can provide new ways of reflecting and relating in our work with young people.

Out of home care

Out of home care (OoHC) refers to formal care provided outside the family home by extended family or kith, volunteer foster carers, or residential care. Statutory authority decisions to remove a child and provide OoHC are typically made due to the child experiencing neglect, physical abuse, sexual abuse, emotional abuse or other adversity. While we need to learn more about the kinds of supports that might be most useful to promote healing and mental health among young people in care, we equally need to consider the ways such supports are offered. Continued development of evidence-based practices for this population is vital, but without attendant attention to engagement and relating, these tools may not be effective. Workers' self-awareness of patterns of relating can be a valuable resource for reducing harm caused to young people in care and offering something that might be helpful.

In this chapter, we'll explore some of the approaches to relating that we've used – or have noticed others using – that we believe support the development of helpful relationships with young people in OoHC, and with others who are involved in their care. We will discuss a fictitious case study 'Mia'. We have developed a fictitious case for ethical reasons: all too often, young people in care become objectified and scrutinised, discussed outside their presence. Despite being invented, both of us feel connected to Mia's fictitious scenario. Mia's emotional pain and difficulties are not going to be resolved in this chapter: that, we believe, would be too trivialising of young people's experiences, and the singularity of each person's journey through care and into adulthood.

A relational frame

Cognitive Analytic Therapy (CAT) suggests that, in childhood, through being related 'to', we develop recurring ways of relating to others. These internalised patterns incorporate a 'childlike' role and a 'caregiver-like' role that are mutually reinforcing. These are described as reciprocal roles (RRs). RRs are often a valuable resource, enabling us to find predictability in our relationships with others. We adopt certain ways of relating – procedures – that reinforce these relational positions. We call these reciprocal role procedures (RRPs). Some people may experience themselves as constrained or trapped by a limited range of RRs and RRPs that inhibit their growth, and sustain pain in their relationships with others. A CAT approach encourages the exploration of new ways of relating.

Recent developments have seen CAT scholars attending to the influence of social, economic, political and cultural contexts in the development of RRs (Lloyd & Pollard, 2018), and we see this as relevant to young people in care. From their particular social context, young people describe experiences of shame and marginalisation associated with being in statutory care. Although some might attribute this to the deleterious effects of childhood abuse and neglect, young people in care equally describe their experiences of social exclusion, judgement and missed opportunities (Dansey *et al*, 2019). A 22-year-old woman with experiences in kinship care, foster care and residential care, said to Katherine: "You're expected to have crappy outcomes if you're a resi kid, that's society's way of thinking about it" (Monson *et al*, 2020).

If we consider legislation and its enactment as a set of relational experiences, then we see that the RRs available to families and young people in contact with the child welfare system might be shaped, confirmed and constrained by particular repeated experiences. Families' first contact with the child welfare system happens when they are struggling, sometimes immensely. Although intended to support them, the child welfare system may exert demands. Without a robust relationship guiding the pathway through the child welfare system, the family may come to experience the relationship as controlling, bureaucratic and unpredictable (Morley, 2022). This might lead to families (and children) experiencing care as conditional and controlling. This might also leave them feeling not good enough and powerless.

This chapter

We are deeply moved and expanded by the work of others, who help us to make sense of how disrupted attachment and relational trauma can shape young people's ways of relating – Judy Atkinson, Dan Hughes, Bruce Perry and Bessel Van Der Kolk. However, to attend to the experiences of young people only – and not the experiences of workers – risks further objectifying young people in OoHC. We might become players in restricted relationships, as drawn in Figure 12.1. Noticing this might help us to avoid repeating prior patterns and confirming them.

Figure 12.1: Common relationship patterns where there is statutory involvement

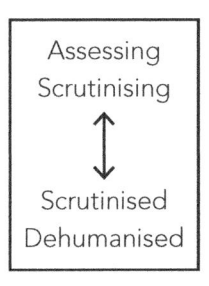

```
┌─────────────────┐
│   Assessing     │
│  Scrutinising   │
│       ↑         │
│       ↓         │
│   Scrutinised   │
│  Dehumanised    │
└─────────────────┘
```

Many young people in OoHC have felt 'forced' to meet with mental health professionals (Tatlow-Golden & McElvaney, 2015; Monson *et al*, 2020). Attention to this sense of disempowerment in supposedly therapeutic encounters demands that mental health professionals have an ethical responsibility to be curious about our own relational procedures, before inviting young people to be curious about theirs.

Steve Potter (2020) suggests that a reasonable rule when noticing and exploring relationship patterns is a 'rule of thirds'. In relating to clients, we should consider about a third of the dynamic as forged by our own relational histories and how these inform recursive relational patterns. A client's relational history and expectations, and practice and social contexts, might each be considered as contributing a further 'third' to any pattern of relating. The large body of theory and practice literature, combined with the context of our organisations (how we receive referrals, consider referral responses, plan work with colleagues), may skew our attention to focus only on the young person's contribution to these dynamics. Yet practitioners may experience the fewest constraints, and the greatest opportunity, to manoeuvre relationally. Our efforts to move into more nurturing ways of relating might enable young people to experiment with new procedures, or nurture and amplify other procedures. Over time, these might be internalised and become a stable part of their repertoire.

Consequently, in this chapter, we focus on how a worker's self-awareness of their own patterns of relating might better position them to create a context for healing. In inviting consideration of our own RRs, we hope you will notice how we might work more flexibly and creatively with others who may be more constrained.

Working directly with young people: relational bids, relational pulls

Referral and assessment

Most referrals include some stories – a story of the young person's history, a story of the particular events that have brought them to the service, or a story of specific kinds of difficulties that have led to the referral. Even before we begin working with a specific young person, their story might stimulate a response that is relational.

Introducing Mia:

> Fourteen-year-old Mia entered care at twelve years old. She does not know her father, and her mum, Lisa, has experienced mental ill-health and substance dependence. In Lisa's care, Mia was sometimes left on

her own. Sometimes, when adults were around, she saw them using drugs and hurting one another. When Mia was five, her grandparents (Lorraine and Trevor) took her to live with them. They felt they needed to protect Mia from Lisa, and so Mia rarely saw her mum. When Mia was twelve, Lorraine died. Trevor felt unable to care for Mia alone. Subsequently, Mia entered residential care.

Mia was referred to Katherine's team because of her care team's concerns about the risks that she was taking, and the possibility of her dying from these. Mia left placement many nights, sometimes to meet adult men who promised her 'ice' (crystal methamphetamine) in exchange for sex. When carers tried to stop Mia from leaving placement, she would sometimes hurt them (hitting and kicking) or sometimes hurt herself (tying things around her neck). When she did leave, Mia sometimes phoned carers to be picked up. Other times, Mia was located by police. On one occasion, while socialising with other young people who had been using 'ice', Mia was in a car accident in a stolen vehicle. The accident led to another young person suffering a brain injury. Mia described to carers that she didn't much care if she lived or died anyway, as other people didn't seem to care too much about this for her.

The young people Katherine works with in OoHC have had dramatically different developmental trajectories from hers. Hearing about Mia before meeting her, Katherine felt a strong desire to protect Mia from further harm.

Figure 12.2: Katherine's 'pulls' when first hearing Mia's story

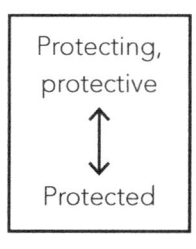

```
┌─────────────────┐
│   Protecting,   │
│    protective   │
│        ↑        │
│        ↓        │
│    Protected    │
└─────────────────┘
```

The protective pull that Katherine felt drew her into a powerful position 'over' Mia.

Relational pulls – such as wanting to be protective – may be shaped as much by agency context as by our own relationship history. The expectations and constraints of the contexts within which we work can lead us to respond in particular ways. As a mental health clinician, Katherine is often expected to engage with young people to assess for mental disorder and to coordinate and provide treatment. But this can lead to a dilemma: framing Mia's experiences as 'symptoms' might validate her emotional pain and facilitate access to (psychiatric) services who might help to 'protect' her. But service access may be experienced by Mia as pathologising and controlling, or even a dismissal of the ways others' actions have hurt her. Mia's experience of having her pain 'assessed' may feel like a re-enactment of past experiences of judgement, and offers of evidence-based treatments may feel to Mia like further efforts from others to control her.

Figure 12.3: Possible relationship 'pulls' when supporting young people in Out of Home Care

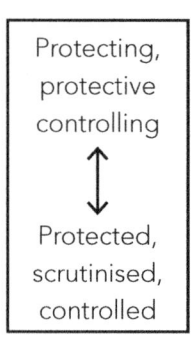

```
┌─────────────┐
│ Protecting, │
│ protective  │
│ controlling │
│      ↑      │
│      ↓      │
│ Protected,  │
│ scrutinised,│
│ controlled  │
└─────────────┘
```

Engagement

Entering into a relationship with a young person with preconceived ideas about what they will want or need from us – such as (only) protection from harm – might inhibit us from developing a more collaborative relationship. This is not to dismiss the importance of theoretical research or practice knowledge. Understanding attachment theory, adolescent development and the impacts of developmental trauma is important, as is some specific knowledge of the young person's development to date. These will shape our considerations about how the young person relates, accepts care or engages with a service, and about how others may relate back. But if we reach conclusions about why the young person is behaving the way that they are, we risk moving ourselves out of connecting and relating with curiosity and collaboration. Holding knowledge 'about' the young person enacts a controlling relationship (and an unreflective one). A nineteen-year-old care-leaver with experiences in residential care described to Katherine that:

> "Some... workers have graduated from college from a good family, and you know, they read all the books, pass and graduate with bachelors, masters, whatever. But what they don't have from all that is ... they would never know how they feel, they would never relate." (Monson, 2020)

'Relating', then, is vital, and may include putting aside book-learning. Harlene Anderson describes the practice of 'bracketing' pre-knowledge (2007), noticing what it might be possible to 'know' but entering into a relationship holding that knowledge lightly.

For the first five weeks after Mia was referred, Katherine did not get to meet her. Mia was often missing from placement. When she was home, Mia was sleeping, or refused to meet someone new. In these situations, we might find ourselves 'pulled' again in a different way: we might feel frustrated and defensive because the young person won't 'let' us help them, or we might begin to feel hopeless that we cannot help.

> *On Katherine's sixth visit to the house, Mia agreed to residential carers inviting Katherine into the lounge of the home. However, she didn't shift her attention from the tablet she was watching. Believing that all engagements – verbal or not – are forms of connection, Katherine seated herself on a nearby couch and explained who she was, her role, and why she had been asked to come and see Mia. Mia said, "Yeah, I know who you are". She didn't look up from the tablet. Peering over, Katherine saw that Mia was watching 'Euphoria' (the US remake of the Israeli series). Katherine found herself making assumptions about why Mia would be drawn to this program: 'Euphoria' explores adolescent sexuality, drug use and child abuse, among other things. It was all too easy for Katherine to assume that Mia found some resonance in the themes, and that she felt drawn to the program in an attempt to make sense of her own experiences.*

Noticing her assumptions, and wanting to draw herself out of the pull to 'assess' and 'formulate' (rather than to 'relate'), Katherine instead said, "That's such amazing eye makeup [on the actor]. I've never really learned to do eye makeup." Mia looked up from the tablet and said (somewhat disparagingly), "Haven't you ever heard of TikTok tutorials?" Katherine and Mia then had a brief conversation about preferred TikTok and YouTuber makeup tutorials, and Mia's preferred places to shop for makeup. Katherine acknowledged the effort Mia had made to meet with her, and indicated she hoped to return to see Mia at the same time each week. On her return a week later, Mia was missing from placement. However, two weeks later Mia was at the placement, and offered to show Katherine a makeup tutorial she'd recently posted to TikTok.

We believe conversations about makeup, fashion, football, preferred fast food outlets for chips, or favourite TikTokers, are all vital to engaging with young people, and can be powerful entry points for engagement. From his research into intimate relationships, Gottman (2001) noted that people may make 'bids' for connection, and that the patterns of their partner's responses to bids impact relationship satisfaction and stability. Gottman's ideas have been translated into concepts for parents, caregivers and workers, aiming to foster nourishing relationships with children and young people (Havighurst *et al*, 2013). These bids might be considered RRPs – strategies undertaken to be in a desired or more tolerable relationship. In response to Mia's query "Haven't you ever heard of TikTok tutorials?", Katherine had a range of available responses:

- She could turn 'away' from the bid. She could fail to notice the bid, or fail to consider it an opportunity for connection. This might happen if Katherine were feeling judged and defensive, anticipating unsuccessful engagement.
- She could turn 'against' this bid. She could respond defensively ("Of course I've heard of TikTok tutorials") or dismissively ("Yes, I've heard of them, but I'm not here to talk about that, I'm here to talk about your mental health"). This might happen if Katherine were focused only on her 'protecting' role, and 'assessing' procedure.
- She could turn 'towards' this bid, assuming it is a bid for connection (or, at least, that there is little relational risk in assuming that it is a bid for connection).

Choosing to consider these interactions as 'bids' creates space for mutual curiosity, rather than linear, clinical inquiry. For us, this stance honours that young people are more than just their difficulties, and that they have expertise in the world.

> *On one visit to Mia, Katherine learned from carers on her arrival that Mia had again been sexually assaulted the night before. Mia declined to talk with Katherine, but tolerated Katherine sitting beside her as she lay on the couch, wrapped in a blanket scrolling TikToks on her tablet. Katherine wondered about letting Mia know that she imagined she felt "awful", that she might feel like she was in some way going to be "blamed" for what had occurred. She wondered about trying to encourage Mia to attend the police station, or access forensic medical care. Katherine noticed these urges to "do something to protect" Mia. Instead, she sat with Mia. After about fifteen minutes, she got up to leave, and said, "I'll see you again next week". Mia looked up at her and scowled, then said, "Your mascara looks pretty shit today. Probably you need a new one."*

Katherine wondered if Mia's comment was a way for her to take up a powerful position (sharing knowledge) that was different from some of her previous powerful positions (hurting carers). Or perhaps it was an effort to take up a position of power (hurting) rather than powerlessness (being hurt). Maybe it was an effort by Mia to show care or connection – a way of leaving a powerless state in response to Katherine's efforts to leave a powerful state. Mia's comment may have had other intended meanings. But rather than reaching some conclusive description of why Mia said what she did, the greatest opportunity Katherine had was to consider how she herself should respond. Katherine and Mia might find themselves doing this dance, or similar, many times. Over time, Mia may find herself feeling more comfortable in this different type of relationship, shaped by care and curiosity (rather than power and control). Over time, we hope this would enable Mia to experience others' efforts to care for her as 'care' rather than as 'control'.

Working indirectly with young people: relational pushes and pulls in teams

Initiating collaboration

'Care teams' of workers supporting young people in OoHC consist of workers in a variety of roles, from a range of organisations. They bring with them a variety of practice frameworks and even legislative contexts. For young people in OoHC, the care team ideally works as a collaborative interdisciplinary team, working together to meet a range of identified needs, addressing the young person's vulnerabilities and supporting their growth into adulthood. Ideally, the care team becomes a site of support for one another, or 'safety net' (Monson et al, 2021), as care team members attempt to find ways to reduce the risk and vulnerability for the specific young person, and/or enhance their strengths and resilience.

> *Mia's care team meets weekly. The meetings are convened by a case manager from statutory child protection services, who has responsibilities for overseeing legal aspects of the care, as well as ensuring that particular tasks are congruent with the overarching care framework. Also in attendance are:*
>
> - *the house supervisor of the house in which Mia lives, who acts as a team leader and supervisor for residential carers*
> - *an alcohol and other drug outreach worker, who has not yet begun to engage with Mia but who has offered some harm-minimisation coaching to residential carers*
> - *a youth justice practitioner with whom Mia is required to maintain fortnightly appointments, following charges for stolen motor vehicles*
> - *a member of the police, who works specifically to engage with young people who are frequent victims of crime, with the aim of improving crime prevention, detection and prosecution*

This diverse care team consists of a variety of practitioners with their own personal and practice experience, approaching work from their own institutional frameworks. These frameworks exert 'pulls' on individual practitioners. These shape the collaboration as much as their individual ways of relating. And, as always, patterns of relating are recursive and reciprocal. Research suggests that care team members' subjective experience of respect and trust among team members contributes to the success of the collaboration (Rumping *et al*, 2019). We believe 'respect' and 'trust' are best fostered through a relationally aware stance.

Child welfare practitioners in interdisciplinary teams can express some ambivalence about their interactions with mental health professionals. At once, they may want the mental health professional to respect their expertise (and fear that it will not be respected), while simultaneously hoping that the mental health professional will share expertise and offer new solutions (Jennings & Evans, 2020). Katherine's awareness of this might shape how she enters into the care team: she might feel pulled to demonstrate her expertise (top-pole), or to demonstrate only her acknowledgement of others' expertise (bottom-pole). Salvator Minuchin described 'joining' systems as "not a skill or technique (rather) a mindset constructed out of respect, empathy, curiosity… and a commitment" (Minuchin *et al*, 2014, p4). Here, Katherine might consider connecting with this team as a 'learner', curious about others' positions and procedures.

Figure 12.4: Approaches to relating for Katherine to consider

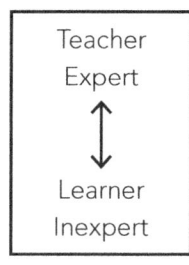

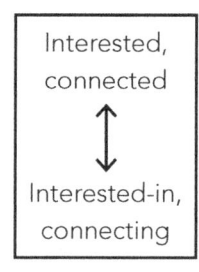

| Teacher / Expert ↕ Learner / Inexpert | Interested, connected ↕ Interested-in, connecting |

We encourage others to overtly take this stance, for example, saying, "I know you all know each other, but do you mind helping me understand everyone's roles in this team?", or "Can you help me understand how we make decisions together in this team?" This may assist other workers in the system to feel confident of their own authority and credibility in the team. But it may also free them up to feel safe in curious or 'not-knowing' positions. Such expressions of curiosity allow team conversations to shift from assumptions and tasks to more reflexive positions that allow attention to the emotional and relational aspects of the work (Greenwood, 2016).

Developing a shared understanding of patterns of relating

We've learned that care team members value the opportunity to develop shared understandings of the history and context of young people's problems, and shared ideas about how to respond (Monson et al, 2021). While our strongest preference is always to centre the young person's voice, this has not always been possible for us. Instead, care teams might attempt to do a good-enough job of trying to make sense of the young person's experiences and needs, and ways we might respond.

We try to escape technical jargon and access 'experience-near' (White, 2007) descriptions of relating. A carer who is describing a concern that Mia is 'becoming dysregulated' is invited to elaborate, to help the team understand that he is referring to times when Mia paces about the house, apparently unable to settle; times when she persistently talks about wanting to get out of the house and 'score' ice. The child protection practitioner familiar with Mia's early childhood development is invited to clarify that (among other things) 'trauma' refers to Mia's experiences of seeing her mum violently beaten by her boyfriend, and either biting and hitting the boyfriend, or hiding in a wardrobe to protect herself. Through these conversations, tentative formulations can be reached. These formulations might be considered 'hypotheses' in the systemic tradition (Bertrando & Lini, 2021) – we have no intention of 'proving' or 'disproving' these hypotheses. Instead, we aim to open up and expand the possible ways of relating. We might offer:

> "It sounds as though Lisa was not always able to meet Mia's needs, and not always able to keep her safe. We've heard that Mia might've felt she had to fight to protect Lisa. It sounds like, at other times, she felt she had to hide and protect herself. Maybe Mia feels that hiding – like being under the covers watching TikTok – is a good way to keep safe. And maybe Mia feels that 'attacking' the world – getting out of the house and taking on every possible threat (drugs, adults, stolen cars) – is a way to be in charge of her own safety... I wonder if there are times Mia doesn't feel intolerably vulnerable, even if she is not hiding or attacking?"

From here, the team might be able to talk about 'exceptions' (White, 2007) to hypothesised relational procedures. Through attention to exceptions – not only to perceived problem procedures – the care team may learn of a wider range of procedures than they had previously been aware.

Continuing to 'relate' in the face of anxiety

After the assault, the care team comes together. The child protection practitioner and the police member are very hopeful that Mia will make a formal report about the incident. The house supervisor wonders if Mia is taking risks so great as to require a period of psychiatric inpatient treatment. The AOD practitioner has suggested that perhaps a period in a residential withdrawal facility would be useful for Mia.

At times when care teams are highly anxious, or in a state of uncertainty about how to move forward, they may find themselves occupying either a strident top-pole, or passive bottom-pole position (not unlike the positions that Katherine felt pulled to with Mia after the assault). Katherine notices how tempted she is to move from feeling powerless around Mia's safety, to taking a top-pole position of powerful and expert. Just as this is unlikely to be helpful with Mia, it is similarly unlikely to be helpful for the care team.

Figure 12.5: Relational 'pulls' in care teams

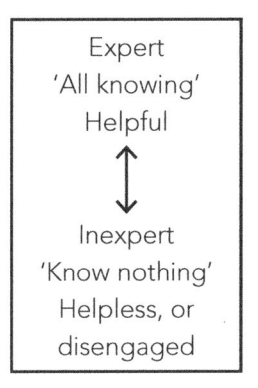

```
┌─────────────────┐
│     Expert      │
│  'All knowing'  │
│     Helpful     │
│        ↑        │
│        ↓        │
│    Inexpert     │
│  'Know nothing' │
│   Helpless, or  │
│   disengaged    │
└─────────────────┘
```

Rather than moving into an either/or powerful/powerless position, it may be possible to reconnect with the 'interested and connected role' described earlier with Mia. Circular questioning as described in Milan systemic therapy (Cecchin, 1987) might be helpful to move to a curious and connected position. Rather than to elicit objective answers, circular questions aim to elicit new information, or bring assumptions from unspoken and implicit to explicit team awareness (Penn, 1982).

- "If Mia were to go to hospital for a week or so, what might we hope would be different for her when she was discharged?"
- "If we were to ask Mia how reporting the assault might help, I wonder what she would say?"
- "Do Lisa and Trevor know what's happened? I wonder what they hope we will do next?"

Figure 12.6: A possible relational approach to care team work

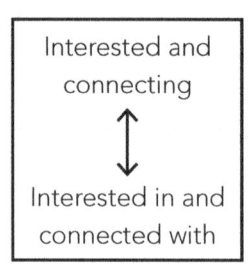

```
┌─────────────────────┐
│   Interested and    │
│     connecting      │
│          ↑          │
│          ↓          │
│  Interested in and  │
│   connected with    │
└─────────────────────┘
```

Taking a curious, 'interested and connecting' stance in the care team might allow the team to enact this with Mia. Ideally, this will provide her with opportunities to experiment with a wider repertoire of ways of relating.

Conclusions

In our efforts to alleviate distress experienced by young people in OoHC, we might slip into restricted and inflexible ways of relating. Our attention may be directed towards the ways in which the young person's developmental experiences might be influencing these patterns of relating. Instead, we encourage similar – or greater! – attention to how practitioners' own experiences, values, beliefs and contexts might shape the relational pattern. As practitioners, we're in more powerful positions and tend to have more freedom to shift how we relate. Here, we have described the adoption of a 'curious and connecting' stance with young people themselves, and their wider system of care. We've found this stance provides us the best chance of being able to engage with young people themselves, and being able to notice and then support patterns of relating that are more healing and less harmful.

Chapter 13:
Burning out and bullying – the need for working relationally within the workplace

Nick Barnes and Lee Crothers

When writing a book about working relationally alongside young people, we were very aware that we would need to ensure there was a chapter that spoke to the needs of those working in this field above and beyond the chapters in which we embrace the multiple and creative opportunities that this way of working provides. Working alongside young people, informed by a relational scaffold and supported by supervisors and colleagues who can think together in a relational manner can be hugely rewarding, but nevertheless it does come with its own demands. After all, this is very much about reciprocity, and through the very nature of relational working, we are in this together. The possibility of being drawn into this relating and finding ourselves overreaching is significant, and hence the need to find a way of working that feels manageable and sustainable, even despite the pushes and pulls that can happen all around. For the risk of burnout and overstretching ourselves, is not just because of the relational dance between us, but also because of what is going on around us, within our services, (eco) systems and society that all contributes to this dance, making it feel more like reaching hands across an uncontrolled mosh pit, rather than a graceful ease across the dancefloor.

As we write this chapter, we are both aware of the escalating pressures on workers in all sectors of health, social care, education and beyond, all impacted not just by the increased workloads within their services. These demands are further entrenched as staff look to manage and negotiate their own struggles with the cost-of-living crisis, the experiences of living through the COVID-19 pandemic, the impact of war and conflicts (such as the wars in Ukraine and Gaza) and the increasing realities of the climate and ecological crisis. It is impossible to avoid the realities of what is happening all around us, especially as these are issues for the young people we are working alongside, as well as for ourselves. Within mental health services specifically, there has been a huge rise in mental health needs since the easing of the COVID lockdowns (RCPsych, 2021), and, as children and young people are being driven to catch up on what they missed educationally and developmentally, it is their emotional well-being that is taking the toll (Holt-White, 2023).

But this is also impacting upon those looking to offer support. All services are working with greatly reduced workforce numbers at a time of massively increased demand. The COVID pandemic lockdowns may have eased, but in our haste to 'get back to normal', a collective denial seems to have descended about the sustained toll of greater absence from work, but also regarding the impact of long COVID. Long COVID has been especially hard on young people where up to one in seven may have developed symptoms that would support a diagnosis (Stephenson, 2023). Other impacts such as increased COVID-attributed morbidity and mortality (Abab, 2022) and the rush to retirement (Partington, 2021), have meant all professionals feel like they are working at half empty, within a system running at half capacity. It is more difficult to think relationally when workers do not feel supported by a stretched system. We all know it's harder to be supportive and not reactive when we believe we are alone in the decision-making.

However, the risks are not isolated to burnout of individuals and loss of capacity within the overall workforce. Increasing demand and pressure and the lack of space for reflection to enable a culture of support within teams, the possibility of sustaining a more toxic culture of workplace bullying becomes firmly established.

Health and social care sectors are often prone to bullying cultures, as there is a need for teamwork and consensus practice, often in high-pressure work environments. Certainly, in the UK, the NHS has struggled to come to terms with the degree of bullying within the workplace, with the 2015 NHS staff survey stating that 25% of staff had experienced bullying within the last twelve months, although with a follow-up survey in 2016 by *The Guardian*, there were suggestions that this was a gross underestimate. This later survey found that 81% of doctors and nurses surveyed had experienced bullying and that, for 44%, this was still ongoing (Johnson, 2016).

In many ways, the COVID-19 pandemic brought a brief pause to this culture within health systems, as frontline health workers were suddenly positioned as frontline heroes, with public gestures of solidarity and support from their doorsteps and balconies being one of the strongest collective memories of the lockdown. Frontline workers were rightly recognised for their remarkable work and bravery, and the working environment, despite being enormously stressful and exhausting, was much more cohesive and connected – where relational support for each other was paramount (Barnes, 2020).

But as the as the restrictions of lockdown eased, and we desired to return to how things were before, the gaps in provision, combined with the overall exhaustion of staff who have had no time to recover, have meant that little has been learnt from what was happening previously, and that non-relational working and bullying have once again become the norm. Pressure, stress and ever-increasing waiting lists have resulted in frontline workers shifting from heroes to villains, as they are now more regularly seen as denying, blocking and/or withholding, rather than brave and sacrificing.

To counter this development, in most services, across most countries, there has been an increased emphasis on considering staff well-being and building resilience. There is an acknowledgement that staff are under considerable pressure within the workplace, and that burnout is becoming an increasing problem that needs to be addressed. Bullying seldom gets articulated within the same blast email sent to all staff, but raising awareness of how staff may be able to access whistleblowing and mediation support has become increasingly common, although there remains little evidence that whistleblowing initiatives are able to overcome some of the more entrenched bullying cultures within larger institutions (Kline, 2023). Rather, it is when the "shit really hits the fan", and a major incident enquiry happens, that senior managers suddenly feel compelled to take notice.

Well-being and resilience-building within the workforce appear to be increasingly used as the tool for managing, or perhaps coping with, the wider systemic failures of a service. If we all just feel a little bit better about ourselves and become a little more resilient, then we might be a little bit more productive on the factory floor. Health workers often feel quite dismissed by these suggestions around well-being and this is sometimes reciprocated by young people who are often directed to self-care and well-being apps as their first point of contact with support, feeling they are being short-changed when a referral to a specialist service results in a recommendation to enhance their self-care.

Is this direction of travel, for both staff and the young people we work alongside, running the risk of further disconnect and alienation? If we fail to think about resilience within a relational framework, then we are simply asking people to show more 'grit' and encouraging people to 'tough it out' (Imtiaz, 2021) – a model so beloved by Conservative ministers in the UK, and one that then encourages us to permit accusations of being a bit 'snowflakey' if we choose to call out the bullying (Grierson, 2023).

Within the resilience research world, there has been a significant shift away from looking to skill up the individual to ensuring they can cope and manage. Rather, a more relational understanding of resilience has emerged in recent times that seeks to recognise that resilience is not just focused on what is within, but also what support and resources may be available around that person. Unger defines resilience as:

> "...more than an individual set of characteristics. It is the structure around the individual, the services the individual receives, the way health knowledge is generated, all of which combine with characteristics of individuals that allow them to overcome the adversity they face and chart pathways to resilience." (Ungar, 2011)

From a relational perspective, we would therefore suggest that resilience needs to be considered "within, between and around", with the work of Angie Hart describing resilience as:

> "Overcoming adversity, whilst also potentially changing, or even dramatically transforming, (aspects of) that adversity." (Hart et al, 2016)

Through movements such as the Resilience Revolution, Hart et al have spoken about the risks of resilience research being focused on the individual, directing the emphasis of interventions on individuals rather than challenging and overcoming profound inequalities and social injustices (Hart et al, 2016). Relational resilience is therefore not just about a way of overcoming adversity through a mastery of skills and developing a sense of agency, but it is also about ensuring there is a capacity and a support of change around the young person – perhaps a reminder that it takes a whole village to raise a child. When we have a sense of support around us, we may develop our skills and find a voice of autonomy that can be contagious, can rally others and/or change the way we see problems or how problems are approached in future. For example, when a manager speaks up as soon as there is undermining of a team member, then other team members can feel more able to do this in future. It can lead to a wider culture of zero tolerance within the environment. In other words, resilience is about "Beating the odds, whilst also changing the odds" (Boing Boing).

Perhaps when we are next invited to a further workplace well-being afternoon, we need to go prepared to attend with a more activist mindset – that building of our resilience needs to be as much about a call to action as it is about a time to de-stress and decompress. The idea that, if we relate to well-being as not just a passive receiver but as deserving of more, then possibly our own well-being is more positively affected.

But how have we got here? How have we become so insensitive to the needs of the workforce, which then can't fail but to impact on the children, young people and their families we work alongside? Why are so many colleagues looking for ways to leave the profession, step out of statutory roles, and find ways of working that are more flexible, adaptive and creative? Why have we lost our compassion and care for each other?

We support many professionals, mostly in the mental health sector in the UK and Australia where they describe a familiar and stuck state of feeling 'demanded upon' and 'responsible' and many have left or adapted their roles so they have less time 'at the coalface'.

Building on some of the previous reflections, perhaps current concerns within the workplace include:

1. Lack of capacity – decreased workforce because of sickness, retirement and underinvestment.
2. Increased demand – especially after the COVID-19 lockdowns and the pandemic effects.
3. Heightened bureaucratisation – more form-filling but without the time to go through them reflectively with the client and others involved.
4. Email saturation – the IT transformation of services allows for greater and greater amounts of information to be shared, and, once sitting in your inbox, becomes your responsibility and a duty to respond.
5. Wider uncertainties – understandable reactions to uncertainty and resulting despair, which then draw us to simplistic solutions and answers such as trying to fit diagnosis with specific interventions rather than considering a more holistic or integrative approach. This often leads to poor engagement, further distress and increasing demands.

6. Services becoming more risk-averse – within a culture of complaint and limitations of capacity, services become more risk-averse and less willing to allow space for creativity and playfulness, the very things that are often effective in building engagement, hope and recovery.

7. Worsening inequalities – rising health inequalities mean greater levels of mental health need and despair (Wilkinson & Pickett, 2010). This then places pressure on an overworked primary care system which is contractually forced to fill the gaps.

8. COVID denial – as noted above, there is a desire for everything to go back to normal, and so the significant levels of long COVID and COVID-caused morbidity need to be collectively ignored, otherwise we would be forced to reflect on what "back to normal" looks like.

9. Bullying – or perhaps a more honest statement might be the failure to acknowledge bullying in our desperate attempts to just complete the task in front of us, and how current whistleblowing opportunities feel as though they are swept under the carpet.

10. Discrimination, prejudice and inequity – after all, there are only so many times we can be dismissed, overlooked or disregarded within a service, experiencing repeated microaggressions, before coming to the conclusion that this is about power and privilege.

We will all burn out more quickly if we continue to feel demanded upon and alone in our responsibilities, especially if we don't take a step back to consider how we are responding and reacting to these pressures, and how others are responding and reacting to us. Reflecting on the listed difficulties above may be useful in being more realistic about what we can achieve in the current setting while clarifying what power we have to help the wider system. Working within a system that is seemingly unsupportive can breed intense emotions and we would encourage all workers to reflect on relational responses, but also to consider where we might need to increase their agency and control.

In our working environments, especially when working alongside young people and families, it is easy for us to be pulled in different directions. On the one side, we can get drawn into the more heroic stance, where we seek to offer the perfect care plan and attend to all the young people as best we can. This might mean needing to stay way beyond our work hours to ensure all the tasks of risk assessment, safety planning and care planning are in place. This working above and beyond our hours is taken for granted within the health sector, and it is well known that mental health professionals are particularly prone to working more than their contractual hours and recommended caseloads. The risk here is that we get drawn into a rescuing dance, where we start to feel that we are the only ones who are going to be able to meet the needs of the young person, and hence it is entirely down to us to manage their crisis or presentation. Being drawn into rescue mode quickly invites a sense of resentment towards others for not pulling their weight, and at management for failing to provide the staff needed, and we rapidly move to a position of exhaustion and fatigue, with burnout just around the corner.

Alternatively, we might recognise where our colleagues are getting drawn into this rescuing position and decide that we are not going to make the same mistake. Here, we might offer a position of resistance, something that feels a more limited and shut-off side of ourselves to colleagues, or to the young person – presenting as distant and dismissive – which the young person is highly attuned to and can quickly interpret as yet another rejection in their lives. Our colleagues, too, can see it as a dismissal, of not wanting to be part of the team or, worse still, sitting back so others can take the hit. This in turn may lead others to become resentful with a risk that more pressurising and even bullying are used to get more from team members. Here we become more detached, disconnecting from the work we have loved and enjoyed, and begin to wonder whether it is time to look elsewhere for work. Once again, burnout starts to take its toll.

But working within a context in which there may be multiple pressures and demands upon a worker's time, their own capacity for a kind and compassionate response and engagement can be limited. Working in an emergency department where this young person may be the first of five that all need to be seen – and discharged, as no one wants a young person with mental health needs admitted to a physical health setting, despite us claiming that children are entitled to have a right to health care – it becomes hard enough to remember each presentation of need, never mind whether they will receive the care that they need or seek.

Fundamentally, whether we take the rescuing stance or become increasingly shut off and detached – or perhaps end up doing a bit of both – without a relational awareness of what is going on, it becomes hard to disentangle what is me, what may be something I am picking up from the young person, and what is the impact of what is going on around us. We are back to the within, between, around.

We need to be thinking relationally about ourselves, drawing our own maps and being honest about our own relational responses in supervision, formally and informally within the dialogues we have with team members, to ensure we can find some middle ground that might help us feel able to manage and cope, while at the same time challenge the failings of the system(s), from services through to governments, to ensure we have a sense of agency in our work-life balance. We, too, need to be "beating the odds, whilst also changing the odds" (Boing Boing).

Figure 13.1: A common pattern of 'demanded upon'

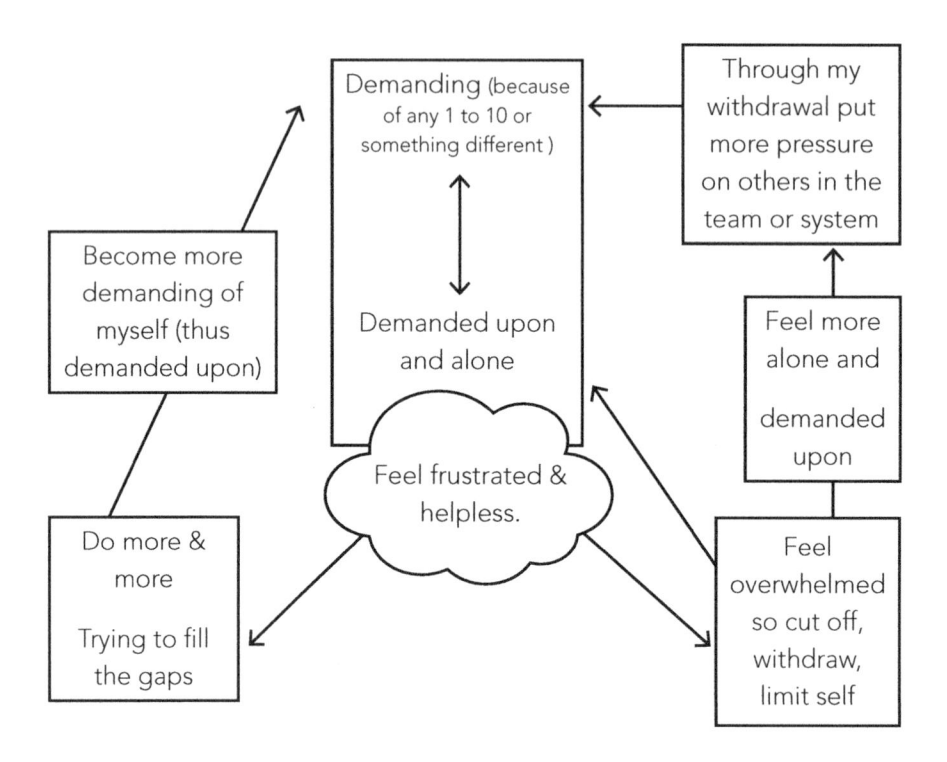

```
                    Demanding (because          Through my
                    of any 1 to 10 or           withdrawal put
                    something different )  ←    more pressure
                            ↑                   on others in the
                            ↓                   team or system
Become more                                              ↑
demanding of
myself (thus        Demanded upon           Feel more
demanded upon)      and alone               alone and
                                            demanded
                                            upon
            Feel frustrated &
            helpless.
Do more &                                   Feel
more                                        overwhelmed
                                            so cut off,
Trying to fill                              withdraw,
the gaps                                    limit self
```

Being reflective together, with a colleague, manager, team and/or young person, can help move a worker from feeling alone and demanded upon to feeling "in this together". The very act of thinking together about the pressures and demands on us or considering what is going on between people, is one of joining together and connecting. This collaborative reflection allows for our energy to be joined and together "push where it moves", to quote Tony Ryle the originator of CAT (2010). A map of these relational positions of 'alone and demanded upon' can lead to a consideration of what may reasonably and realistically help. A map of when we are feeling lost helps locate where we are and then makes space for plans on how to get to where we want to be. The helper's dance list by Potter (2019) can help us reflect on some of the positions we hold as helpers.

Figure 13.1 is a map that is a start to finding a more collaborative and supported/supportive stance. Of course, reflecting together and thus working more effectively together is not that simple and is not quickly effective. But, recognising the loops and confirmatory cycles we find ourselves in can move us to a different position where we can feel more empowered to do something different.

CAT and relational working allow space for a dialogue and a level of understanding that helps us consider our own sense of agency and possibilities for taking control; for enabling change. Services in many countries have seen the evolution of a drive towards leadership programmes as a way of addressing crises within their settings and contexts. The desire for leadership roles has perhaps been widely embraced by health care staff in particular, as it represents other exits on their map – an exit from the exhaustion of being on the frontline, but also an opportunity to bring about some of the change so clearly needed and noted through their own experience. While there are many examples of times people have progressed into managerial and leadership roles and have gone on to have a significant impact on the day-to-day delivery of their service, there frequently remains a disconnect between the leadership and the shop floor that might reflect widening inequalities elsewhere within society and becomes easily translated into quite polarised positions within the service.

Many senior managers and health service leaders find themselves repeatedly caught in the trap of needing to connect with the realities of the lived experience of those who access services, as well as the pressures of those who deliver these services on the ground, with a need to demonstrate to commissioners and governmental departments the transformative impact of their work. Dashboards and outcome indices speak to a remarkable transformation in delivery which simply doesn't marry with the realities of people's experiences on the frontline. This disconnect becomes alienating and exhausting for the young person and the worker, and is perhaps where relational working and thinking is most urgently required.

If we look to engage in a relational understanding of what the lived experience of services is really like, and how it feels, as a member of a team to continuously offer a limited and/or exhausted version of yourself and your skill set, then we need to embrace ways of working that look to overcome the hierarchies within our services, and enhance a culture of democratisation and dialogue. CAT, and more specifically mapping, has the tools to enable these types of conversations, as they are and will be uncomfortable, as they will speak to the realities of power and privilege, as much as they voice concerns about hopelessness and despair. If we are looking to genuinely address concerns around burnout, as well as acknowledge how we so easily get drawn into positions of workplace bullying, then we need to create a space for dialogue that allows for collaboration, coproduction and compassion. Collaboration needs us all to find a way of being at the table and being part of the conversation, but to be truly collaborative we also need to find the means for coproduction. For too long coproduction has been hijacked by a form of faux production, where young people, service users, staff and wider stakeholder groups are repeatedly consulted about a service but are seldom the agents of change within that service. It is only through genuine co-production that we will enable the systemic change needed to overcome burnout and bullying.

Being compassionate and caring within a healthcare setting should be a given and not just stored up for the young people and the families we work alongside. But if we work in a toxic environment, then we are often looking out for ourselves more than we might be looking out for others. There have been many frameworks used to ensure a compassionate approach within service delivery and management, as the work on Intelligent Kindness can testify (Campling, 2015). However, our argument remains that, by embracing relational working in our practice and within our systems for support and supervision, we are allowing the space to understand where we are getting drawn into an unhelpful dance within and between ourselves and others. But more than this, we are also allowing ourselves to question not only what is going on within and between, but also what might be going on around us and its relational impacts. Relational working allows us to develop an understanding and consider opportunities for change for the young people we work alongside – it is perhaps time we recognise that this is also what we need to be doing for ourselves. But we can't do this in isolation – it is only through working relationally together that we can perceive and believe that things could be different, and that there can be change. It is only through connecting and being together that we can 'be the change'.

Chapter 14: CAT in education – reflections on the spaces between the 'cogs in the machine'

Claire Regan and Leah O'Toole

Introduction

In the introductory chapter of this book, Nick Barnes and Lee Crothers explore how the pervading neoliberalism in most Western societies has in recent decades contributed to a sense of alienation, individualism and reductionist understandings of young people. Our schools, higher educational institutions and early childhood educational settings are also embedded within this same socio-political context. CAT can inform and support relational approaches to education in theory and in practice, offering hope for a more inclusive, socially just educational system that supports the mental health and well-being of both our teachers and our young people.

Education in context

Decades of theory and research show how educational relationships are influenced by the contexts in which they take place, in terms of both the immediate local environment and wider policy-based and societal concerns (Hayes *et al*, 2023). Vygotskian (1978) theory on the social formation of the mind helps us to understand how children and young people internalise their experience of the learning relationship through their engagement with (or exclusion from) these educational systems. In many countries, neoliberal educational systems are built on a three-legged foundation of narrowing of curriculum, standardisation of assessment, and inspection systems seeking 'accountability' and 'value for money' (O'Toole *et al*, 2019). Curricula are narrowed to focus on those subjects considered valuable in a global economy, namely literacy, numeracy and science. If young people only experience educational situations where particular areas of human skill, interest and endeavour are valued, like in classrooms focussed solely on literacy and numeracy scores to the neglect of the arts, physical education etc., those whose skills and interests are underappreciated tend to disengage from learning generally, and reduce effort accordingly with predictably damaging effects on achievement and on self-esteem (Bandura, 1994).

Schools, teachers and pupils are pitted against each other in this system and are measured through standardised testing and international rankings. Learning environments become competitive, not collaborative, generating high levels of stress and anxiety. At the surface level, the aim is to maintain high standards in education, through standardised teachers teaching standardised lessons to the standard child/young person. All pupils are to be brought to a predetermined fixed point, irrespective of experience, (dis)ability, background or culture. Those who get there are applauded, while those who do not may be judged, devalued or excluded. This approach does not acknowledge that 'success' as a destination looks very different for different human beings. Those in favour of standardised testing often refer to ideas of fairness and objectivity, but the injustice of this is shown in evidence, dating back decades, of significant bias within standardised tests based on social class, linguistic background and race (MacRuairc, 2009; Roberts & DeBlassie, 1983). Diversity is not celebrated or welcomed, at least not in the evaluative processes.

The process of 'norming' means that failure is built in: each individual child's scores are compared against the scores of large groups of children of similar age, and the quality of performance is judged by where a score falls within the curve of performance (Renbarger & Norman, 2018). It is not mathematically possible for all children to be 'above average', and so the requirement for some children to fail is built into the construction of standardised tests. Yet the system devalues and stigmatises those who do poorly, as though doing poorly was ultimately avoidable for all, but there is no such thing as 'levelling up'. If children as a whole begin to score more highly, the norms are shifted so that the 'bell curve' still exists, rendering it impossible for some children to ever succeed. Within this system, children and young people are likely to internalise fractured ideas of success and learning: if I am 'successful' I am 'good enough' and possibly even 'better than'; if I fail, I am devalued as 'not good enough', potentially disillusioned and alienated.

When schools are viewed through the lens of a business model, seeking 'accountability' and 'value for money', a school is like a factory assembly line, and with high-quality input ('good' teaching) and efficient systems (clear behaviour policies, standardised lesson planning and assessment) the outcome should be a high-quality product (children with high test scores who do what adults tell them to). If inspection systems evaluate the 'product' as flawed (i.e. children either do not score highly or do not behave 'well'), then the problem must be the teacher, a lack of efficiency, or the child. This easily sold 'blaming and shaming' narrative, which neglects to acknowledge relational or socio-political context, comes at a very high price: that of the mental health and well-being of large swathes of pupils and teachers today. At the extreme, recent tragic events in the UK in which a school principal took her own life in the aftermath of a deeply bruising Ofsted inspection, may be the appalling but inevitable conclusion of a neoliberal educational system.

Perhaps the most insidious element of this is that neoliberalism has become the dominant discourse in education in many countries worldwide, to the extent that it can guide policy-making, and therefore practice, without ever being explicitly named (O'Toole *et al*, 2023). Drawing on the old joke of the fish who asks, 'What's water?', in many jurisdictions neoliberalism has become the water in which we swim – the unquestioned, dominant paradigm that directs all decision-making without ever being challenged or even acknowledged. Young people and their teachers know that the picture painted above does not capture the complexity of their work, their relationships, their learning or their lives. They do not want to be reduced and polarised in this way. A relational approach to education, with its emphasis on the fundamental importance of learning relationships in context offers an antidote to this polarising neoliberal paradigm. It offers a more dynamic and empowering relationship in learning institutions and thus within children and young people. It offers hope for the future of our educational systems to be more inclusive, respectful and compassionate, where everyone, in all their diversity, can be welcomed and can feel like they belong. It also offers the possibility of a systemic resolution to the 'epidemic' of stress and mental health difficulties reported in our children, young people and teachers today.

Conceptualising relational education

The tools and insights of CAT can be used to develop an alternative conceptualisation of education which centres the role of dynamic human relationships. Figure 14.1 shows how early relationships can impact educational dynamics. The bottom axis of the image shows the developing person over time. Above, the key relationships in the person's development are highlighted, and above that again there is a summary of factors impacting their life-long dispositions and ability to learn. In the first quadrant, primary attachment relationships are key to the child's development and engagement in learning, and these relationships have long-term impacts. Moving into the second quadrant, the child's life influences include their relationships with their early childhood educators and primary school teachers. Early educational experiences are about the *process* of learning as much or more than they are about the *content*; in early childhood, we are 'learning how to learn' through the development of 'dispositions for learning' (Carr *et al*, 2010). The child is developing their relationship with education, and the relationship that the educator has with the child will impact how the child engages with learning in the future (Hill, 2020).

Figure 14.1: The impact of relationships on development

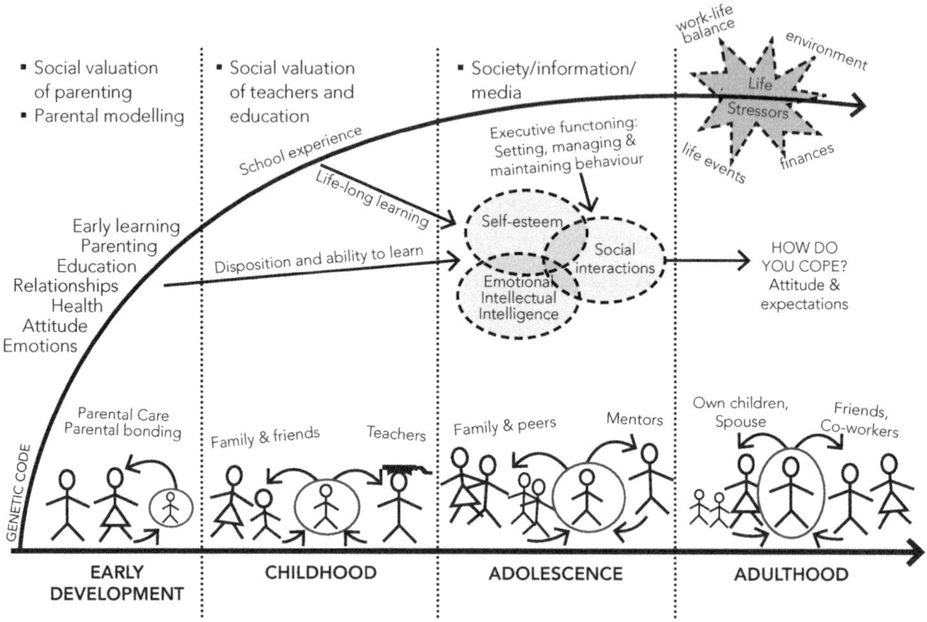

This impact is mediated by a multitude of other factors, including health, peers, socioeconomics, family educational engagement and the demands of the educational system (Hayes *et al*, 2023). How a child has learned to engage with learning has an ongoing impact in their adolescence, shaping their sense of self and their self-esteem, impacting their brain development, attention, ability to plan, manage and monitor their own behaviour, indeed on overall executive functioning (O'Toole & Hayes, 2020). How a child engages with learning also impacts their social functioning, peer relationships and their work and personal developmental opportunities. Educational relationships can be enabling and encouraging or disabling and destructive, and they can have profound, life-long impacts (O'Toole & Hayes, 2020).

Tony Ryle's work is rooted in an understanding of the individual in the context of relationships and societies. The complex relational dynamics underpinning teaching and learning can only truly be understood in the context of the systems within which they reside. Bronfenbrenner's bioecological model of human development (Bronfenbrenner & Morris, 2006) gives us a visual model that can support this understanding (see Figure 14.2).

Figure 14.2: Bronfenbrenner's Bioecological Model of Human Development

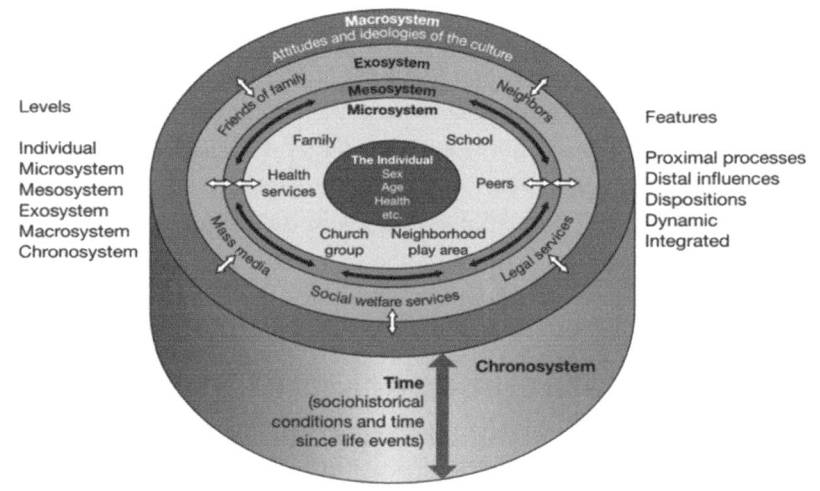

(Hayes, O'Toole & Halpenny, 2023, p14)

Bronfenbrenner (1979) identified how contexts play a crucial role in learning and development, from direct environmental impacts ('micro-system') to broader cultural factors ('macro-system'). He also emphasised the interactions between these different levels of systems ('meso-system' and 'exo-system'). The most recent version of the bioecological model incorporates the child's agency and time (socio-historical and personal – 'chrono-system'), and emphasises reciprocal, dynamic, non-linear relationships (Bronfenbrenner & Morris, 2006; Hayes *et al*, 2023). Relationships are not simply enacted upon children or upon educators; rather, children and educators both comprise active participants in their development, nature and quality (Hayes *et al*, 2023), consistent with the reciprocity of relationships emphasised in CAT. Bronfenbrenner and CAT agree that different people elicit different reactions from us depending on our own personal histories and our own cultural and social norms. All educational processes are underpinned by the resulting relationships.

This conceptualisation allows us to explore with educators how the incessant and often intolerable pressures of neoliberal expectations can impact on their engagement with children and their families, and colour their understanding of what their job is supposed be. This framework views learning not simply as a function of individual ability and effort, or of the standard of teaching, or of school standards, but rather as a relational experience between children/young people and their teachers, classmates and school community, which is influenced in an ongoing way by their social and cultural contexts (Nowak-Łojewska *et al*, 2019). Furthermore, it acknowledges that learners/children/young people internalise messages about themselves and their capabilities that are developed in these educational relationships that will shape their ongoing engagement with education and thus their future prospects through these dynamic interactions. The relational insights of CAT, supported by a bioecological framework, provide an important alternative conceptualisation of education to that which is dominant today.

Enacting relational education: Relational Reflective Practice using the 'map and talk' approach

This leads us to two important questions:

1. Can we support the improvement of educational relationships in practical ways without losing any of the complexity of the relational dance?

2. Can people who work in educational systems become more relationally aware in a way that enables greater flexibility with children and young people?

The tools and concepts of CAT are critically important in helping us to answer these questions in the affirmative.

CAT mapping is the essential tool to enact these changes in educational settings, through Relational Reflective Practice. In recent years, reflective practice has increasingly been presented as the gold standard in education with benefits for educators, children, parents and communities (McDonagh *et al*, 2020). Multiple reflective practice 'models' have emerged (e.g. Borton, 1970; Kolb, 1984; Gibbs, 1988), but many existing models encourage a procedural approach to reflection, focused on solving a perceived problem in educational practice. Children/young people may be reduced to a simplistic version of themselves and seen as a problem to be solved. Such reductionist approaches do not allow for relational complexities to be unpacked. Using CAT mapping, staff in educational settings can reflect on the dynamic of an ongoing relationship with a child, a parent or the system, and, simultaneously, on their role within this relational 'dance'. This opens up the possibility of change by enabling us to describe, understand and alter educational relationships for the better, while supporting staff in this process. It renders describable the often frustratingly intangible concept of the 'quality' of relationships (Nowak-Łojewska *et al*, 2019).

The use of CAT mapping as an aid to multidisciplinary team reflection has been practised in mental health settings for the past 20 years and in forensic settings for at least ten years (Marshall & Kirkland, 2021). It has variously been referred to as 'relational mapping', 'reflective mapping' or 'map and talk' (Potter, 2021a), and a more detailed description of CAT-informed relational mapping can be found in Potter (2020; 2021a; 2021b) and Kemp *et al* (2017). Briefly, this form of reflective practice is done using pen and paper, ideally large A3 sheets, working in pairs, teams or as a group with a facilitator. We identify and map in words and images the dynamic, felt reciprocity of a relationship, known as the reciprocal roles.

Relational Reflective Practice using mapping is not only about our thoughts or feelings. It is about trying to understand how the other person is thinking or feeling based on our understanding of relationships as two-way, dynamic processes in context; we want to understand 'the dance' of the relationship. As we sketch the reciprocal roles and procedures that come from them, they grow into a relational 'map', aiding our reflection on the dynamics of the relationship. For example, if we are getting stuck in an unhelpful way of relating with a child, mapping allows us to sit together and wonder, to 'hover' over what is happening. We can critically reflect on what pressures come from external systems, what assumptions come from personal histories, and where our own educational values truly lie. Thus, we can think differently about situations and potentially choose other 'steps' (or exits) in the relational 'dance', that we may not have been apparent before. We may also be able to see more clearly what our work in education is actually *for*, beyond the requirements of standardisation and 'accountability'.

Potter (2020) emphasises a non-judgemental approach to seeing our own role in relationships. He urges us to 'name the dance, don't blame the dancer'. Thus, we can see our role in the relationship without fault or blame being attributed. This allows a deeper, less critical relational reflection and potentially more flexibility in response. Mapping can improve educational relationships and thereby educational practice. It is about recognising that it is not just what we do that matters, but how we feel about what we do. By naming our own emotional responses to children/young people/parents/colleagues and our observation of their responses to us, we step into the relational space in a different way and begin to describe the often-ineffable push and pull. This broadens our perspective and increases our capacity for compassionate understanding. If we want to get a different outcome in the relationship, this opens up the possibility of choosing different 'steps' in the 'dance'.

The process of relational mapping is an important technique. The map that is created is a tool that can be returned to time and again in working with a particular young person. It can also be amended to allow for changing positions and increased understanding. Mapping enables confusion to be contained, complexity to be held and strong emotions to be safely expressed, owned and understood in context. 'Not knowing' can be valued as a useful step towards greater understanding, and this is important because educators (like children) are often given the strong message that they are only successful if they have the 'right' answer. Mapping allows for deeper understandings to be generated because many options can be 'hovered over' at once and we can 'shimmer' between multiple perspectives (Potter, 2020). It opens possibilities for increased empathy and perspective taking, learning together to be facilitated and personal growth at individual and group levels. Importantly, there is no such thing as a 'correct' map, only one that is useful and facilitates a deeper understanding (Potter, 2020).

The THRIECE Project: an example of CAT in education

In 2017, we launched an international research project called Teaching for Holistic, Relational and Inclusive Early Childhood Education, or THRIECE

(Nowak-Łojewska *et al*, 2019; O'Toole, 2020). This was a two-year project, run across three countries (Ireland, Poland and Portugal) funded under Erasmus + . Within each country, we had partners across three educational levels: early childhood education and care (ECEC); primary school; and higher educational institutions (HEIs). Our aim was to provide an alternative to the 'all powerful' or 'all powerless' polarisations of the dominant neoliberal voice, and to support a different conceptualisation of 'quality' education. In Ireland, we introduced Relational Reflective Practice using the 'map and talk' approach outlined above. We worked with one primary school and two early childhood education settings to explore the impact on staff collaboration, relationships with students, teaching styles, approaches to behaviour management, and partnership with families.

We began this work with a three-day interactive workshop for all staff of our three partner sites, using a whole-system approach (Shannon *et al*, 2016; 2017). We offered an invitation to each person to choose their own level of participation. We developed and engaged participants with a suite of training materials, which included insights on the dynamic nature of relationships in the context informed by Bronfenbrenner, and on CAT concepts including reciprocal roles. We discussed reflective practice and Steve Potter taught relational mapping using the 'map and talk' approach (Kemp *et al*, 2017; Marshall & Kirkland, 2021). We encouraged staff to use the language of CAT and to begin to 'map' together, where useful.

Following the workshops, we established a 'Map Club', a one-hour Relational Reflective Practice group that ran monthly for nine months. Participation was voluntary. Staff attended during their CPD time. On average, we had 12 to 15 participants. This group was facilitated by the first author, an experienced CAT supervisor. Mapping between sessions was scaffolded by colleagues with significant exposure to CAT through the THRIECE project. Participants were encouraged to bring their maps, struggles and reflections to Map Club where we worked through them together. Semi-structured interviews were conducted with educators at the end of the project.

Participants indicated that engaging with mapping *improved their relational awareness*. In particular, children's behaviour began to make more sense to them and their ability to locate behaviour in context was significantly developed through mapping. *Increased reflection* was particularly evident in their ability to recognise their own contribution to the relational dynamic. The increased insight and understanding that came from this reflection helped them to develop practical solutions and to feel better equipped to know what to do in tricky situations.

One reason that relationships are often undervalued is that they are notoriously difficult to measure, and the terms used to describe them are often imprecise, leaving room for lack of clarity. Our participants reported that mapping together gave them *a common language for understanding and explaining complex relational events and dynamics in context*. On an individual level, this deepened reflection, and at a team level, it also empowered them to support each other through educational dilemmas. They further found that their strengthened relational awareness and reflection and their developing common language led to *increased psychological safety*, with consequent *improvements in team functioning*. The blame-free culture emphasised by Potter (2021) was highlighted by these educators. Unsurprisingly, the participants reported how the development of such psychological safety broke down barriers between different categories of staff (e.g. teachers and SNAs) and supported staff to recognise each other's strengths and potential contributions. They also found that this improvement in staff relationships supported them to *improve relationships with parents*.

In summary, thematic analysis of the content of these interviews identified six areas of change: increased relational awareness, increased reflection, creation of a common language, improved relationships with parents, increased sense of psychological safety and improved staff relationships.

Below, we share testimony of the experience of engaging in Relational Reflective Practice from two teachers involved in the THRIECE project.

Emily, a primary school teacher, talked about how CAT mapping impacted her teacher–pupil relationships

It has definitely impacted me and the way I teach, especially with behaviours of concern. There is a particular child in my class who had proved very challenging. I did several maps and this has helped me with the way that I think before I respond to his actions. He does the same things on a weekly basis. This way I've had time to reflect differently. When I map it out, I can see some other options for my response that I couldn't see before. Sometimes it works, and sometimes it doesn't, but now I always try to stop and reflect. →

It has also helped me with the reserved kids. There were some that I found it hard to have a relationship with. Through mapping, I've changed the way I interact with them. Now I make a big effort to get to know them and to know their interests. I start the day by trying to engage them in what they are interested in, to get them out of their shells. I build the relationship based on where they are coming from, not waiting for them to bring something forward. It can take a while, but it has made a big difference.

Suzanne, a learning support teacher, reflected on how CAT mapping has helped her blame herself less and be more open

Mapping is a useful thing to do. We often think of the negatives in what we've done. I think "I could have done much better". Through the reflection and the mapping, we can see all the good that we do. It's not that we can't do any better. Of course we can. But it allows me to acknowledge that I did my best in that situation at that particular time. I can also see that, if it happens again, I could try a different approach. Mapping allows me to wonder what different approaches might work. I know that in the next instance, I won't, for example, allow the child's frustration levels to get that high. I can accept my part in either augmenting the frustration or relieving it, coming from a positive place of learning, not blaming myself. I can acknowledge that, yes, maybe I could have done better, but in that particular situation I wasn't armed with the tools to do any better. By mapping, we are giving ourselves the tools to see that, if it happens again, I can change my tack and that might lead us to a different, better outcome."

The future of CAT in education

What CAT has to offer to education is new and innovative. The fundamental role of early attachment relationships for the developing person has been well understood and widely accepted in the psychology literature and in broader popular culture for many decades. Early childhood educators and teachers are 'in loco parentis' for large portions of time for the vast majority of childhoods and are mandated to be so by our states. In academic circles, there is a strong, well-established literature on relational pedagogy (Bingham & Sidorkin, 2004), but this has sometimes been translated into utilitarian, outcome-based provision in practice, consistent with the culture of the system. In daily practice, there is an ongoing awareness of the importance of 'good' relationships, but a deeper reflective recognition of the significance of relationships in education is long overdue in many systems. A good, supportive teacher-pupil relationship can change the course of a person's life. CAT provides the insights, and most importantly the tools, to support an increasing relational reflective capacity for teachers. This can empower teachers to create micro-moments of social justice for children and young people within our system, where they can 'hover over' situations and understand all of the elements at play. This is particularly important for children/young people who may be disenfranchised by systemic expectations for behaviour or attainment demands outside of their reach. There is significant scope for a CAT relational mapping approach to understanding and managing behaviours of concern within educational settings. We are particularly interested in how relational reflective practice can be integrated into school behaviour management policies.

This kind of Relational Reflective Practice, stepping outside of our roles and wondering about all elements at play, is counter-cultural in our educational systems as they stand. However, in our experience, it speaks to the felt sense of what is wise and already known by our teachers. It creates space for what many teachers already feel within themselves to be important, and it provides a language and a method for discussing the dynamics of relationships. By understanding their own roles in a situation, educators can see where their power resides in a system that can feel otherwise disempowering. The improvement in relationships at all levels, along with the increased sense of psychological safety generated within staff teams that we saw in THRIECE, provide potential antidotes to the stress and anxiety created by a demanding and competitive system. The use of CAT in educational systems, as elsewhere, may well lead to an improvement in the mental health and well-being of teaching staff and students alike. In this way, CAT provides a systemic, relational approach to well-being.

However, CAT in education can also be so much more. When we emphasise relationships in this way, when we provide language, support and space for that which has been disavowed, and when what we value resonates with the values and beliefs of teachers and students who are overwhelmed and/or disillusioned, we provide the preconditions for cultural change. CAT in education could be a powerful vehicle to support the development of a more inclusive, holistic and socially just educational system, reaching into the space that lies between us.

Case study 3: Excluded, disengaged and on the outside – reconnecting through 'Learning to Learn'

Donna Lockett

The following case studies look to demonstrate a way of working that has evolved over many years of working with children and young people who, for a multiplicity of reasons, find themselves on the outside, in a position of exclusion from mainstream education provision and support. This work has evolved through supporting young people who may have physical and/or emotional health needs (such as being diagnosed with cancer or experiencing a depressive episode), that have impacted on their capacity to access and engage with their education and who might be excluded, disengaged and/or outside of educational (and wider) support, unable to attend an alternative setting (such as a pupil referral unit). In essence, this practice evolved into a home and community tuition service for those young people unable to engage with the formal offer of mainstream and alternative educational provision.

Outward facing anxiety: Ryan

Mainstream education became increasingly unable to support Ryan (fictitious name) because of concerns about his behaviour, and he fell through the gaps in support within his first year of transition to secondary school. Ryan had no formal diagnosis and, likewise there was no understanding of his cognitive strengths or needs. His parents were reluctant for him to attend a pupil referral unit for fear he would be "recruited into local gangs" (given the experiences of some of his peer group), and hence Ryan spent the following two years at home, not attending any schooling, until he was referred for home tuition.

At the time of this referral Ryan was unable to leave the family home for fear of exposure to violence and the threat of knife crime in his housing estate, and so failed to attend appointments or engage with professionals, despite there being a large network around him. There were multiple professionals' meetings about Ryan, but nobody actively engaging him in any youth work activities, substance misuse support, social care interventions, education or therapeutic input. Hence, the likelihood for engagement with home tuition was limited.

On the first visit I laid out the teaching materials on the kitchen table and invited Ryan to write his name on both his maths and English books. An agenda for the next forty-five minutes was agreed using a visual timetable on the whiteboard. Without the need for introductions of the topic, Ryan was then shown how to rule up a margin and asked to complete four more pages. He copied the heading from the whiteboard into his book and looked at the first example: $a + a + a + a = 4a$. Another example was given, and Ryan completed the task independently. A grade was assigned in the margin using highlighter pen, and it was acknowledged that Ryan had just started their GCSE (school leaving exam) maths course, preparing for an exam in eight months' time. The remaining time was used to build the subject up from a grade 1 to grade 3.

Word problems were not tackled, in order to avoid possible confusion and opportunities to reject the task. Over the years it has been frequently demonstrated that the risk of feeling exposed, and the experiencing of possible humiliation, are significant drivers for refusing to engage with an educational task – hence the need to stay in a space where the young person perceives minimal threat and danger. With barely any spoken instructions Ryan was actively learning, and attainment was being captured, offering a glimmer of hope that the sessions may be worth investing in, and that failure, exposure and humiliation were not certainties. Along with the hope came trust that the level of learning would be visual, broken down so it was accessible with minimal auditory information to navigate.

Due to high levels of anxiety and his hypervigilance to any possible threat, Ryan self-medicated using cannabis to enable him to be calm enough to engage and have sufficient screen area on his (internal) working desktop to enable him to think and process visual information. Within a few minutes he had achieved, without the cost of humiliation – he was engaged.

Tutoring continued for three sessions a week, with Ryan engaging and demonstrating basic maths skills and a natural talent for creative writing.

Despite this progress, he was unable to extend the trust or make sense of any of the other support offered within the network. But through beginning a process of learning, more reflective of learning to learn, Ryan continued to engage with his education, acknowledging that the cannabis was interfering with the learning, and gradually beginning to consider there was a world he could engage with outside of the home. Education, attuned learning to learn, was giving a window of normality, offering him an exit for the first time in over five years.

Perhaps what this case study most clearly articulates is the need to step away from seeing young people as "hard to reach"; after all, it wasn't hard to reach Ryan. Rather, the task is to think about teaching to engage first, to allow space for learning to learn, and the wider curriculum comes second.

Inward facing anxiety: Mel

Mel (fictitious name) stopped attending school in her first year of secondary school, at the age of eleven. By the time she was referred for tuition aged sixteen, she had a diagnosis of severe obsessive-compulsive disorder (OCD) and had not been able to access education for the last four years. Her sensory needs, linked to her OCD, meant that engaging with people from outside or within the family home was challenging, especially with her fears of contamination. Touching anything from outside the home, being exposed to new smells such as perfumes, or sharing a space with an unfamiliar person were all triggers for anxiety and distress. As a result, Mel had not been able to leave the home to access help and support from other professionals. Nor could she access professionals coming into the home, leaving her isolated and without the opportunity to be included in education.

Following a referral for home tuition, once again at the kitchen table, I laid out what was needed for today's lesson, writing out a visual timetable. Mel was not in the room at this point, but her curiosity was noted as she sat on the stairs out of sight. I started to read 'An Inspector Calls' aloud (taking on all the different characters of J.B. Priestley's modern morality play, a set text for the English Literature curriculum). By the end of this first session, Mel was still on the stairs, but within sight, listening and commenting on characters. We were on task, focused on a core curriculum text without the need for awkward introductions or icebreakers.

At the next session, Mel was looking over my shoulder at the text – and by the third lesson she was taking on two of the characters from her own book placed on the table away from me. We began to analyse the characters, and we had conversations about what text we might need to read next to ensure that Mel could achieve a qualification in English. Some Dickens perhaps? How appropriate to be thinking and reflecting on the Victorian chronicler of inequality, poverty and exclusion.

Analysis

Ryan and Mel are in the same position, even if their initial presenting needs are quite different. One externalises their anxieties and worries to the extent that they end up being excluded; the other experiences their distress in a way that forces them to turn in on themselves and retreat. But the end result is that they are both on the outside, excluded from and unable to engage in education. Nor can they access wider support – from social care, from mental health services or from youth work.

Enabling them to engage with learning needed to be presented as a stripped-down, no-nonsense approach to education and attainment. This approach is a relational one, recognising that the young person needs a positive relationship with learning, at first within their safe space, their home. The approach provides an environment where threats and anxiety triggering moments are minimised or removed so that learning can occur. For young people in these types of situations, there is a risk of too much time being given to face-to-face introductions, exploring how we have arrived at this point, over-explaining and over-teaching points, with delays in recognising and recording attainment and progress, all providing opportunities to give up on the tutor. To prevent this feeling of high pressure and the understandable sabotaging procedure of the young person (often a long-established way of dealing with any risk of failure or humiliation), clarity and directness in expectation, without being patronising or dismissive of the contextual complexity, provides a relational experience for the young person of succeeding from the start.

Ryan and Mel exemplify the type of young person who are referred for our support. They no longer leave their home or often even their bedrooms, and they don't engage with family or professionals, despite having been offered a wide menu of interventions by school and the wider networks. The combined expense and expertise involved seems to offer limited scope for change. The system grinds to a halt and everything can feel very stuck, with parents often feeling powerless to create change. The young people themselves are then in a position of retreating into a place of disconnect and hopelessness – one that can be communicated equally by inward- and outward-facing distress and/or actions.

Relational learning

In effect, the work going on at the kitchen table offers a triangulation of the developing relationship between the young person and the tutor – where we might draw the attention away from the direct, face to face connection, and allow the learning to become a focus, or dare I say, a distraction.

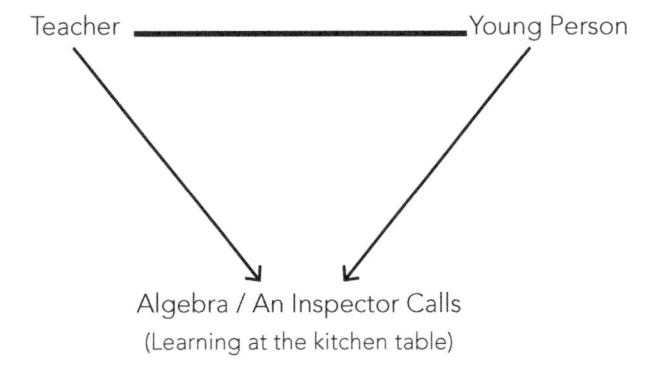

```
Teacher ────────────────── Young Person
         \                /
          \              /
           \            /
            ↘          ↙
         Algebra / An Inspector Calls
          (Learning at the kitchen table)
```

We are two people co-existing, sharing a space, sitting side by side, both with a focus that is being directed away from anything that feels too personal, which has been so unsafe for the young person, and directed entirely towards the learning in a scaffolded way. But this is also about taking away the wider distractions and threats – limited direct eye contact, no unnecessary small talk, minimising the possibility of sensory overload, and simply ensuring that the right climate for learning is being set, allowing for mentalisation to occur within the room. We are here to achieve and attain, but the young person needs to believe that they can attain, and they need to experience that attainment.

On the surface, I would argue that what is offered is incredibly simple, but I fear that such a lens might negate the complexity of the needs of the young person. After all, this is fundamentally about Vygotsky's theory of learning socially, and about working where a young person is at and seeing where they can be in the future with the right support. Young people who have been socially excluded for so long have such hugely pronounced anxieties and fears about connecting with any professional that any encounter with education and learning can be perceived as a threat. If one doesn't act in a threatening or pressuring manner, but rather in a matter of fact, "let's do this together" kind of way, it helps young people consider themselves as capable enough.

This approach differs from many of the more trauma-informed approaches, which tend to be much more focused on raising awareness and understanding, and ensuring that we don't tread on the toes of emotions – which can be perceived by the young person as just as alienating. In many ways, taking a less direct and more softly trodden approach may feel even more threatening, as the young person remains uncertain about the professional's agenda.

The task is to be clear and concise, and to provide clarity about expectations and outcomes, relating in an almost businesslike way that can feel safe for the young person. The focus is to re-engage with learning, to expect and have education as a window of normality amongst a set of circumstances that don't provide normality. By doing so, a message is conveyed to the young people that we are here to achieve, to build trust through the experience of attainment, and to allow the young person to consider space for hope and explore a possibility for change. In many ways, the tutor's role is to provide a clear signal that they are the adults leading the session and it is safe for the young person to be the learner without feeling judged. This gives the young person and the tutor the confidence to remain on task, and to avoid straying into unchartered waters.

Enabling possibilities for change through 'Learning to Learn'

For many young people in situations similar to those of Ryan and Mel, the dialogue is so often about the need to manage their mental health and emotional wellbeing first and foremost, with education to come later. Experience has shown that for some, this needs approach could be challenged and reversed. For some young people, they need to have a sense of themselves through an experience of attaining and achievement, rather than through an exploration of emotions and a language of anxiety that does not resonate with them. This is not disregarding their emotional state, but rather providing a space for regulating their emotional states through prizing the relationship of trust that is developing between the young person and tutor. Tuning in and being aware of the emotional need remains important, but it doesn't mean stepping away from the tutoring role and professional purpose.

Over the last few years our team have worked with others in exploring this approach to engagement and learning with young people as a way to enable change. Working with other relationally aware practitioners – be they educational psychologists, psychiatrists, youth justice practitioners or speech and language therapists – it has been possible to articulate this relationally-aware approach as 'Learning to Learn'.

The young people who are referred to me have missed so much of their educational experience, through exclusion or significant mental health difficulties, that when faced with the prospect of reconnecting with their learning it feels terrifying to them – it carries a huge risk of humiliation, shame and failure. For a child who has locked themselves in their room for the last two years or has been exploited through county lines, they usually expect others to offer further humiliation or shame. To stay and engage is taking a huge risk. 'Learning to Learn' is therefore about acknowledging the need to work with where the child is at (in their ZPD) but at pace, and with a focus that allows success and the emergence of self-respect, even pride, within the first minutes of connecting with their tutor. At that first connection over the kitchen table, the clock is ticking – by the end of that first lesson they need to believe for themselves that they can achieve. They don't need me to believe for them.

'Learning to Learn' is a relationally based way of educating in that it takes a consideration of self and other from a position that allows space to think about what is going on within, what is happening between, and what may be going on around. Through this approach, we are not simply looking to support a young person to achieve end of school qualifications. Rather, 'Learning to Learn' allows a young person to explore the possibility of change – a changing of platforms. For some time, the young person has been on a learning journey where the train has been taking them further and further away from their family and friends, and from an understanding of themselves. When the train lands at the platform, that part of the journey is over, and the young person needs to cross the platform, with carefully planned and executed interventions, so they can board a new train travelling in a new and more positive direction.

Through 'Learning to Learn', young people can begin to believe in themselves, allow themselves to connect with others, and begin to consider how and where they might want to see themselves in the future – something we think is needed to learn.

PART 4: Relational approaches to communities and society

Chapter 15: From Hellblade to Game Group – relating and connecting in digital spaces

Alex Bretherton and Nick Barnes

Our aim in this chapter is to help those working alongside young people to have an insight into and understanding of the potentials within the gaming world, and to reflect on the possibilities that this could become a tool or medium for working relationally. Gaming and gaming communities can create sufficient space for dialogue and a sense of connection that can be both helpful and supportive for some young people. Our hope is that practitioners may explore this possible dialogue with young people from a more relational perspective and recognise that the positive reciprocal roles of connecting-to-connected are accessible through this digital space. Alex's journey, articulated in this chapter, leading us to his co-creation of Game Group, is all about this possibility of relating and connecting in digital spaces.

For many professionals working in young people's services, it can often be difficult to consider the possibilities of gaming and the utilisation of digital platforms as anything other than a marker for social isolation and disconnect. Admittedly, this will predominantly be a generational concern, with many more recently qualified professionals having been brought up within a digital world, and therefore feeling more comfortable engaging in conversations that are drawn into digital spaces. Even so, with so much focus on the negative impacts of social media and fears about over-reliance, dependence, and even internet addiction, engagement within the digital world – especially the world of gaming – is often used as a (subjective) marker of the impact on a person's capacity to function outside of the home, or outside of the bedroom, and is seldom seen as a scaffold for relating, connecting and enabling a sense of community (Young Minds, 2020).

We have written this chapter as a dialogue between gamer and curious clinician, both looking to explore our capacity to connect and relate through gaming and digital platforms through a CAT lens, seeking to consider what a relationally informed approach to mental health can learn from gamers, and vice versa. Through Alex's lived experience of significant emotional and mental health needs, he will share his journey of engagement with the gaming platform 'Hellblade: Senua's Sacrifice' (Ninja Theory, 2017), in the hope that this narrative may help others understand the value and potential benefit of this type of gaming, and how this has the potential to be embraced within a context of relational mental health.

Alex

My name's Alex. I'm a novelist, a poet, a classical music composer and a gamer; I've survived psychosis and understood myself through a journey of clinical diagnoses that include severe depression, anxiety, OCD, social anxiety and paranoid schizophrenia. This journey began when I was five. I long ago discovered that my demons know how to swim and can't be drowned, which led me to learn to live both with and above them.

I'm now stable, fully functioning, holding down a full-time job in mental healthcare, socialising, and maintaining my mental health within the context of the above experiences. I'm supported by people around me, my daily routine, self-awareness and medication. I work as a Senior Peer Support Worker in an Early Intervention Service in London and use my lived experience of significant emotional and mental health needs to help and provide hope to the next individual using the service, a service from which I personally benefited.

During my experiences, I've managed to find several things that have helped, one of which is gaming. This is a huge topic and gaming has many pros and cons, with positive, negative, additive, and subtractive qualities. But through my experiences, I will hopefully shed some insight into the gaming world's impact and interconnectivity, offering a conversation on whether gaming can be a force for good, especially for young people.

When looking into the ever-expanding field of gaming and its relation to mental health, we were immediately struck by how the dialogue across this field is shifting so rapidly. For so long, the discourse has been focused on how detrimental gaming has been to people's mental health, and especially to that of children and young people, and subsequently why so much of the media attention has been on a growing awareness of Gaming Disorder. The decision by the World Health Organization to include Gaming Disorder in the International Classification of Diseases, Version 11, has not been universally welcomed, as many argue that there has been insufficient evidence to determine whether the constellation of symptoms allows it to fall within its own classification category, and in particular falling within the wider grouping of Addictive Disorders. Even the Diagnostic and Statistical Manual of Mental Disorders, Fifth Edition (DSM-5) has withheld from naming Internet Gaming Disorder as a specific disorder, being of the view that further research and time is required before a firmer decision can be made (Darvesh, 2020)

However, we do then wonder whether this discourse on gaming and mental health being focused so firmly on the need for psycho-pathologising has had a profound impact on clinical perceptions of gaming as a whole and skewed our questioning towards gaming being seen within the realms of problematic behaviour, blinding us to any possible positives that may emerge from this digital space.

Within the field of child and adolescent mental health services, this bias might also reflect a generational difference, not only for the clinicians, as hinted at earlier, but also for the parents, who have felt out of touch with the rapidly expanding digital world. Recognition that the gaming world has now overtaken the video and music industry combined (BBC, 2019) in terms of capital generation is perhaps one of the best markers of this profound cultural shift and explains gaps in understanding that might be present between parent and child.

But with the current average age of gamers now falling within the 29 to 31-year-old age group, and with a marked increase in female and non-binary identifying gamers, rapidly catching up on what two decades ago was a much more male-dominated activity, we are perhaps at a time, and in a space, where we are seeing a profound shift in the world of gaming, alongside how we relate and connect with digital platforms in general.

This shift in perspective was possibly reinforced during the COVID-19 pandemic, when connecting through digital platforms became the norm for the majority, with organisations such as the Campaign Against Living Miserably creating the slogan "When the world is on pause games can help keep you connected" (Robertson, A 2020).

But we are not in denial that there can be risks involved, and that the online world can be a hugely exploitative and abusive space. The online world can be profoundly threatening, intimidating and exploitative, and cause many young people to feel anxious and overwhelmed, while their parents or carers feel impotent in the face of such challenges.

> ## Alex
>
> First off, it is unarguable that gaming, and potential addictions therein, can pertain to serious and debilitating problems, of which I have often experienced. The risks of the digital and online worlds can lead to exploitative and abusive reaches, even with the best of intentions and safeguards in place. Such risks could originate from online trolls or unbridled aggression, encouragement of self-harm, suicidal acts or sexual exploitation. Again, even with the best safeguards in place, anyone can be placed at risk while online, leading to prolonged or lifelong experiences of trauma, abuse and anxiety, rendering parents or carers to feel helpless in the face of such anonymity and seclusion. I have experienced a lot of these risks first hand and observed it in friends. There have been times when over-immersion in online worlds and fantasy lands has constructed an unstable scaffolding perched atop a semi-solid foundation, resulting in isolation, even to the point of not leaving my bedroom. Over-reliance on these worlds of false accomplishment can lead to dependence or addiction. I am keen to explore, however, the possible impact that certain types of gaming could have on young people, especially when discussing the topics of relating, connecting and discovering an enabling community, consuming content from games that inspire a dialogue regarding sensitive topics instead of leading towards social isolation and disconnect.

Many of those within the gaming world have sought to try and engage with the topic of mental health, and likewise many clinicians have wondered if there may be a therapeutic avenue that could be explored through gaming's capacity to connect and engage some young people (Fitzgerald, 2020). After all, if we are considering gaming from a Vygotskian perspective, then, for some young people, this is very much about working within their Zone of Proximal Development (ZPD) with gaming offering a clear example of scaffolded learning, seeking mastery and attainment to reach the next level.

Through the University of Auckland, child and adolescent psychiatrist Professor Sally Merry was able to co-develop a fantasy role-playing game, SPARX, ('Smart, Positive, Active, Realistic, X-factor thoughts') which looked to offer an interactive form of computerised Cognitive Behavioural Therapy (cCBT) for children and young people with mild to moderate depression (Merry *et al*, 2012). Recognising that many children were not able to access support and services – whether through barriers of stigma, or lack of capacity – this game was promoted as one way in which early action, mental health support could be accessed. This approach has been taken up in Australia and Japan, and interestingly, the format has allowed for considerable adaptations to address needs and reflect cultural context. For example, in the game Finding Hope, the inclusion of the Tui bird - a cultural representation of hope – resonated with many young people within this population. Developing this sense of connection further, young people from the LGBTQI community, found considerable safety and security in being able to explore this space as a solitary figure initially, and then gradually connecting with others, through the world of Rainbow SPARX (Lucassen *et al*, 2015).

Perhaps what we are aware of is that gaming needs to be given the space to sit alongside other tools and media for engaging young people, and not immediately be seen through the prejudicial lens that has been a predominant perspective to date. There are worries about huge amounts of time being taken up engaged with gaming activities, but if this amount of time were being taken up by playing football would there be a similar outcry? Admittedly, football would mean being active and outside for much of the time, but many of those who have sought to recast the world of gaming in a more positive and potentially helpful/supportive light would argue that we should only be seeking to problematise gaming when it starts to impact on functioning, socialising and wider realms of emotional development. After all, it may not be the gaming itself that is the motivation to spend more and more time locked away on a console, but rather it is the manifestation of other more contextualised problems for the young person – at home, in school or in the community – and gaming becomes one of the few safe spaces to truly explore and let one's guard down.

Alex

In a short summary, I experienced a psychosis in late adolescence, following my mother's diagnosis of terminal cancer. I was admitted to A&E with psychotic symptoms, but my mania was entirely internalised. I was in a waking coma, on a saline drip for hydration, lying like a sleeping vampire on a hospital bed for at least three days before I could speak, capable solely of the word 'sorry'. This was the first time in years I achieved a sense of quiet from voices and internal monologue. For six months, I expanded my vocabulary, powering through an OCD which lasted for over eleven hours, then reduced to two seconds, now practically non-existent.

My recovery was supported through the Early Intervention Service, allowing me to test the waters of my anxiety and depression, seeing what worked and what didn't, trialling and co-creating personalised coping mechanisms.

Playing on games was far too stimulating for me in the beginning months of my recovery, setting off what I called 'screeching violins' in my head, the best possible way to describe that intense sensation of anxiety. I found solace, instead, in films and creative writing and music and exercise.

Sometime later, I managed to get back into gaming and the fantastical worlds and immersive escapism it could provide. I delved too deep, noticing through self-awareness that I was isolating myself, leading me to reengage with my other daily routines, turning habits into second-nature acts embedded in my mind, reading up on Occupational Therapy techniques and Socratic conversational methods that I could apply to conversing kindly with myself. In the end, I created a healthy and symbiotic balance with gaming, providing a sense of community with online gaming, boundaries with the online world, as well as hosting game nights with friends.

While I am aware that gaming can be a marker of a lack of capacity or a sign of regression – both of which have been valid in my case – I have also had a thoroughly positive experience with the gaming world. I have made lifelong friends, and a digital environment certainly helped me through the COVID lockdowns. My imagination is keen and, at times, →

> rampant, leading to paranoid thoughts. But, through the medium of gaming and the engagement with others that it can provide, I have been able to hone my imagination into wider areas of creativity, such as composing classical pieces of music, writing poetry and novels – but, most recently, I have focused my gaming on playing through Hellblade.

So, what is Hellblade? It is a fantasy action-adventure game, designed by Ninja Theory, and released in 2017, that engages you in the journey of a Celtic Warrior, Senua, who is on a quest to retrieve the soul of her sacrificed lover. The story of this journey is told from the perspective of Senua, who also experiences auditory hallucinations and delusions. Senua is not defined by these unusual experiences, but rather, these are part of her way of perceiving the world around her, and hence how she, and subsequently the gamer, then experience the journey of her quest.

Hellblade is not a game that seeks to explain or psycho-educate people about psychosis, or unusual experiences, but rather seeks to allow the gamer to share an understanding with the character what this experience is like, perhaps generating a capacity to empathise with Senua, and thus with themselves and the voices and unusual experiences they may hold. The development and design of this game built on considerable experience of gaming in previous attempts to explore mental health through digital platforms but also demonstrated a considerable degree of collaboration and coproduction, working alongside scientists, academics, clinicians and, most importantly, services users, to create a game that many with significant and enduring mental health needs completely connect with and relate to (University of Cambridge, 2018).

> ### Alex
> Hellblade's design has led it to be respectful of my experience of mental illness. I personified easily – one could argue too easily – with the game's expression of auditory hallucinations, vis-a-vis voices, and pareidolia, the perception of patterns in the subjectively mundane. I wore headphones, as suggested by the game, and the nine-hour experience was exhilarating. Upon initiating the game, I found the accessibility options to be inclusive, one could say minimalist, and the controls to be very intuitive. It was very easy to mechanically play the game; emotionally, I found that the game plucked emotions out →

of me and drew me into the experience, allowing me to personify and empathise with the protagonist's – Senua's – journey. There's a vast feeling of symbology throughout the game, amongst themes of darkness and danger and a descent beyond Dante's. One can relate very easily with the experience of Senua, her crucible, her odyssey; Senua has many characteristics to which one can relate, and many that could very well be alien to one's own experience of mental health. The gameplay was fantastic and alluring to me as someone who experiences challenges with mental health, the complexity of other games' heads-up displays minimised so that the focus is dedicated to Senua. Tribal themes and Norse mythology contribute to a fantasy landscape, all the while permitting someone from our reality to delve into Senua's journey. In a lot of role-playing games, immersion is a strong factor. I've not played many games that have this particular allusion and immersion, an enthralling descent into someone else's madness and love-fuelled purpose, the gameplay allowing the gamer to engage first-hand with Senua's experience of psychosis.

The camera angles keep you focused on the path as though you are Senua, while also retaining the perception that you could very well be one of the voices in her mind. I found myself feeling slightly triggered for a few, fleeting seconds, and then safe, secure in the essence that I was among a fellow sufferer/survivor. I engaged with my coping mechanisms, just in case I would feel triggered deeper, but I found my empathy, coupled with immersion, to be my saving grace, willingly choosing to descend this rabbit hole into another's reality, to follow the river that is Senua's lifepath.

I personally use the essence of darkness in a lot of my writings, defining and reflecting on my experience very binarily and universally, but I function not in absolutes, residing in between darkness and light, to walk only in the light, above my darkness. Throughout the game, I found there to be a lot of questions revolving around 'what is real?' and 'what has happened before this point to Senua?', which leads to a very effective type of storytelling by the game designers, both with quick flashes to the past and with past strands taking root in the present. Words as thoughts, Nordic, tribal, mystical, dimensional, hellscape, resurrection, closure, these words all lingered on the tip of my tongue as I journeyed through Senua's odyssey. At times, it was like watching a one-person play; the experience was fascinatingly dark and light. →

> It could easily be argued that, through games such as these, self-comprehension, self-love and a caring dialogue with oneself and others could be initiated after – or during – playing. While it can be proffered that a lot of commercialised games may not focus so heavily on mental illness as Hellblade does, an expansion of awareness and education across the industry is gradually becoming more apparent to me, contributing to a hopeful reduction in fear, misinformation and miseducation. Using games, be they parallel, liminal or abstract to Hellblade's playstyle and experience, to connect with young people could revolutionise methodology in self-comprehension for young people experiencing mental illness and increase understanding for those trying to help young people in their care. Games would not be the only source of co-creating a relational approach in a digital world or online spectrum, but it would be a great place for many to start, perhaps further supported within the digital realms using (some) social media, online counselling, mental health apps, and more. But that requires a book of its own.

Relating and connecting: Mapping and gaming

When reflecting on this narrative about gaming, from the perspectives of both the gamer and the practitioner, we have both been struck by the ease with which we can be drawn into binary arguments about whether gaming can be seen positively or negatively within the realm of mental health and mental health services. In fairness, most of us would accept that we would look to find some middle ground, seeking to accept gaming for the recreational and social value it can bring, but cautious about the risks of being drawn into a place of dependence and social isolation, reinforced through a narrative of being caught up in constructs such as diagnosis and/or aggressive and bullying behaviour that can so easily then justify the stance of those who dismiss the world of gaming.

Chapter 15: From Hellblade to Game Group – relating and connecting in digital spaces

Figure 15.1: Seeking a middle ground

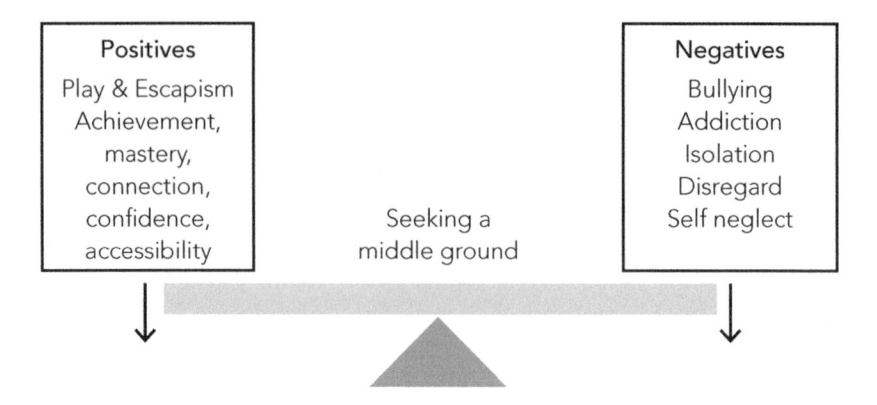

Positives
Play & Escapism
Achievement,
mastery,
connection,
confidence,
accessibility

Negatives
Bullying
Addiction
Isolation
Disregard
Self neglect

Seeking a middle ground

Thinking together about Alex's experience of gaming, we reflected on both the times when gaming was felt to be a helpful and safe place for Alex, a place where he felt connected and could achieve despite everything else going on in his life, through to times when it simply became all-consuming and overwhelming, trapping him in a place where he would fail to take care and look after himself.

Figure 15.2: Moving between helpful and less helpful connections with gaming

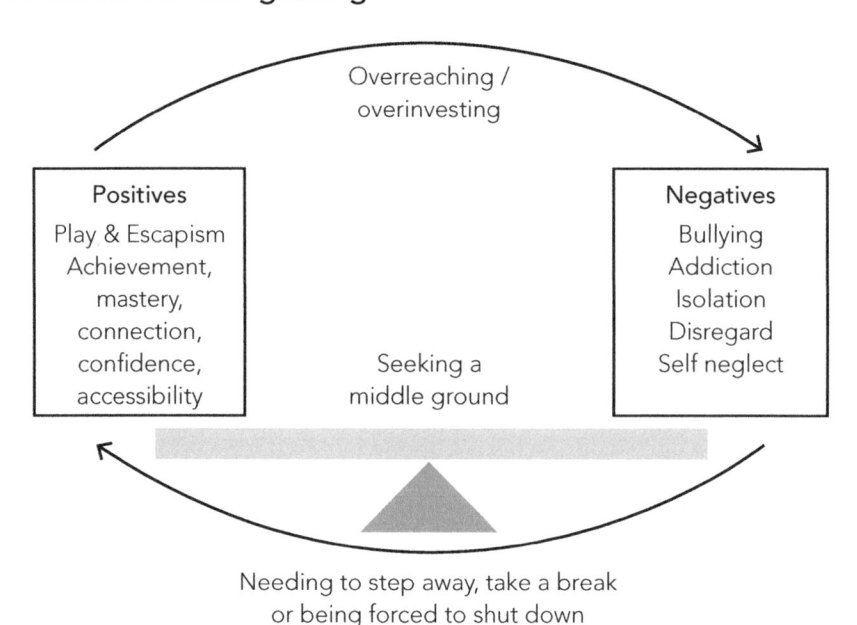

Overreaching / overinvesting

Positives
Play & Escapism
Achievement,
mastery,
connection,
confidence,
accessibility

Negatives
Bullying
Addiction
Isolation
Disregard
Self neglect

Seeking a middle ground

Needing to step away, take a break or being forced to shut down

Over time, Alex learnt the need to step away, shutting down his access to gaming when it became too much, finding a way of reconnecting online only once he felt he was back in a better place.

However, despite learning of the risk, it remained the case that he would simply be drawn into a repeating cycle in which he strove to find that (perfect and idealised) place where he would be acknowledged and feel wonderfully connected, but very quickly overreaching and overcommitting himself, and therefore falling back onto the dependence on gaming and the risks of self-neglect. The cycle itself could become exhausting, and reinforced the possibility that his mental health would suffer further, rather than it being a space for feeling supported and connected with others.

Figure 15.3: Understanding of the repeating patterns of Alex's relationship with gaming

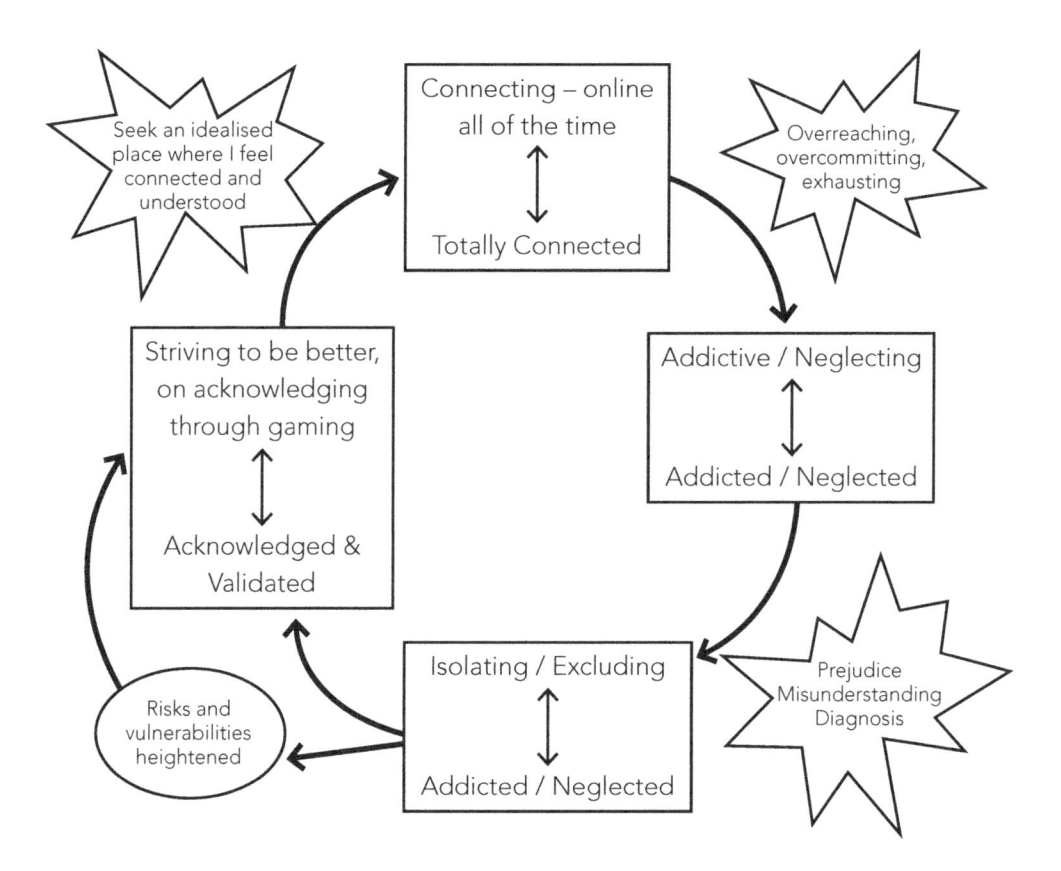

```
        Seek an idealised              Connecting – online              Overreaching,
        place where I feel             all of the time                  overcommitting,
        connected and                      ↑                            exhausting
        understood                         ↓
                                      Totally Connected

        Striving to be better,                                    Addictive / Neglecting
        on acknowledging                                                 ↑
        through gaming                                                   ↓
              ↑                                                   Addicted / Neglected
              ↓
        Acknowledged &
        Validated
                                                                        Prejudice
                                      Isolating / Excluding             Misunderstanding
        Risks and                            ↑                          Diagnosis
        vulnerabilities                      ↓
        heightened                    Addicted / Neglected
```

Chapter 15: From Hellblade to Game Group – relating and connecting in digital spaces

The cycle represents not just Alex's own relationship with gaming, but also maps how professionals can get caught in a dance with gaming and the gamer, where they simply see the signs and symptoms of distress and need – isolation, neglect, dependence, aggression etc – that then draws the practitioner into reaching for the latest copy of ICD-11.

But through learning how to care for himself, and in particular through his relationship with games such as Hellblade, which offered an understanding, a sense of connection and an experience of empathy that was accessible to Alex at this stage of his recovery, gaming enabled Alex to find this middle ground, a place where he began to experience the need for connecting with and caring for self and others. His gaming allowed him to access a place of compassion and self-care, and, likewise, be able to share this with others around him. Gaming had created a space for connecting and caring for self and others: self to self, self to other, other to self.

Figure 15.4: Finding Exits – a more manageable middle ground

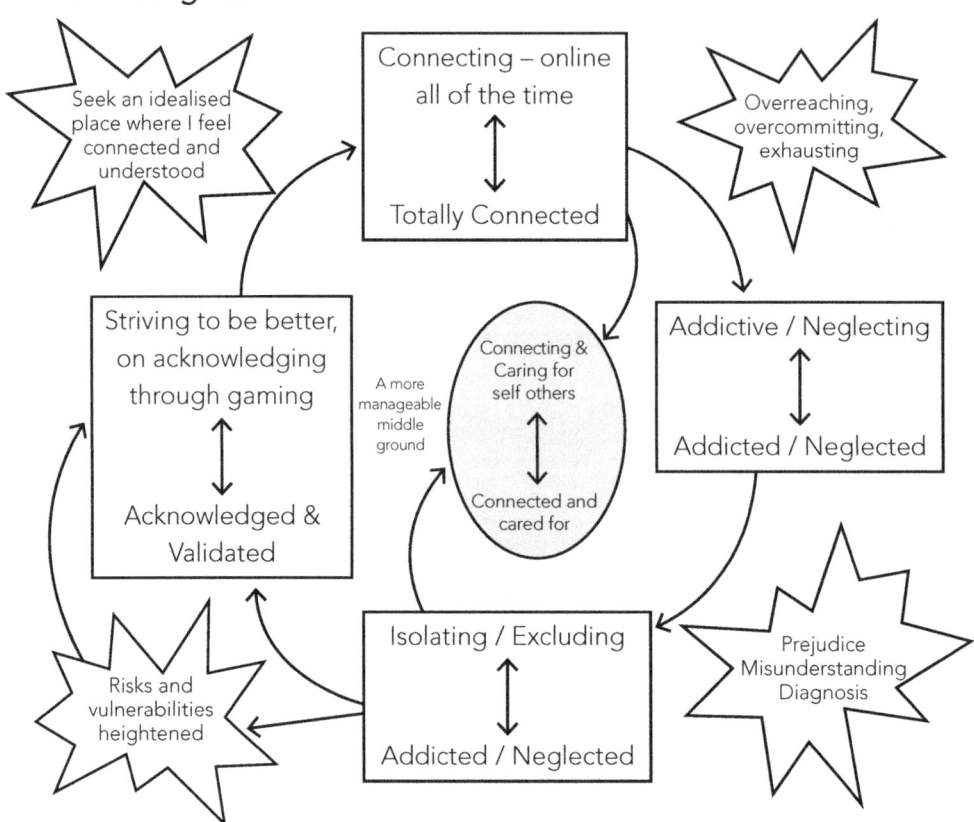

[Diagram showing a cycle with the following elements:]

- **Connecting – online all of the time** ↕ **Totally Connected**
- **Striving to be better, on acknowledging through gaming** ↕ **Acknowledged & Validated**
- **Addictive / Neglecting** ↕ **Addicted / Neglected**
- **Isolating / Excluding** ↕ **Addicted / Neglected**
- Central: **A more manageable middle ground** — *Connecting & Caring for self others* / *Connected and cared for*

Surrounding callouts:
- Seek an idealised place where I feel connected and understood
- Overreaching, overcommitting, exhausting
- Prejudice Misunderstanding Diagnosis
- Risks and vulnerabilities heightened

But it was perhaps from this learning that Alex was able to have the self-belief that he had something he might be able to offer. It seems almost inevitable that Alex was able to take on the role of a Peer Support Worker and share his lived experience with others facing similar struggles. But he has taken this learning to the next level. Learning from his experiences with gaming, he has taken the need for connecting and caring for self and others and collaborated with two colleagues to set up Game Group within his workplace, his local Early Intervention Service, offering a space for his peers that allows a safe place for recovery and growth – within, between and around.

> ## Pausing for reflection – Nick and Alex
>
> As we journeyed through the co-creation of this chapter, we were both struck by the relational way of working that emerged between, a dialogue that allowed for a sharing of experiences and expertise, that resulted in this shared contribution to the overall book.
>
> For Nick, the world of gaming had always been quite remote, until an introduction to Hellblade at the Manchester Science Museum back in 2018.
>
> "Until coming across Hellblade, gaming had always been a place for another generation, but a meeting with Ninja Theory really challenged that position, and I've remained curious about the potential of gaming ever since. Collaborating with Alex in writing this chapter has really reminded me of the world of possibilities that gaming opens up. Talking together, mapping together and hearing how he has found a way of connecting and relating within and beyond digital spaces, with online communities, through spaces offered up by games like Hellblade has been so heartening."
>
> With Alex being very much in the expert for this chapter, it was perhaps the invitation to explore this narrative through mapping that tweaked his curiosity.
>
> "Experiencing mapping in CAT was like watching my thoughts come to life, conceptualised on paper. The experience was rather surreal, being able to follow the flow of my thoughts on a surface. Beyond it being thoroughly useful, I enjoyed the process and would recommend it to those who seek to map out their thoughts, actions and understandings."   →

Chapter 15: From Hellblade to Game Group – relating and connecting in digital spaces

> "Perhaps what mapping gave us was a way of connecting and relating over our own digital platform. We wrote this chapter from different ends of the United Kingdom, and yet, despite coming from such different places and experiences, it felt as though we were always, very much on the same page."

Figure 15.5: From a more manageable middle ground – the evolution of Game Group

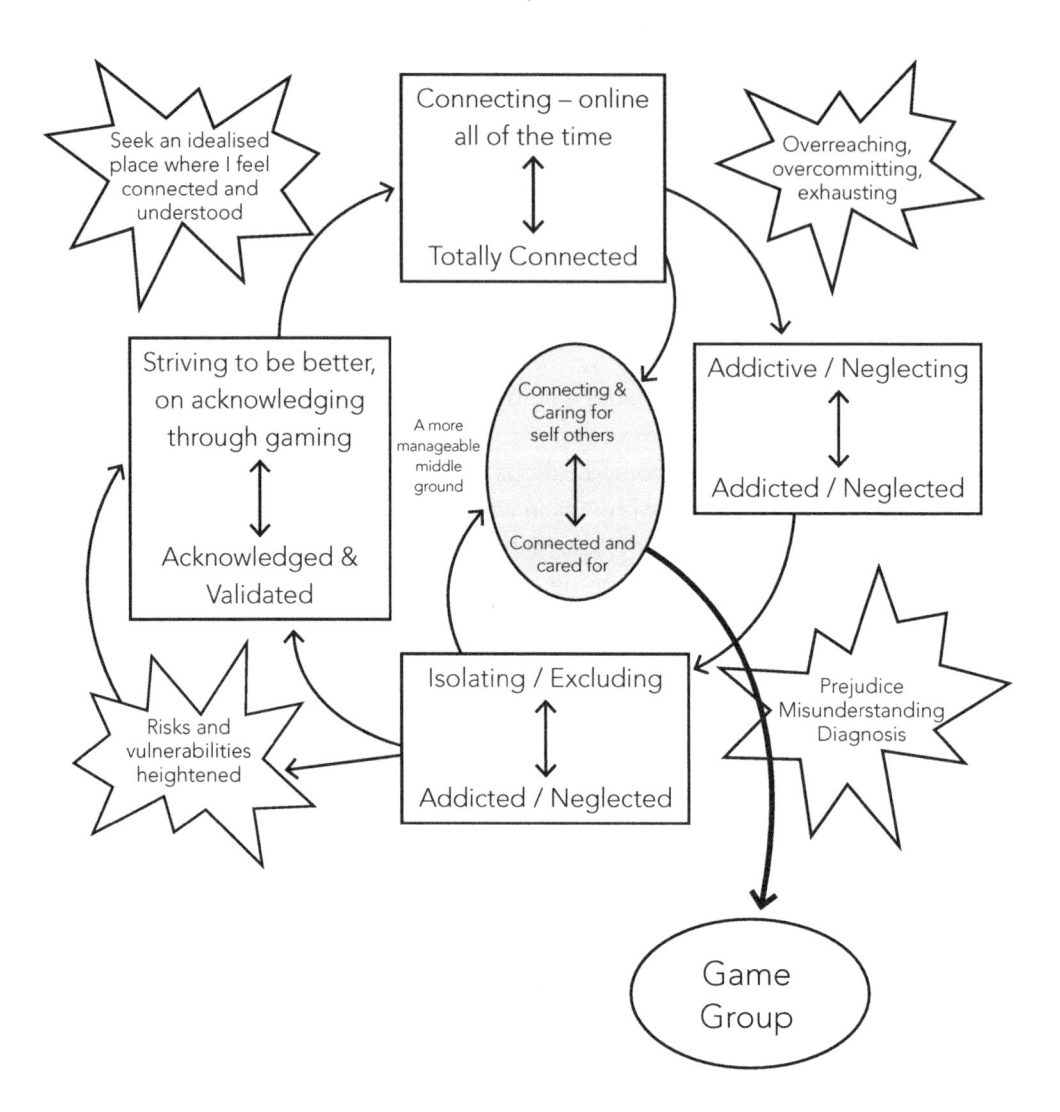

- Seek an idealised place where I feel connected and understood
- Connecting – online all of the time ↕ Totally Connected
- Overreaching, overcommitting, exhausting
- Striving to be better, on acknowledging through gaming ↕ Acknowledged & Validated
- A more manageable middle ground
- Connecting & Caring for self / others ↕ Connected and cared for
- Addictive / Neglecting ↕ Addicted / Neglected
- Risks and vulnerabilities heightened
- Isolating / Excluding ↕ Addicted / Neglected
- Prejudice, Misunderstanding, Diagnosis
- Game Group

Game Group

The Game Group began when a staff member commented that I [Alex] would suit running a group with board games for service users, which interested me, but only if we could include digital games! From a suggestion to an idea, from an idea into a space for connection, I now co-run the group with two other colleagues alongside service users. The aim of the group is to bring people together, to enjoy the elements of socialising and friendly competition alongside peers who have gone through similar experiences, myself included, but all within the safety of a shared engagement and connection with gaming.

We didn't want the group to be run top-down; we wanted it to be created from the ground-up, co-produced with service users, something about which I'm very passionate, so that is what we have done since day one. Service users are involved in every aspect of the group's decision making and planning, ranging from what we play to what we eat to ground rules of what is said in the group, of it being a safe space where we can talk about topics with the common denominator of gaming, food and socialising with peers as a catalyst for connection. We agreed that all ideas will be heard, but recognise that not all can be implemented, and that we decide on things together.

The group has become one of the most successful and repeatedly attended groups in our service, helping to engage with service users who may not want to otherwise engage in other groups. I found it beneficial, also, in helping bridge gaps where service users were not keen to engage with the Early Intervention Service, the NHS, or with the wider community. Being among peers has led to normalisation, self-comprehension, and hopefulness, allowing people to be themselves and enjoy time spent with peers. Banter in the group arises in a friendly manner, driven by friendly competition with both digital and tabletop games. The dangers of online and digital gaming, such as various types of abuse and social isolation and self-neglect, are not seen in our group. Instead, we share stories of recovery, discuss struggles with staff and fellow service users, attending the group as part of our routine, supporting and befriending one another, allowing a coming together, a sense of community.

Who knows where the group will lead, where its potential will guide its trajectory? This group offers a space within services that feels like a safe haven, with room for respect and equity, all through gaming, as demonstrated by the voices of those involved:

"Game Group is fun and helps to escape voices in my head. It's cool to have a place to hang out, opposed to staying in bed suffering from mental health."

"Game Group is a wonderful window of well-being. I am extremely proud of how Alex and the service users come together and have fun and togetherness in the group. To see all the smiles and happiness in people's faces is absolutely marvellous."

"Game Group is well good for socialising and chilling with good energy people. Good fun games, I have a lovely time."

Chapter 16:
Dear Planet Earth – the climate and ecological emergency through a relational lens

Angie Phong, Reem Ramadan and Nick Barnes

"We can no longer let the people in power decide what is politically possible. We can no longer let the people in power decide what hope is. Hope is not passive. Hope is not blah, blah, blah. Hope is telling the truth. Hope is taking action. And hope always comes from the people."
Greta Thunberg, Youth4Climate summit, Milan, Italy, September 2021

Dear Planet Earth

We write this letter knowing that we start from a position of apology and guilt. From a place of deep, deep shame and embarrassment for what we have allowed to happen, and continue to do to you and all the wonders of the natural world that you hold within your biosphere. The Anthropocene now clearly defines your geological age (Crutzen, 2002), as it speaks of how our activity, our relationship with you, has become the dominant influence on the climate and the environment. Our need to extract, exploit and consume, has left you in a state of such depletion and loss of biodiversity, that we can only now talk about mitigation and adaptation to address the existential threats to life on you, Planet Earth – the days of prevention and early intervention are well and truly over. "No matter what we do now, it's too late to avoid climate change" (Attenborough, 2021). We are so sorry.

As we begin to write, there has to be a question about how you might even receive these thoughts as you might rightly note that we are only reaching out at the point at which our own survival is in danger, simply reinforcing how selfish we can be, and how our relentless demand for economic growth has brought us to the edge of extinction (Raworth, 2017).

Who are 'we'?

But when we, the authors of this letter, refer to 'we', perhaps there needs to be a note of clarification. Are we really talking about all of humankind? If we think about the historical and current drivers of our collective crisis, how we have got where we are today? Do we really see the major shareholders of global banks (Harvey, 2023) as equally complicit as a First Nations Elder living on reclaimed land in the centre of Australia? Are those in the industrialised West benefiting from the extraction and burning of your coal, oil and gas for centuries on the same footing as children in Kenya or Uganda who join their peers every Friday for #SchoolStrikesforClimate?

When we talk about 'we', there is a need to speak to the realities of people's experiences of the climate and ecological crisis, and how this informs our reactions and responses. How our relationships with you, with your lands, your waters and your air, affect how we then seek to act, or fail to act, when the evidence of how we have destroyed you becomes irrefutable (IPCC, 2023). We might now all be in this fight together, but we aren't equally responsible for causing this crisis, and we certainly aren't equally responsible for, or able to, make amends.

Relating to power and privilege

We do not intend to talk on behalf of others. This letter speaks from the collective voice of its three authors. But we recognise that, if there is a need to understand our relationship with you, Planet Earth, and begin to explore what is needed to ensure we can make a transition towards a sustainable life hosted by you, then we need to speak to the inequalities and social injustices that have perpetuated the exploitation of your resources, leading us to where we are today.

If we fail to acknowledge the need for a Just Transition (UNDP, 2023) to economic and political systems that allow for more green, blue and sustainable lifestyles for all, then we will fail to ever find the balance needed to ensure an ongoing relationship. A Just Transition requires the participation and involvement of all – an equity of access and a recognition that no one can be left behind. While multibillionaires can play with their fantasies of colonial explorations to Mars, our Western governments invest massively (economically and electorally) in ensuring migrants from the Global South can't cross treacherous waters in search of a more secure life for their families (Vince, 2022). And yet it is these multibillionaires that are being entertained by governments and economic forums (such as the World Economic Forum) as potential investors in seeking solutions to the very problems they have contributed to – the ultimate form of climate iatrogenesis.

These entrenched systemic inequalities within most Western societies were further accentuated during the COVID-19 pandemic (Marmot, 2020a). In this context, it can be of no surprise that the #BlackLivesMatters movement found its loudest voice across the globe. Likewise, the #MeToo movement rallied to the support of survivors of sexual violence, demanding #EnoughisEnough. And now, in countries like the UK, the very act of public protest is denied by governments that seek to crack down on voices of dissent, through the criminalisation of the right to protest (Horton, 2022).

If we are to find a way of overcoming the devastation we have caused you, and the profound act of self-injury that we have inflicted on ourselves, we need to recognise that the solutions lie in equity through the collective rather than continuing to deify the individual. There is a need for a collective that embraces and values our relationship with ourselves, with each other, and with you, Planet Earth. We need to recognise how privileged we are to be hosted by you.

> **Angie**
>
> Privilege. A word that weighs heavily.
>
> My parents immigrated to Australia so that my sister and I could have a better life. It was because of this that I had the opportunity to learn, grow, play and work in a community in which I could flourish. It meant I had all the access in the world to infinite knowledge to help me learn about myself and my passions, but also the frightening truths that extended beyond me: the deterioration of you, our one and only home, Earth.
>
> I am privileged because I am lucky to have the energy and capacity to fight for climate justice. This is in comparison to governments and corporations leaving large carbon footprints, who have failed to act →

with urgency to the climate crisis. Seeing people's livelihoods and young people's futures being shelved away for economic gain leaves me feeling stressed, powerless, angry and confused. Yet, I also feel guilt.

I am able to satisfy my thirst for climate justice in all settings that occupy my life: activism on social media, advocacy at work and in my personal daily choices. However, I never feel that I'm doing enough. My family's financial circumstances mean that I can't invest in solar panels and other sustainable technologies. My anxiety holds me back from participating in social protests. And when I feel overwhelmed and powerless to do anything more, I push all worries to the back of my mind and continue living life as usual. This is also a privilege – to be able to switch off – when there are communities worldwide that can't escape the direct and inequitable impacts of the climate crisis.

In these times, I feel like a hypocrite and immediately worry that people will judge me. This anxiety repeatedly cycles as I continue to criticise and pressure myself to do more, to be better. Ultimately, these expectations become increasingly higher, leaving me feeling stressed, hopeless and never doing enough. It takes support to be pulled out of this anxious cycle, and that is when I met Reem who helped me to see that, rather than criticising myself, I could be more compassionate, caring and respectful in how I relate to myself.

I can now see how I can have more agency to channel my worries and passions for climate change through seeking volunteering roles, like co-writing this chapter; advocating for climate considerations whenever I can on other policies beyond my work; and listening and learning from the wisdom of First Nations communities on how we tackle climate action. While I am not the most powerful person, I feel empowered that I can use my privilege to advocate for stronger climate action within my control.

There is also comfort in knowing that there is a community of people out there who may resonate with my feelings and are ready to act collectively. As individuals in the community, we are not alone and it is not our sole responsibility to fight this climate crisis. It is this thought that energises me with hope.

Left with difficult emotions: mapping our relationships

Engaging with the climate and ecological crisis, and the resulting inequalities and injustices, can't help but bring up difficult and painful emotions. And this is perhaps even more pronounced for young people across the globe, aware that it is their future (and your Planet Earth) that will ultimately be impacted the most by this crisis. It has been young people who have needed to take on the burden of awareness for this climate crisis, with no equivalent level of demonstration or action among adults that can compare with the millions that took to the streets for the #SchoolStrikeforClimate in May 2019, with young people in over 125 countries taking part.

But this awareness comes at a price, with so many young people expressing a range of feelings from despair to rage, from guilt to anxiety, from exhaustion to an overriding sense of hopelessness. With so much evidence demonstrating the sense of eco-distress and despair being expressed by young people (Hickman, 2021), this is further compounded by media sources that offer contemptuous reactions, dismissing those who might seek to care for you as 'snowflakes' (Hickman, 2022). Leaving one of the few alternative places left for people to go to, when faced with the realities of what we have done to you – denial.

Within this space, there are different positions for denial. Fuelled by the likes of Donald Trump, denialism has been an essential tool in sowing doubt about the science, marginalising and denigrating credible voices of the scientific community, with their declarations of Fake News (Ward, 2018). But, as noted above, denial can also become a place where we seek a negation of what we have done to you, a protective place (for ourselves) to buy time to think about the impact on self and community. This negation is more about the loss of our relationship with you – and speaks about the different places we can go, such as shock, acceptance, a hope for innovation, as well as denial. As with all relational encounters, our relationship with the climate and ecological crisis, and with you, Planet Earth, may move through many different places, many different states – from times when we feel overwhelmed and hopeless, to times when we might feel more resilient and hopeful – with many places in between…

Figure 16.1: Mapping our relationships within the climate and ecological crisis

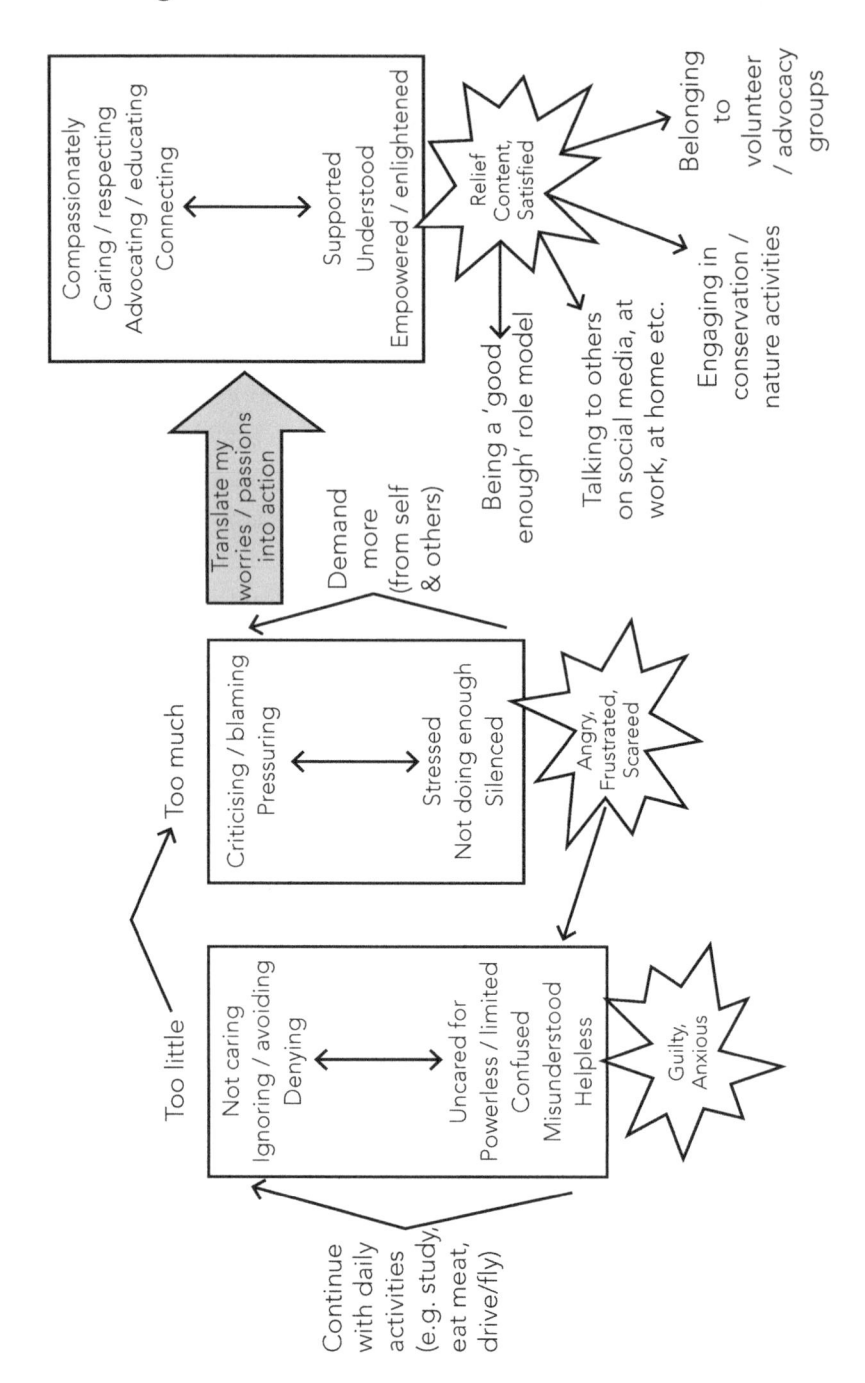

Looking to map these difficult feelings, and where these feelings take us, is what Cognitive Analytic Therapy (CAT) and relational ways of working have to offer for those engaged in this dialogue. The map above, developed through a dialogue of the shared experiences between Reem and Angie, allows us to align with all positions on the map, offering a way of showing how we can take on many different positions and perspectives on the climate crisis, depending on what might be going on for ourselves, or with others around us. We might feel hopeless one minute, or hopeful a short while later, but we don't need to remain stuck in one place – this is a dynamic and dialogical process. And the map may help to loosen some of the hold of these positions.

The role of mapping has proven to be enormously helpful in creating opportunities for dialogue and new insights, and for seeking ways of generating a discussion with those who might hold very different views or perspectives from our own (Potter, 2022). After all, it is those who are more 'climate crisis ambivalent' who we really need to get on board, to become part of the solution.

Engaging others in conversations about the climate crisis feels so important in these current times. Relational mapping is one tool that might allow these conversations to happen safely in public spaces, such as climate cafes or even on demonstrations and acts of civil disobedience. Be it with pen and paper, or chalk on a pavement, community conversations can be mapped and explored to recognise that we all have complex feelings, and attitudes about how we can help restore you, Planet Earth. There are many ways we can contribute to saving and protecting you. We don't necessarily need to take action by blockading an oil depot; rather, all forms of action and activism are valid and valued, especially if we act locally, and think globally.

But as relationally aware workers and practitioners, we also need to ensure we are not only looking out and ensuring we are supporting young people to feel able to take action. We also need to ensure we are there for each other. The challenges we face in seeking to create a more just, equitable and sustainable society that restores our relationship with you, preventing further loss in biodiversity, can be exhausting and draining, and it is easy for us to fall into a place of hopelessness and despair. Approaches such as Active Hope (see Resources and Support) or spaces offered such as the CAT Climate Special Interest Group (ICATA, 2023) are necessary, not just for raising awareness and understanding. If we are to help you recover and regenerate, then we also need to better know how to do this for ourselves, only this time we mustn't finish with just thinking about ourselves. This time we need to think within, between and all around.

From anxiety to activism

It is only through understanding our emotional responses and reactions to what we have done and to how we have impacted you, Planet Earth, that we might then be able to consider what we might be able to do – how we might take action.

For many young people who feel overwhelmed by what is going on, we need to think about what support they need and are asking for, in order to have any sense of hope for their future. This is not to pathologise their distress – feeling anxious or overwhelmed by the climate and ecological crisis is an appropriate reaction to a profound trauma and loss that we are causing – and we need to recognise these difficult emotions for what they are. If anything, the position of climate denial is much more a psychopathological response than the healthier and more honest position of climate distress.

But this is not about binary places of distress or denial. This is perhaps more a recognition of 'how to be both'. If we think about this with a therapeutic and relational lens, then what is it that we offer through our work alongside young people that makes sense and feels appropriate in this context? Wherever we seek to explore change in therapy, we know that we need to ensure there is a trusted and supportive relationship with another to work alongside, and that to foster a sense of hope for the future, we need to promote agency through finding exits and new possibilities – ways of stepping out of our repeated patterns, and testing out new ways of being and feeling.

Is this what we need to be exploring for those who seek to improve our relationship with you, Planet Earth, and yet feel trapped and overwhelmed by the limitations being placed upon them? For someone who needs a sense of agency to overcome their anxiety, is enabling someone to move to a position of action and activism a possible exit? (Schwartz, 2022). And if we do empower someone to find a position of activism, how do we then ensure that they feel they are not alone or isolated, from where they may easily fall into a position of despair?

Working alongside, finding the space for peer support and ensuring that young people don't believe that it is all being left to them to sort out, are all essential aspects of any support that is established within the space of climate justice and activism. But just as we noted previously – that the origins of this crisis are entrenched in inequality and social injustice, reinforced by a colonial exploitation of people and resources across the globe – we need to allow the space for activism to articulate authentic and representative voices of all and not just the few.

Reem

For mental health practitioners and services – working relationally within the climate and ecological crisis.

My passion for addressing social injustice and supporting people experiencing distress developed from my own personal experiences, and, ultimately, this led me to become a clinical psychologist. Similarly, my experiences of spending time connecting to nature, which have filled me with joy, curiosity and containment, combined with recognising the social injustices that have precipitated and perpetuated the climate and ecological crisis, led me to become a climate activist.

For a while, my personal involvement in climate activism was very much separate from my professional identity as a clinical psychologist. However, this separation has always felt uncomfortable, perhaps more so because I work with young people. I questioned what my role as a mental health practitioner in relation to the climate and ecological crisis was. The prevailing view has been that the role of mental health practitioners is to help people learn how to cope with climate change. Increasingly, there has been more emphasis on developing tools to measure climate distress, resources for people to identify strategies they can use, and encouraging practitioners to understand climate distress better. These are all very important and necessary things that are needed to support young people who are experiencing eco-distress. Health practitioners are not used to having to deal with politics, and traditionally have been tasked with responding to the problems resulting from social injustice, but when we are facing a global situation that is becoming increasingly more serious and →

distressing, is this adequate? I worry, Planet Earth, that we are simply colluding with the notion that we can carry on with 'business as usual'. Does our silence make us in some way complicit?

I have felt professional pressure as a mental health practitioner (perceived and overt) to not get involved in climate advocacy or even in developing climate distress interventions that sit outside of the conventional 'therapeutic approaches' we already employ. However, as health practitioners/services, we are both scientists and social advocates, so when asked how we help young people manage their eco-distress, surely our first response should be: "By stopping the ongoing destruction of 'you', our planet". This is the single, most important action needed to address the crisis we are facing and achieve a low-energy, sustainable, zero-carbon world, and to prevent a global (mental) health, humanitarian and ecological disaster. So why are we feeling so pressured to stay silent on the issue of climate action, despite the overwhelming evidence that this is what is needed? Why are we discouraged from developing interventions that empower young people to advocate and protest for climate action or that support connection to and conservation of your natural environment despite the evidence demonstrating that these strategies are effective in addressing eco-distress for many young people? Is this another form of denial being enacted on you, Planet Earth?

It has taken time for me to be able to connect my personal and professional roles in relation to the climate and ecological crisis; to end the dissociation between my professional practice and activism, but doing so has empowered me to become bolder with what I do and what I can hope to achieve. This integration has enabled me to connect more with young people, like Angie, who have helped me to better understand what they want and need from health professionals and services. Collaborating with young people has also influenced what and how I talk to others about climate action and their relationship to you. By encouraging open discussion of clinical, advocacy and sustainable practices in relation to the climate and ecological crisis in my organisation, and to other mental health practitioners and researchers at conferences and in publications, I have felt more confident in how to be both – both a clinician who supports young people explore and manage their distress, by talking about their distress and by →

> experiencing connection with others and with nature, and an advocate that highlights the need for urgent systemic action, as our duty and responsibility to future generations, to you as our home and planet, as well as being alongside young people.

Addressing inequality through accessing green (and blue) spaces

For too long it has been possible for the right-wing media to throw insults at the youth climate activist movement by declaring it to be only representative of the "woke, white middle-class intelligentsia" and that the very inequalities that they proclaim to redress are repeatedly reinforced within their privileged opportunity to take action. Activist movements are constantly on the backfoot as politicians appeal to the "honest working [man]" whose journey to earn a day's living is impacted by some eco-warrior hanging off a bridge. If we are to enable participation and engagement in actions and activism that seek to highlight the realities of this crisis, then we also need to demonstrate how we can overcome the societal inequalities through our relationships with our natural world.

One of the reasons why it has become so possible for us to ravage and destroy you, Planet Earth, is because of our sense of disconnect from nature. If we no longer feel a part of your natural world, then it becomes so much easier to exploit you and extract as we please. Just as within our own neighbourhoods, if we have a greater sense of connection and community, it becomes harder for us to feel able to, or even want to, take advantage of others within our locality. The same applies to how our sense of connection with nature impacts how we look to care for you, Planet Earth.

There is considerable evidence that enabling people to spend time out in nature, in the outdoors, allows us to foster a greater appreciation of your natural beauty, and brings about some of the changes in behaviour needed to work towards net zero communities and enhance carbon capture (Whitburn, 2020). But even more than this, actively engaging in restoration and conservation work, through programmes such as rewilding initiatives, helps to raise awareness and much-needed climate action. Additionally, actively engaging with green and blue spaces, and encouraging people "to get their hands dirty" in restoration work, has a significant impact on health inequalities and social injustices (Rogerson, 2017).

Most importantly, access to green and blue spaces, and engaging in restoration and rewilding activities, that impact biodiversity are equigenic – i.e., they enable opportunities to level the playing field and overcome inequality (Public Health England, 2020). And yet, as practitioners, working alongside young people, how many of us seek to go outside the therapy room and allow our work to occur in spaces that embrace our relationship with you, Planet Earth, and all the wonders of nature that you provide?

This has to be the other side of what we can offer as practitioners who work alongside young people within the climate space (Mellor, 2022). As noted above, we can validate the feelings that emerge within this space and how devastated we are about the loss of our relationship with you, Planet Earth, and also how we might enable young people to feel able to take action, offering windows of hope. But alongside this, we also have the opportunity to directly impact entrenched inequalities by taking this work outside and allowing ourselves and others to reconnect with nature.

Rewilding ourselves

But this step outside needs a shift within, as well as closing the clinic door behind us. Under the name of progress and improvement, enabled by our insatiable appetite for growth and prosperity, we have failed to notice how impoverished we have become through our domestication of the world around us. As we have enclosed the land, and removed the possibility of risks from our surroundings, we have also alienated ourselves from each other and from nature, leaving us in a place where we are othering, or feel othered, in our relationship with the natural world.

Societies that have been able to hold on to their sense of connection with the land are much more aware of how they don't own or control the land, but rather they are its custodians. The Western colonial mindset has usurped this position, at a horrendous cost to First Nations communities and cultures, with a desperate need to be in control, to exploit and extract. Throughout human history, from the origins of slavery to the establishment of empire, the disconnection from 'others' – be they different cultures or different ecologies and environments – has led us to detach ourselves from you, Planet Earth, and your natural world. We have lost our capacity to have both "a fear and a longing contained within the idea of running wild" (Trotton, 2021).

Our task as relational practitioners, working alongside young people, might be to help us rekindle this connection – with each other, but also with you, Planet Earth. Rewilding the planet, enabling us to restore some of the green and blue spaces available for all, is an essential task for all of us, both now and in the years to come (Monbiot, 2013). But to achieve this, we need to begin to rewild ourselves. We need to learn from those who have learnt ways of living with and alongside you that were sustainable and respectful. We need to learn from the wisdom of First Nations societies that recognise the limitations of consumption and exploitation in the relationship between their culture and you, Planet Earth. But to allow ourselves to learn, we must be brave, and courageous, and avoid being drawn to easy, simplistic solutions.

Planet Earth, you are a wonderfully complex world with so much going on about which we understand so little – despite our pretence to say otherwise. But what we do know is that, if we are to sustain our relationship with you, then we need to embrace the uncertainties that lie ahead, to recognise the complexity of your natural world and to have the courage to rewild ourselves in how we relate to ourselves, to each other, to nature and to you. Perhaps, through rewilding ourselves, we are then seeding hope for young people and for your future connection and relationship with them.

"In Wildness is the preservation of the world" (Thoreau, 1865)

Further support and resources for young people and practitioners

Active Hope – www.activehope.info/
Connecting climate minds – www.connectingclimateminds.org/
Force of nature – www.forceofnature.xyz/
Eco anxious stories – https://ecoanxious.ca/
Seed Indigenous Youth Climate Network – www.seedmob.org.au/
Australian Youth Climate Coalition – www.aycc.org.au/
Extinction Rebellion Global website – https://rebellion.global/
Children and Nature Network – www.childrenandnature.org
Schools Strikes for Climate – https://fridaysforfuture.org/

Chapter 17:
Dancing in the spaces between – reflections on proximity and power when working alongside communities

Nick Barnes and Rhona Brown

Over the last forty years, the neoliberal orthodoxy among Western governments has led to the most profound and significant rise in inequality, with more and more children, young people and their families being forced into poverty and social deprivation (The Equality Trust, 2023). This has been further entrenched by its impact on health and social isolation (Marmot, 2020b). The COVID pandemic reinforced the realities of people's experience of inequality and social injustice, with far higher proportions of people from poorer and more marginalised communities suffering far greater rates of loss and enduring health needs through conditions such as long COVID (Pilkington, 2022).

Not surprisingly, given the social and economic context of the last few years, and especially with the current cost-of-living crisis, we are now seeing an escalating demand for mental health support and services against a backdrop of marked underfunding and inadequate resourcing. Services, such as the NHS in the UK, then become the focus of people's frustration, rather than the source of pride with which the NHS has been held for so long.

As mental health practitioners, we bear witness to the impact of inequalities and social injustices within and across our societies through the stories of those whom we are privileged to work alongside. We are frequently drawn to explore ways of working in spaces that may allow for these inequalities and injustices to be named and seek ways for them to be addressed. In the world of cognitive analytic therapy (CAT), there has always been concern and commitment to change in the social, cultural and political context of understandings of emotional distress. Tony Ryle's egalitarian personal values run through the model, and his writings have encouraged proponents of CAT to remain engaged, thoughtful and articulate about social determinants of distress (Ryle, 2010). This chapter therefore looks to explore how CAT, and other relationally informed approaches, have been able to establish themselves in community settings and reflect on how this way of working can be perceived by and within such contexts. We think particularly about the ideas raised by Darren McGarvey (2022) on the social distance between, and how power and proximity can influence meaningful connection within a community.

Equality is the best therapy

Inequality is recognised as one of the fundamental drivers of mental health needs and emotional distress (Pickett & Wilkinson, 2020). If our role as mental health practitioners is to help alleviate a young person's distress, then surely part of our work needs to be focused on calling out the need for addressing the causes of their distress, tackling the inequalities that people face, and the social injustices and discrimination that cause, sustain and perpetuate these inequalities. Within a health system and political culture that encourages us to focus on the individual rather than the collective, it can be difficult for practitioners to feel empowered to address the political, beyond supportive actions such as letters for the housing department or applications for benefits. These may be hugely valuable interventions to the individual and their family, but at the same time may represent a means of working within the system, rather than feeling able to challenge and change it.

For many professionals working within the health sector, alongside social care and education, we may feel we are offering a mop to clean the floor, rather than all working together to empower communities to turn off the running tap. "Equality is the best therapy" is the rallying cry of Psychologists for Social Change. Yet many feel limited in being able to work towards the goal of equality when we work within systems that are often perpetuating and sustaining the status quo. To counter this, some practitioners are drawn to working within community settings, often embedded within or working alongside community and voluntary sector (CVS) organisations. These may be better positioned to understand and articulate the needs of communities, offering interventions that can be as much about the collective and communal as they are about the individual.

Powerful to powerless: controlling – controlled/out of control

All relationally aware therapeutic approaches have the capacity to ensure that a person's lived experience of social injustice and inequality finds a place within the therapeutic space. However, whether this is actualised or not is perhaps more of a reflection of the power differential within the room. For many young people, simply engaging with services within the confines of the clinical space immediately introduces an imbalance of power and an institutionally reinforced inequality. This might be experienced and enacted even before stepping into the room. Introduce further intersections with gender, race, sexuality and class, alongside wider determinants of identity, and the potential barriers to access and engagement become even more entrenched. Within the field of children and young people's services, there is also the dynamic of adult-to-child, and the possibility for competition between the voice of the parent and the voice of the child. We may find ourselves in the reciprocal roles of Controlling – Controlled, with the bottom pole often becoming a presenting complaint of the young person either being or feeling 'out of control'.

The field of CAT is no stranger to speaking to power. In CAT's early days, Ryle argued for a 'powerful-to-powerless' reciprocal role to be included on all CAT diagrams in order to foreground the influence of power as an inevitable feature of experiences and their impact. A narrative around power features strongly in contemporary CAT literature (for example, Brown, 2018; Brown, in press; Ryle, 2010). Being curious about people's experiences, the CAT approach has always been interested in the story of 'what happened to you?' More recently, the Power Threat Meaning Framework (Johnstone & Boyle 2018) has built on preceding therapeutic approaches that actively challenge a predominantly medical paradigm of mental ill health, more often focused on 'what's wrong with you?', and framing distress within the paradigm of mental disorder. By framing our enquiry in a problem-focused manner, we run the risk of falling back into the reciprocal roles of Judging – Feeling Judged, with Shaming – Feeling Ashamed being a close destination.

In many services, a greater emphasis is placed on the social and environmental determinants of emotional distress, and the Power Threat Meaning Framework (PTMF) is a further collaborative way of exploring and understanding distress. While the PTMF offers discrete and organised categorisations of power and its damaging impacts, the relational approach, encouraged through models like CAT, offers something that can be understood alongside the individual's specific context with an emphasis on how meaning is derived from experience. Working relationally allows for a 'not-one-size-fits-all' and an encouragement of a horizontal gaze, perhaps fitting more with the 'a thousand ways to therapy' model (Sefi, 2018). CAT more strongly leans towards exploring and describing the impacts of personal and societal abuses of power in ideographic terms, within the individual's own unique meaning-making framework.

Reaching communities

Offering a wider, more community-based lens has provided a greater articulation of the social and environmental determinants of distress, without being too prescriptive on adherence to specific models or theories. Rather, by ensuring there is a relationally informed approach that looks to scaffold support and thinking across networks within the community, it has been possible to make significant contributions to supporting marginalised and excluded young people. The process of dialogue and respectful engagement may be at least as important as the 'brand' of therapeutic approach, be it mentalisation-based therapy (MBT), trauma-informed practice (e.g. see Scottish Violence Reduction Unit), or CAT-informed practice.

Organisations such as MAC-UK (https://mac-uk.org/) have used MBT to offer systems-based approaches to working alongside young people impacted by and/or experiencing serious and significant violence, and has been able to demonstrate a profound impact within these communities (Stubbs, 2017). This work not only explores possibilities for peer-led change for young people, but also works alongside the very systems that so often perpetuate cycles of exclusion and alienation in order to bring about change. After all, excluding or alienating systems may increase vulnerabilities and potentiate the chances that young people become drawn to crime, repeating cycles of violence, especially if associated relational gains outweigh the risks of further disconnect from mainstream society.

However, working within and alongside communities requires open collaboration and co-creation. As mental health professionals, there can be concerns about our role and title that some may find alienating or othering, reinforcing fears of things being 'done to' rather than 'done with'. Actively collaborative community engagement allows for relationships to be very much at the heart of practice, irrespective of the brand of the scaffolding therapeutic model. We seldom hear people asking for a particular therapeutic model to be delivered within their community. Rather, what we do hear is people saying that they want things to be different. They want there to be change, but they also want 'to be the change', to maintain ownership and agency in that process. It is through coproduction, peer support, and a valuing of lived experience alongside an emphasis on relational working that enables a space for dialogue, offers challenge and informs possibilities for change.

CAT in the community

So how does CAT and CAT-informed relational working find its place within this dialogue? How may it embrace and contribute to the broader narrative of community engagement and empowerment? The CAT model has been used in a variety of settings and contexts, firstly through descriptions of contextual reformulation in the 1990s (Ryle, 2002) to help understand the ways in which teams and systems around individuals mirror, maintain and perpetuate damaging reciprocal roles. In more recent years, examples have flourished of the use of CAT to help understand and reformulate patterns of systemic exclusion and the positioning of people in systemically silenced or marginalised places (Varela & Franks, 2018; Shannon *et al*, 2017; Welch, 2020). However, CAT not only speaks to the power imbalance that can exist within the therapeutic space but also within the wider system.

With increasingly entrenched inequalities in most countries, it is inevitable that those already marginalised within society find themselves even less likely to be able to access support. In both material and psychological ways, we see a reinforcement of the impact of exclusion and isolation. (e.g. see Brown's (in press) CAT-informed diagrammatic reworking of the Austerity Ailments (McGrath *et al*, 2016)).

For children and young people, the experience of exclusion is most clearly articulated through school exclusion, often the gateway to further marginalisation and alienation from mainstream opportunities. Young people who have been excluded from school in the UK are 20 times more likely to have contact with social services, four times more likely to live in poverty, seven times more likely to have special needs and ten times more likely to have a mental health issue. Black Caribbean and children from other minority groups are disproportionately affected (The Difference, 2022). While significant work is done by organisations such as The Difference, support for these groups is currently too little too late, reflected by a high level of contact with the youth justice systems and the police (Lammy, 2017).

We suggest that a relational approach is required to engage with this lived experience of inequality, social injustice and exclusion. But this engagement needs to be authentic, meaningful and accessible, and aware of the power imbalances that could reinforce feelings of shame and guilt. Looking to avoid risk of further embarrassment and humiliation, such work needs scaffolded spaces allowing for authentic recognition of lived experience. We suggest this can be most effectively and compassionately offered through peer support, promoting a culture of coproduction, and being mindful of the "social distance between us" (McGarvey, 2022).

McGarvey offers a perspective for thinking about community work that is focused on the idea of 'proximity'. Passionate about inequalities in our society and the failures of statutory services and governments to offer realistic possibilities for change, he rails against the experience of being:

> "...frozen out by an opaque administrative maze populated by faceless desk-killers... An organisational jigsaw puzzle where decisions with life-and-death implications are made behind a curtain of unaccountable officialdom." (McGarvey, 2022)

Garvey talks about the "social distance between us" as an awareness of "proximity", and how:

> "...even at a local level, power tends to operate far away from the people it kicks around and manipulates. When it comes to the central state, moreover, decision-making turns even more cold and cruel, largely because in Westminster and Whitehall, the domination of political and administrative matters by privileged cliques is at its worst."

From a CAT perspective this dialogue about proximity – be it local or governmental – speaks of the contribution of Vygotsky to CAT theory and the need for us to be working within the zone of proximal development (ZPD) (ACAT Public Engagement Team, 2020). But we suggest that the idea of ZPD should extend beyond the individual's personal and individual development to encompass a sense of proximity by geography, by community or through a broader sense of connection. Any individual's ZPD is inevitably limited (or extended) by the environment within which the person exists, in that space or time.

By considering this concept of proximity, and the spaces between us, we can begin to construct a scaffold that allows for the possibility and consideration of change through ladders of connection and co-recognition, working towards a scaffold that allows and enables exits. With collaboration at its heart, a key aspect of both CAT's therapeutic and consultative stance is to be 'alongside' the young person (or a service or network). It could be argued that the greater the 'social distance between' client/service and CAT collaborator, the more the 'space between' needs to be acknowledged and negotiated, and if there is contact, this can be negotiated through close listening and collaborative tools such as mapping (e.g. as outlined in the torchlight model (Jeffries *et al*, 2020)).

However, with increasing aspects of difference contributing to social distances, there may be more work to be done to reach a place of sufficient and secure enough alliance to create a space in which creative collaboration can take place. Even as co-authors, we became increasingly aware of our own points of connection and distance as we wrote this chapter. Reflecting on how we may come to this work from perspectives informed by our own class, gender, sexuality or professions, we wondered if we had sufficient common ground in the space between us to offer something meaningful and accessible to us both, and then to share. The distance between us, in CAT-informed working, remains a key consideration when we seek to explore change – for an individual, for an organisation, for a system, or when we reflect on wider political and ecological challenges.

Risk of community colonisation

Any community-based relational approach needs to be mindful of the risks of community colonisation, avoiding taking an imposing, expert or 'doing to' position, and starting where the young people, the community or even an agency 'is at' (Durcan, 2017). Guidelines for practitioners recognise the need to be aware of relationships with power, privilege and discrimination which impact any potential partnership building within a community setting (for example, British Psychological Society, 2018). This guidance talks particularly to the need for the practitioner to find a different language, as the words used and manner of delivery will contribute to characterising potential distance between.

Yet, with a professional hat on, we can all find it hard to step away from our roles and ways of being. Likewise, if we remain fixed in our own models and ways of working – believing our approach to be the best – we run the risk of promoting an ideology of exceptionalism, reinforcing an expert position, and negating possibilities for building trust and meaningful conversation. Within the CAT world, we also need to be aware of our vulnerability to centring a privileged practitioner perspective. Even though CAT and relationally informed practitioners may see themselves as being neutrally 'outside', they nevertheless still embody and perpetuate social inequalities and bias.

The risk of colonisation of community engagement has also been considered by Nargis Islam, who notes how professional knowledge and models regarding mental health may be imported into an international context – with due cognisance of power issues (Islam, 2019). This risk speaks to an assumption of epistemic superiority of the professionalised (Western) 'expert' perspective – with assumed inferiority of 'local' third-sector models, although Prabalkumari, in her chapter in this book (Chapter 7), cautions against broad generalisations.

Describing his own path to change from problematic alcohol use, McGarvey (BBC, 2022) comments that the personal and experiential qualities of those 'alongside' were not available in the professionals around him:

> *"Instead, I got well in rooms where the advice dispensed came from other sufferers of the problem and not from medical men and women, or well-meaning theorists. Mutual-aid groups where there are no hierarchies, no professional titles, and no state or private*

> *funding. I learned how to traverse the greatest challenge I have ever faced as an individual – the illness of addiction – merely by following the suggestions of those who had gone before me. I did this in a community where it is understood that we could only ever hope to be of any meaningful or lasting use to that community by first making ourselves accountable. Accountable for whatever part we play in our adverse circumstances, accountable for the harms we have caused, for our dishonesties, our attitudes and our behaviours, and committing to living by certain principles in all of our affairs."*

The proximity described in this context allowed McGarvey to move on from a reciprocal relationship with the professional that might have been more 'Judging to Judged', more meaningfully to a place of 'Caring for to Cared for', which may then have allowed 'Connecting to Connected'.

For children and young people, there is an inherent distance between themselves and helpers and staff who are older than them, and this is a generational gulf that cannot be avoided. Indeed, attempts to get alongside by the use of supposedly credible language or gestures, looking to get 'down with the youth', can easily backfire, as many parents of teenagers can attest. Multiple opportunities for consultation with young people about the types of support that they seek highlight not only a wish for better-resourced and more accessible services, but also a recognition of the value and importance of relationships with people who can make sense of where they are coming from. This may be realised through the availability of practitioners who are representative of their own backgrounds (perhaps through identifications of gender, race or sexuality) or through a recognition of a sideways, peer-based relationship more defined by age and/or lived experience.

Within the CAT community, the development of the 'My Social Self File' (Brown, in press) offers a possible useful starting point for considering the proximity between parties in interactions. This draft tool builds on CAT's existing Psychosocial Checklist (Pollard & Toye 2006) but incorporates identity markers named in Burnham & Roper Hall's Social Graces framework (Burnham, 2012). While the latter was developed within a systemic therapy tradition, it has much overlap with CAT ideas as a tool for reflective practice. The 'My Social Self File' can be used as a tool and focus for reflection on aspects of self as a worker, professional, or one's sense of proximity within a team, a service, or a community. Self-to-self reflections may help to bring to a more explicit awareness of:

- where there may be comfort or discomfort
- where tensions may lie
- where there may be fluidity or rigidity
- which aspects of self we amplify or de-emphasise in different settings and with different people.

As an internal reflective dialogue, this may help to open up conversations between, with others, with curiosity about how others see aspects of themselves and ourselves. In any clinical or service setting, we often make assumptions about clients, service users, colleagues or a team's or organisation's culture, touching on such aspects of identity. Reciprocally, assumptions may be made about us as potential helpers by others. Inviting others to consider these aspects in themselves and what closeness/overlap or distance/divergence may exist, may heighten the chances of articulating and bringing them into dialogue.

Minding the gap

We have all had moments when we have become aware, often through error and hindsight, that the distance between has been too great, or not noticed. For those occasions where we have failed to pick up on the gap, we perhaps might do better to look at those situations where young people have disengaged or DNA'd, rather than focus on their overall motivation to attend therapy. Frequently, services talk about some children and families in need of support as 'hard to reach', implying we have no idea where they are – as if they are lost within the wilds of a council estate. Perhaps the phrase 'hard to engage' may be more fitting – but only provided this comes with a self-reflective caveat – 'hard to engage with what we offered and/or the way it has been offered'. The stance and approach of the service itself, or the helper, may represent the greatest obstacle to engagement.

When thinking about community approaches, the gaps between are often not just with the young people, but also with the community organisations we seek to connect and work alongside. Partnership working is one of the hallmarks of effective delivery in communities, recognising that Community and Voluntary Sector (CVS) organisations often have a credibility and connection with communities that the statutory sectors simply do not. CVS organisations are often staffed with people from within the community, people who are trusted, able to stick around, with an understanding of the lived experience of some young people that may mirror their own journeys. As McGarvey noted, most help for him came through mutual aid groups, and not from those with titles and positions of professional privilege.

But even within carefully co-constructed collaborative working, without regular reflection and dialogue, it can be easy to continue to miss noticing the spaces between. When we have made a mistake, an assumption, or a clumsy or ill-informed response, we may feel uncomfortable and ashamed. It is easy to steer away from such discomfort and avoid, or perhaps deflect and blame, the other party. However, learning best through our mistakes, and with the space and sense of connection with others to reflect on what we have done, such ruptures and repairs allow us to grow and develop in our role – we don't need to continue beating ourselves up.

Dialogue in the space between: a role for peer support

Just as McGarvey encourages us to think about proximity and how, within the CAT community we consider Vygotsky and working in the ZPD to help us locate this proximity, we also need to consider Bakhtin's contribution to CAT theory, where dialogism helps us consider what is going on in the space between. Through addressing proximity, we are allowing for the space between – often liminal spaces – to be a place in which dialogue can occur, and possibilities for 'new truths', for possibilities of change, to emerge.

Recently, there has been considerable interest in services about the role of peer support. Peer support speaks to the distance between, whether this reflects age, identity or lived experience, often finding a way of spanning the gap(s) that the expert (powerful) position of the professional may fail to bridge. But just as with professional therapeutic support, there is a risk the role becomes hostage to the needs of the service, with the peer support worker feeling the need to justify the stance of the service, rather than being more alongside, offering more of an advocacy-type role, as much as it might be about support and recovery.

Our experience of peer support and peer mentoring that has been effective and meaningful for young people, such as the Time 2 Talk project (HSJ Awards 2015), has mostly been when a relational approach has informed the core values of the training for mentors. This has been further reinforced by supervisory support for the mentors facilitated through relational mapping, and an introduction to constructs such as reciprocal roles (Barnes, 2019). Progress has been further sustained by the development of the "5 core principles of peer support" (Barnes, 2018) which reinforces the need for a "focus on relationships" and for young people to have a sense of ownership and agency within the development and delivery of a peer support programme.

One of the most important comments heard in evaluation (Stapley, 2022) from both mentors and mentees involved in this type of programme, is the recognition of the value of this approach for both mentor and mentee – a genuine sense of reciprocation through connection. The opportunity for the mentor to volunteer their time, to support another young person, who may be struggling in a similar way to what they might have experienced, may have a profound impact on both, and speaks more honestly about the impact and strengths of sideways support.

From sideways support to relational autonomy

Through sideways support there is an opportunity to step aside from needs defined within the parameters of a service, allowing dialogue to emerge that is much more where the young person is at, rather than where the services want them to be at. This is perhaps best highlighted by Case Study 4 aligned to this chapter – Shifting the gaze – which demonstrates how peer support delivered within a relationally informed context through creativity and meaningful/purposeful activity can have the most profound and moving effect on the participants and those around. Wolff has offered this work as a case study of Relational Autonomy, a philosophical construct developed within a dialogue on the mitigation of social inequalities.

> *"Such interventions work towards the development of relational autonomy, chip away at social inequality by enhancing confidence and self-expression of individuals and provide recognition of their achievements in the eyes of others. Although micro-steps of this nature will not transform society in themselves, they can transform the lives of particular individuals, and those around them."* (Wolff, 2021)

What CAT and relational working offers: and a need for honesty

It is our view, informed by CAT theory and relational practice, that it is only through:

- the recognition of a need for proximity
- an awareness of the interface and intersections of relationships with power
- a playful working through creativity and meaningful activities
- the complete valuing and commitment to the importance of relationships

that we can then co-create, with individuals, services and communities, spaces in which trust and agency can be safely tested, and a belief in the possibility of change can be realised.

To be able to apply CAT tools, and work within a CAT-informed and relational way, within the space between, in these liminal spaces, we need to be profoundly aware of who we are, and what we bring to this space. Fundamentally, we need to ask ourselves, honestly, whether we are the right people to do so. This can sometimes feel very uncomfortable, but the authors doubt it is a feeling that none of us have had in the therapy room, or out in the community. At times, upon reflection, we can recognise there may be parties far more aligned or appropriate to take on helping roles. The right response may not be to persevere but instead to reposition, stand aside, remove oneself from someone else's path and potentially facilitate access if they face obstacles. CAT offers a huge amount to the dialogue of community approaches and offers tools for considering and exploring change in many different contexts. But we need to be aware of all the possible barriers that we might impose – consciously or not – on opportunities for engagement. Fundamentally, we need to recognise that, if we are to genuinely enable and empower communities, then there is a need for localised and democratised support – as it is only by co-creating the opportunities for dancing in the spaces in-between that we might ever entertain the possibilities of change – both individually and collectively.

> *"If the building of a bridge does not enrich the awareness of those who work on it, then the bridge ought not to be built."*
> Franz Fanon, *The Dammed*, 1963

Case Study 4: Shifting the gaze – creativity for Recovery and Emotional Well-being (CREW)

Nick Barnes and Jon Hall

Stepping into the community centre that warm summer evening, you could be forgiven for thinking you were in a paid venue, awaiting the arrival of the latest 'bright young things' to jump on stage and blow you away with sound or energy, or simply just with their arrogance and attitude. There was such a buzz to the place, an excitement attendant to those intimate gigs or launches that you look back on and say, "I was there when…". And yet the anticipation was for a night of performance, that looked to "amuse and amaze" (Lotter, 2011), the very embodiment of relational working and possibly a working definition of enabling agency.

This event was the first open performance night of the CREW project, an initiative aligned to mental health services in North London delivered by music producer and music therapist Jon Hall (Outsider Music) and artist Ben Wakeling (Outsider Gallery). On show that night was the culmination of ten weeks of work, one-to-one and in groups, through music and art on canvas, that facilitated the emergence of a group of young people with lived experience of mental health difficulties and distress that had forged a profound sense of connection, belonging and support between each other.

We were surrounded by huge canvases of work, a blending of oils and aerosols, that shared a visual representation of a narrative towards recovery and spoke more through a visual dialogue than could ever be navigated through language and words. Ben had been able to choreograph a dance on canvas that gave voice to the experiences of the young people involved. What initially may have appeared as simple in its representation soon gave way and revealed its underlying complexity, acknowledging the layers and depths of the textures captured on canvas. This was an encounter that allowed the observer to just see the simplistic if that is as far as they wished to gaze. But take a look further, and you might be able to embrace the complexity, and reconcile with the uncertainty.

As the evening progressed, live music took centre stage. At times as individuals, on other occasions in groups, songs and spoken word were performed that filled the space and demanded your attention. Thrash chords were hammered out on a guitar played by a young person who had failed to leave his bedroom for the last two years. Fronted by one of the mentors for the project, scream vocals offered the first meaningful naming of this young person's rage at the world around him, all the while asking whether this fury might be also directed at himself. Multiple genres of music were shared, with Jon offering a good enough fit for all music tastes, ensuring each performer felt an authenticity with what they performed, and pride in themselves for being able to hold the room.

For this performance evening was about agency and authenticity. This was a group of young people with profound and enduring mental health needs, who, within the space of a few weeks with the support of each other, and scaffolded on the expertise of Jon and Ben, had been able to believe that they could stand up in front of 250 people and share some of their most personal and intimate experiences with an audience of family, friends and professionals. All, if asked at the start of the project, whether they believed this might be possible would have laughed (or cried) at the very thought, but none would have believed it. Likewise, if the audience had been asked the same question of the performers, most would have doubted they had the confidence to overcome their anxieties and fears to find such capacity for open expression, for such a public dialogue. This was a step beyond their capacity to amuse and amaze – this was an evening where there was a noticeable shifting of the gaze.

Exploring what makes this type of project have such a profound impact, on both the attendee as well as the participant, one is frequently drawn to this idea of a shifting of the gaze. The performers offer something that is both moving and relatable, as the energy and dialogue within the space seem to speak to the connection and the collective. So often mental health is observed in terms of isolation and distress, and the sufferer is seen from a place of deficit and disorder, often contextualised within a diagnostic formulation. Perhaps what has been occurring within this way of working is a sharing and offering of something that is so fundamentally humane that we all find a way of being drawn in with a need to connect. As one analysis of this work suggested:

> *"We have thus argued elsewhere that CREW should be seen as a 'mode of engagement' rather than a model; a way of working which maintains open possibility, invites rather than instructs, placing participants and showcase attendees on a shared footing of common humanity, or 'communitas'"* (Laver, 2021)

Are we therefore asking the question whether genuine relational working is less about offering a model of working and more about a mode of engagement?

This also raises the question of whether this 'mode of engagement' is translatable to other settings and contexts. Both Jon and Ben have positioned themselves and their work on the fringes of statutory services – perhaps in the liminal space that might exist between the Insider and the Outsider. But there also needs to be close attention to this way of working. It would be easy to underestimate the sophistication of their craft, and how they enable relationships to be at the heart of their delivery. Jon brings a credibility to his music through his journey within the industry, and his training as a musician, producer and as a Nordoff-Robbins (https://www.nordoff-robbins.org.uk/) trained therapist. But this needs to also be seen in parallel to the lived experience that Ben brings to all his artwork, sharing much of his own childhood trauma through a visual representation that allows participants to connect with him as a peer, as much as with him as an artist.

The CREW approach has had many different iterations over the last few years – and even adapted to being online during the COVID-19 lockdowns. There are times when Jon and Ben are working alongside each other, and times when Jon may be on his own, but each adaptation appears to demonstrate a significant impact on all involved (Galaxy House, 2023). Although impossible to prove, I remain doubtful that it is just the music or the art that is the driver of creating such a collective and relational experience. I absolutely believe that the creativity is a constituent part, without which the project would fall apart. But I am always left with a question about whether there is something about Jon and Ben that makes this work hold together.

Wolff describes a CREW performance and being completely in awe of the performance and the impact of the event, appreciating the sense of agency and empowerment that this experience held for the participants, framing this within a construct of relational autonomy, and seeing this 'mode of engagement' as a vehicle for navigating towards a society of equals (Wolff, 2021).

Was it this demonstration of the possibility of equality being shown and performed within this collectivist space that drew the observer in? Could it be that this way of working challenges us to really think about who is the Insider and who is the Outsider, or could we all have connected with both?

Jon suggests:

"Creative works of music give participants something to be proud of, a tangible achievement, which in turn helps them develop an appreciation of their own abilities, fostering self-belief and presenting a view of how they would be as a 'well-functioning' person free of the challenges they face."

As Wolff notes, this suggests an opportunity to see one's liberation through one's [creative] labour, and is reminded of Marx's depiction of a non-alienated society:

"Our products would be so many mirrors in which we saw reflected our essential... My work would be a free manifestation of life, hence an enjoyment of life... Secondly, the specific nature of my individuality, therefore, would be affirmed in my labour, since the latter would be an affirmation of my individual life."

Perhaps CREW has taken this utopian perspective of the individual, of the self, and made it entirely relational? For just one night, one performance, does CREW offer us the possibility of a society of equals? Through creativity and peer support, CREW has enabled an experience of relational empowerment.

For further information, see:

Outsider Music – www.outsidermusic.org.uk/

Outside Gallery – www.facebook.com/OutsiderGalleryLondon

Ben Wakeling – https://benwakeling.wixsite.com/mysite

Conclusion

Chapter 18: Closing thoughts – common threads

Nick Barnes and Lee Crothers

As we draw this book to a close, we are mindful of the many common threads that have emerged throughout, and particularly through the dialogues that have emerged in the spaces between contributors and editors and the process of shared learning and creating.

Some of the commonalities will be of little surprise to most readers, as they speak to the scaffold that Cognitive Analytic Therapy (CAT) has provided for most, but not necessarily all of us involved in the book's co-creation. CAT has brought with it a culture of collaboration, of being alongside, embracing or going beyond a transdiagnostic perspective and supporting us in finding ways to bring together many different aspects of ourselves and our experiences so that a more integrated whole can be shared in the final edit.

Likewise, many of the chapters reference the core tools of our CAT practice, bringing our letters and mapping to the table, and we have all communicated through "the mother of all ideas" (Potter, 2018), Tony Ryle's construct of reciprocal roles, being aware that, wherever we find ourselves in the active doing, we are so easily left in a place of reciprocated being and feeling.

But we are not all CAT therapists, and we are not all versed in the language of the therapist, and we also never anticipated that the reader would necessarily need to be fully up to scratch with our CAT jargon, and our CAT ways of doing and being.

Our emphasis has been to ensure that the relationship in all its variations is very much at the heart of all our thinking and being, within each chapter, and through how this book is read and experienced.

Working relationally has been the core premise of engagement within this book, and while we recognise that CAT offers a way of holding this premise, we have not been of the view that this is the only way of being and working relationally.

The pushes and pulls of co-creating this book

The very writing of this book has been a relational exercise. Where possible we have looked to encourage contributors to write alongside others, to be in dialogue with each other, and see this as a collaboration and coming together of minds and experiences. Where this hasn't been possible, we, as editors have tried to connect with contributors to share ideas and reflections, and to allow for there to be enough space, to enable some important examples of relational ways of working to emerge.

Likewise, there has also been a dialogue between ourselves as editors, trying to work out how we might create a safe-enough space to be able to work collaboratively from opposite sides of the world. Just as Alex and Nick in Chapter 15 ('From Hellblade to Game Group') spoke about finding a way to develop a shared understanding through mapping over Zoom across the length of the UK, we as editors have needed to find a way of co-working and co-creating that fits for both, keeping the need for dialogue and open curiosity as a key motivation behind the development of the book.

We have probably moved between places of feeling excited and enthused about the book, through to feeling overwhelmed and doubting ourselves and our ability to complete the tasks ahead. We have also needed to be mindful that the contributors have felt similarly torn at times, and hence our wish to remain as supportive as possible through connecting. In between these positions of feeling overwhelmed or energised, there have also been times when we might be seeking recognition from others, or fearful of embarrassment and of being a fraud, simply not up to the task. For all of us, there will have been many pushes and pulls in the relational dance that has emerged in the writing of each chapter, each case study and with the eventual evolution of the whole book.

Voices of young people, voices of lived experience

There is always a balance, when looking to involve the voice of young people in writing, especially when that topic may be mental health. Our wish is to ensure that what is offered through this book is authentic and representative of those that we have had the privilege to work alongside in our years as clinicians and practitioners. But this badge of approval can so easily become a brand of exploitation if this is not managed in a way that is respectful, ensures informed consent and offers a level playing field for co-creation and co-production.

We are enormously grateful to the young people and those with lived experience of services and support for contributing to this book, as it is our view that their stories really bring the whole book alive in another way and speak to what we mean when we talk about working relationally alongside young people. As editors, we have learnt a huge amount from all who have contributed to the book, but the stories of the young people and those with lived experience have added most to our working and thinking as the book has developed.

Finding the space for dialogue

As this book goes to print, it is not lost on either of us that there is a considerable change in direction emerging that seeks to welcome a more dialogic and relational way of being and thinking. Within the field of mental health, the importance of relationships is starting to be recognised, with models of care such as the Open Dialogue Approach (https://open-dialogue.net/) for working with those experiencing psychosis, and trauma-informed care that recognises relationships can be both damaging and healing.

Even within the more institutionalised settings such as the Royal College of Psychiatry in the UK, a new role has been developed to offer a presidential lead for compassionate and relational care (RCPsych, 2023), which marries developments in other fields of care, such as general practitioners reconnecting over the impact and value of continuity of care and the power of relationships (RCGP, 2021).

These shifts are also noted outside of health care. In education, the academic literature and pedagogic research increasingly speaks to the importance of relationships between teacher and pupil. A thematic analysis of reflections of current educators highlights:

> *"Relationships are more than just knowing the student's names; they encompass mutual respect, building trust, and feelings of safety. Relationships can make or break a student's experience at school; in fact, student success hinges on a teacher's ability to build effective relationships with students."* (MacKay et al, 2021)

There are parallel shifts within social care, a discipline in which all practitioners would aspire to build meaningful relationships with their clients, but most would recognise the challenges that can become a barrier (Wise, 2019). But if there is already a recognition within all sectors working alongside children and young people, then why did we feel the need to write this book?

The space between and proximity

As several contributors have mentioned in their chapters, there is often a fundamental disconnect between the worker or the service provider, and those that they are looking to support which makes it increasingly difficult to find the space and time for conversations that matter, for relationships to occur, for trust to develop.

One of the key themes that has been repeatedly used throughout all the chapters has been the need to find a space where conversations and connections can happen. Drawing on McGarvey's notion of the social distance between us (McGarvey, 2022), it occurs to us, as editors of the book, that proximity – whether this is physical and geographical or articulated through a shared lived experience – is pivotal in ensuring the efficacy of relational working. We can all be mindful of the meaning of the relationship between ourselves and the young person that we are working alongside, but without the capacity for and experience of connection, this awareness falls on empty ground.

As discussed in Chapter 17 (Dancing in the spaces between) the development of relationally informed tools, such as the My Social Self File, might enable an awareness and reflection on this construct of proximity. However, an alternative approach might be through a scaffold of conversational awareness proposed by Steve Potter in *Talking with a Map* (2022). Here, Steve Potter has devised a 16-item grid that explores the variety of ways a conversation can open up within, between, around and beyond us. His key themes are awareness of the human capacity to be simultaneously speaking within to oneself, while speaking intimately, interpersonally, socially and contextually to the wider natural and spiritual context. The qualities he defines are the shared capacity for shimmering between mixed qualities and intensities of feeling and hovering here and there among contrasting ideas and viewpoints in search of moments of shared authorship and agency.

One could argue that the very need for institutions to spell out the need to prioritise relationships within our care models speaks to the void of connection within what is currently on offer. This void is brought about by a lack of resources, lack of time, and a demand for targets that are indicative of a conveyor belt of care, that mirrors the alienation and dislocation that many people feel and experience in the current polarised political and economic climate that accentuates inequalities and reinforces social injustices.

Being relational is not just about being 'nice'

When we call out the need for relational working, we are increasingly aware of the risk that this somehow becomes diluted into a way of being with others that is simply about being kind to one another. Not for a minute are we rejecting the need for kindness and compassion in our care – very much the opposite, in fact – but we are also aware that to be working relationally is not only about moments of kindness, but also about recognising how we find ourselves and the systems that we are working within and represent, being drawn into the relational dances that exist in the worlds within, between and around the young people we are working alongside. It is about being aware of the relationship repeats we could enact and through this awareness and, often with the use of compassionate candour, reflect with systems, professionals and young people about these repeats to do something more helpful.

This book has offered many ways of exploring relational working, in many different settings and contexts, but all have demonstrated the need for us to be attuned to the movements and dances that we are either invited or drawn into that then help inform how the work may develop and progress. Values of respect and being kind to all are integral but are not the totality.

Relational working: Relational justice and relational empowerment?

The strength of CAT is in its flexibility, adaptability and creativity, as it allows for a respectful and collaborative approach to be supported by a willingness to recognise and work with the relational – the self to self, the self to other and other to self – illuminated through tools such as mapping and letter writing, and explore the possibilities of, and the barriers to, an authentic sense of connection. It may or may not be possible to speak to the multiple intersections, such as class, gender, race, ethnicity, or sexuality, that might allow or prevent a sense of connection, but by holding to our scaffold of Vygotsky's Zone of Proximal Development, and aligning this with this broader construct of proximity, we have a genuine opportunity to develop a shared understanding – within, between and around – that may enable a sense of agency, perhaps a relational autonomy (Wolff, 2021), challenging entrenched inequalities and offering a space for relational systemic change.

This dialogue about space feels reminiscent of Soja's work on spatial justice (Soja, 2013) who offered an innovative way of understanding and changing the unjust geographies in which we live. Soja argued that justice has a geography and that the equitable distribution of resources, services and access is a basic human right. Perhaps what we have been sharing throughout this book is a way of helping people make meaning, perhaps through mapping, of their unjust geographies, enabling an awareness of spatial justice, and starting to conceptualise a construct of relational justice?

The theme of social justice and empowerment has repeated itself throughout the book, and, as co-editors, we have found ourselves pushing back against an orthodoxy, particularly within services, that speaks critically about a dialogue of dependence. While we are not necessarily seeking to foster a dependence upon clinicians, we all very much want to promote a sense of relational dependence that enables young people to feel connected with those and the world around them. It is through a sense of dependence that young people may feel able to share their vulnerabilities without fear of exposure and humiliation, to better understand their needs within the context of what may be going on around them, and to feel held, heard and connected. To feel a sense of belonging. Surely what we are all seeking to promote, encourage and enable is a culture of dependence through the realisation of relational empowerment.

How to be both

Within the spaces that have been highlighted throughout the book, there has also been an appreciation of our capacity for plurality – a 'how to be both' – and how a relationally informed approach allows us to step away from feeling trapped within fixed binary positions and embrace a way of being that might be more dynamic, more fluid. We live in profoundly polarised societies, which can be so easily reinforced within our own social media bubbles and the repeated shouts of fake news or the possible challenges of artificial intelligence, all offering simplistic and tokenistic solutions that are inadequately containing and that contribute to a lack of clarity and our overall sense of uncertainty. Within this climate, we are often drawn to solutions that make things feel easier and clearer, but especially simpler – "Just tell me what I need to do". A relational approach won't necessarily offer a quick fix and may indeed open up more questions. But here it is simple: being in a curious and open stance does stop or at least pause the binary thinking, allowing us to step away from the 'Us and Them' thinking.

Acknowledging complexity

In a culture in which we seek immediate responses, in which we struggle to wait or process how we might feel, but desire a sense of gratification, or even just reassurance, then we repeat this request within our own services and the support that we offer. People's distress becomes increasingly defined by pathways that are more and more streamlined, encouraging us all to see our discomfort and alienation with the world around us through a diagnostic paradigm that has a clearly defined care package and evidence base – even if there isn't the capacity to be able to deliver this care plan.

What we hope the chapters in this book have shown is that we don't necessarily need to leap into the dance and seek to find solutions immediately. Sometimes there needs to be a sitting together in the messiness before we can begin to think about how we might find a way forward, to test out different ways of being or experiencing, to consider exits. A quick and easy answer might be appealing but could be yet another item of single-use plastic that gets discarded and adds to the wider problems surrounding us. We might be drawn to simplicity, but we do have to acknowledge there can be complexity, but, as we said in the opening chapter, we can't allow that complexity to be yet another barrier to support and recovery.

Embracing uncertainty

Rather, by recognising the complexity, to speak of the intersections in people's lives that then impact their lived experiences and how they might then see themselves, others and the world around them, and to acknowledge that we don't need to be wedded to binary positions and stances but can embrace our fluidity, we may be enabling the relational tools to tolerate, and perhaps embrace the surrounding uncertainties.

In his study of four great Russian writers, Saunders notes:

"It's hard to be alive. The anxiety of living makes us want to judge, be sure, have a stance, definitively decide. Having a fixed, rigid system of belief can be a great relief.

"In a world full of people who seem to know everything, passionately, based on little (often slanted) information, where certainty is often mistaken for power, what a relief it is to be in the company of someone confident enough to stay unsure (that is, perpetually curious)." (Saunders, 2022)

Saunders, through his reflections on the writing of Chekov, encourages us to embrace "reconsideration" – that there may be another point of view, another mind, another perspective. Chekov (and therefore Saunders) is perhaps inviting us to allow for reconsideration, for us to remain open. But perhaps also speaks to how our dialogues – within us, between us and around us – will, as Bakhtin stated in his study of another Russian great, always remain unfinalised (Bakhtin, 1984). In a world where it seems we are constantly being asked to take up a fixed and often opposing opinion or even identity to another group, this idea of reconsidering, being grey in a black-and-white thinking world, can be done with integrity and courage.

Access and engaging through creativity

Creativity is a common thread that weaves its way throughout this book, and just as Chekov may encourage us to remain open, the examples shared have likewise demonstrated how art or music or any other creative media has the capacity to allow access to these spaces for dialogue. Here, the space doesn't need to rely on the verbal, not everyone's a talker, but through creativity, there is a way to enable proximity, and hence connection.

But there is also something about creativity that allows us to no longer be captive to our traumatised selves. The rising awareness of trauma and attachment, and how this has informed the development of services and best practice has allowed for an important shift in how we perceive many of the more vulnerable children and young people we seek to work alongside, perhaps being most evident for those in the youth justice system. But even with a shift in perspective from "what is wrong with you?" to "what happened to you?", there is little room for then being able to find a way forward and prevent your story and narrative from being defined by your experience of trauma.

Relational ways of working, and especially through access to creativity, allow for a validation of the experience, but also for a consideration – or even a reconsideration – of what might be possible. In Susan Sontag's letter to Jorge Louis Borges on the tenth anniversary of his death (Sontag, 1996), she quotes him:

> "A writer – and, I believe, generally all persons – must think that whatever happens to him or her is a resource. All things have been given to us for a purpose, and an artist must feel this more intensely. All that happens to us, including our humiliations, our misfortunes, our embarrassments, all is given to us as raw material, as clay, so that we may shape our art."

This does not seek to embrace and celebrate people's misfortunes, but rather seeks to empower people to move between victim and survivor, to being both, and to be open to the possibility of journeying from survivor to a more agentic place. But this journey is only possible through feeling safe, having sufficient space and having an authentic experience of connection.

Spaces, localities and stepping out

The chapters in this book have all given clear examples of how to create the spaces needed, what the spaces might look like, and who could facilitate these spaces. The various authors acknowledge that, if a young person will not engage with a service, then it might be that the service needs to be made more accessible, not only through creativity but through location or approach. The contributors have also reflected on where these spaces can develop and evolve. Sometimes, these spaces exist within the clinic and in more formal or traditional healthcare settings; other times these spaces are in schools, or on the streets, starting more where young people are at, rather than where services expect them to be. For if we are to consider proximity in general, then we also need to consider locality, and ensure that the spaces available are friendly and accessible to young people – especially as safe spaces for young people seem to be increasingly cut (Hill, 2021).

The decimation of youth services over the last decade speaks to the complete disregard that those in power have for young people and future generations, reinforcing the sense of alienation and disconnect many young people experience. Yet it is those very same people in positions of power who will cry out when this societal neglect becomes articulated through increasingly antisocial and/or disruptive behaviours – begging the question of where is the modelling of pro-social behaviour by those in governments (local, regional or national) for young people to learn from? If we are serious in our desire to address issues of children and young people's mental health and their contacts with youth justice services, then we need to prioritise the role of youth work and community-held youth centres in enabling safe, accessible and friendly spaces for children and young people.

If there is one thing the COVID-19 pandemic has achieved, it is the consolidation of a broad awareness that stepping outside, being in the fresh air, and connecting with natural environments and green (and blue) spaces is good for our mental health and well-being (McCrorie *et al*, 2021). But at the same time, the pandemic also highlighted the structural inequalities in being able to access green spaces (Gray & Kellas, 2020). Moving out of lockdown and with a growing awareness of the need for more climate-aware and sustainable practice within health services, we are starting to see a profound shift in how and where we practice – stepping into spaces that allow us to explore our relationship with land and nature, for some, enabling nature to be the co-therapist within this space. Moving our practice into the outdoors can feel quite uncertain for many practitioners, although we can learn much from our colleagues within youth services, but it is crucial that this shift in locality is guided by collaboration and coproduction with young people. The desire to work in green and blue settings can be enormously appealing to the climate and environmentally aware clinician but be the stuff of nightmares for a young person. Hence, stepping out of the clinic needs to be very much within the young person's ZPD.

This often very literal shift in location, combined with an embracing of the natural world around us, is encouraging a wider exploration of our relational being and our sense of belonging. Taking our relational triad of thinking about relationships within us, between us and around us, many are now considering the ecological alongside (and within) the biological, the psychological and social. With growing evidence of the benefits of this way of working, for both the young person and the practitioner, we are undoubtedly going to see more services stepping out of the clinic, and working much more in the outdoors, in (green and blue) localities that are accessible and hopefully meaningful for young people and their communities.

The bigger picture

No matter how support services and wider (global) societies develop and evolve over the coming years, we believe that relationships and relational ways of working will be crucial to enabling and ensuring meaningful transitions, resilient communities, and sustainable living. All the chapters in this book are aware of the value and potential of relational working, but they also acknowledge that this is an ongoing dialogue.

When we work alongside young people, their families or the wider systems, we are being invited to consider what change might be needed and/or possible to overcome their difficulties or distress. But we need to be mindful that this distress is also a product of the disconnect and alienation that they experience through inequalities and social injustices at so many levels in their lives. Our task is not only to think about change within, but also between and around, and that around must now speak not only to the political and economic drivers of this alienation and inequalities, but also to the resultant climate and ecological crisis. If we are to work relationally alongside young people, we need to consider their journey from a place of disconnect and alienation, through to a place of connection and belonging, a place of being within the community.

Enabling self – enabling communities – it's all about relationships

We draw this book to a close noting the need for ongoing dialogue: it is never-ending and there is no final word. The writing of this book has been a journey for which we both feel hugely privileged, having the opportunity to connect with and work alongside such wonderful contributors, young people and those with lived experience, who have all offered remarkable insights into the meaning of relational working, and how this way of working is possible.

As we go to press, there has recently been a joint report released by Liberty in the UK reflecting on young people's experiences of serious youth violence and the impact this has on their lives and their communities. *Holding Our Own: A guide to non-policing solutions to serious youth violence* (Liberty, 2023) is a challenge to us all, and not just the police and youth justice systems in the UK. This is the articulation of people's pain and distress, brought together through groups and organisations that allow for experiences to be shared and heard. It offers a dialogue about space, proximity, complexity, uncertainty, creativity and plurality. But most of all, this report talks about community. By prioritising relationships and relational working, this is about enabling communities to 'Hold Our Own'. Is this not what we all need to be doing in our practice, in our services and within our systems and societies?

References

Abab P et al. (2022). Comorbidities and COVID-19. BMJ 2022; 377 to 341 doi: https://doi.org/10.1136/bmj.o1431

ACAT Public Engagement Team (2020) Are you in the zone for change? Blog posting at https://www.engage.acat.org.uk/are-you-in-the-zone-for-change/ (accessed September 2023)

Allen KL, O'Hara CB, Bartholdy S, Renwick B, Keyes A, Lose A, Kenyon M, DeJong H, Broadbent H, Loomes R, McClelland J, Serpell L, Richards L, Johnson-Sabine E, Boughton N, Whitehead L, Treasure J, Wade T & Schmidt U (2016), Written case formulations in the treatment of anorexia nervosa: Evidence for therapeutic benefits. Int. *J. Eat. Disord.*, 49: 874-882. https://doi.org/10.1002/eat.22561

Anderson H & Goolishian HA (1998). "Human systems as linguistic systems: Preliminary and evolving ideas about the implications for clinical theory." *Family process* 27, no. 4: 371-393.

Anderson H & Gehart D (Eds). (2007). *Collaborative therapy: Relationships and conversations that make a difference*. Routledge/Taylor & Francis Group.

Antoine S (2023) https://www.sciencedirect.com/science/article/abs/pii/S016517812300077X

Attenborough D (2021). YouTube - https://youtu.be/Sswe4iNJQjs (accessed September 2023)

Australian Institute of Family Studies (2022). *LGBTIQA + glossary of common terms*. Child Family Community Australia.

Bakhtin MM (1984). Problems of Dostoevsky's Poetics . Edited and Translated by Caryl Emerson. Theory and History of Literature, Volume 8, page 68. University of Minnesota Press, Minneapolis & London.

Bakhtin MM (1981). Discourse in the novel. In M.M. Bakhtin (Ed.)., The dialogic imagination. Four Essays by M. M. Bakhtin. Austin. University of Texas Press.

Bakhtin M (1987). Problems of Dostoevsky's Poetics. Theory and History of Literature, Volume 8. University of Minesota Press, Minneapolis, London. 1984

Bale T (2015). Epigenetics and Transgenerational Reprogramming of Brain Development. Nature Reviews Neuroscience, 16; 332-44

Balmain N, Melia Y, John C, Dent H & Smith K (2021). Experiences of receiving cognitive analytic therapy for those with complex secondary care mental health difficulties. *Psychol Psychother*. (2021) Mar;94 Suppl 1:120-136. doi: 10.1111/papt.12326. Epub 2021 Jan 23. PMID: 33484005.

Bancroft A, Collins S, Crowley V, Harding C, Kim Y, Lloyd J & Murphy N (2008). Is CAT an Island or Solar System?. *Reformulation*, Summer, 23-25

Bandura A (1994). Self Efficacy. In V. S. Ramachandran (Ed.), *Encyclopedia of Human Behaviour*, 4, 71–81. New York: Academic Press.

Barker M-J (2017). *Gender, Sexual and Relationship Diversity (GSRD)*. British Association for Counselling and Psychotherapy.

Barnes N (2018). Peer Support for Children and Young People's Mental Health and Emotional Wellbeing Programme Facilitator Toolkit. Nick Barnes & Simon Munk. Anna Freud Centre. Available at - https://www.annafreud.org/media/10015/new-toolkit_afc-3-003.pdf Accessed September 2023

Barnes N (2019). How the More than Mentors Peer Mentoring Programme is aligned with the THRIVE Framework for system change. Available via - http://implementingthrive.org/implemented/case-studies-2/how-the-more-than-mentors-peer-mentoring-programme-is-aligned-with-the-thrive-framework-for-system-change/ Accessed September 2023

Barnes N (2020) It's All About Relationships: Connecting to connected [online]. Available at: https://relationshipsproject.org/its-all-about-relationships/ (accessed September 2023)

Barr KR, Jewell M, Townsend ML & Grenyer BFS (2020). Living with personality disorder and seeking mental health treatment: patients and family members reflect on their experiences. *Borderline Personal Disord Emot Dysregul.* 7:21. doi: 10.1186/s40479-020-00136-4. PMID: 32944249; PMCID: PMC7487914.

Bates A, Hobman T & Bell BT (2020). "Let Me Do What I Please With It...Don't Decide My Identity For Me": LGBTQ+ Youth Experiences of Social Media in Narrative Identity Development. *Journal of Adolescent Research*, 51-83.

BBC (2019). How the UK became a major player in the gaming world (online). Available at : www.bbc.co.uk/news/newsbeat-46757989 (accessed September 2023)

Bendall S, Phelps A, Browne V, Metcalf O, Cooper J, Rose B & Fava N (2018). *Trauma and young people. Moving toward trauma-informed services and systems*. Melbourne: Orygen, The National Centre of Excellence in Youth Mental Health.

Benton TD, Boyd RC & Njoroge WF (2021). Addressing the Global Crisis of Child and Adolescent Mental Health. *JAMA Pediatr.* 175(11):1108–1110. doi:10.1001/jamapediatrics.2021.2479

Betts J K, Seigerman M R, Hulbert C, McKechnie B, Rayner VK, Jovev M, Cotton SM, McCutcheon LK, McNab C, Burke E & Chanen AM (2023). A randomised controlled trial of a psychoeducational group intervention for family and friends of young people with borderline personality disorder features. *Australian and New Zealand Journal of Psychiatry*, https://doi.org/10.1177/00048674231172108.

Bergner R (2007). Therapeutic Storytelling Revisited, *American Journal of Psychotherapy*, 61 (2): 149-62

Bertrando P & Lini C (2021). "Towards a systemic-dialogical model of therapy." *Human Systems* 1, no. 1: 15-28.

BILD. About Positive Behaviour Support. About PBS | bild Accessed September 2023.

Bingham CW & Sidorkin AM (Eds.). (2004). *No education without relation*. Peter Lang.

Bishop MD, Fish J N, Hammack PL & Russell ST (2020). Sexual Identity Development Milestones in Three Generations of Sexual Minority People: A National Probability Sample. *Dev Psychol*, 2177-2193.

Boing Boing (2023) What is Resilience? Definitions of resilience [online]. Available at: www.boingboing.org.uk/resilience/definitions-resilience/ (accessed September 2023)

Bork N & Varela J (in press) In: L Brummer, M Cavieres and R Tan (Eds), The Oxford Handbook of Cognitive Analytic Therapy (2022) https://doi.org/10.1093/oxfordhb/9780198866572.001.0001 (accessed September 2023)

Borton T (1970). *Reach, Teach and Touch*. London: Mcgraw Hill.

Bostock L & Newlands F (2020) Scaling and Deepening the Reclaiming Social Work Model: Longitudinal follow up evaluation report [online]. Department For Education. Available at: www.gov.uk/government/publications/scaling-and-deepening-the-reclaiming-social-work-model (accessed September 2023)

Bowlby J (1988). *A secure base: clinical applications of attachment theory*. Routledge

Boydell K, Stasiulis E, Gladstone B, Vople T, Addington J, Goering P, Krupa T & McCay E, (2012) Recognition of Psychosis in the Pathway to Mental Health Care Ch 1 in Boydell K, Ferguson HB [eds] K.A. Boydell and W.B. Ferguson (Eds), *Hearing Voices: Qualitative Inquiry in Early Psychosis*. Wilfred Laurier University Press.

BPS (2018). Guidance for psychologists on working with community organisations. ISBN (print): 978-1-85433-765-8 Published: 05-2018 DOI: https://doi.org/10.53841/bpsrep.2018.rep121

BPS (2021). *Working with autism – Best practice guidelines for psychologists*. https://www.bps.org.uk/guideline/working-autism-best-practice-guidelines-psychologists (accessed September 2023)

Brabban A, Byrne R, Longden E & Morrison A (2016) *The importance of human relationships, ethics and recovery-orientated values in the delivery of CBT for people with psychosis. Psychosis: Social and Integrative Approaches*. Routledge Taylor and Francis Group.

Bronfenbrenner U (1979). *The ecology of human development: Experiments by nature and design*. Harvard university press.

Bronfenbrenner U & Morris PA (2006). The bioecological model of human development. In R. M. Lerner and W. E. Damon (Eds), *Handbook of Child Psychology: Vol 1, Theoretical Models of Human Development*, (6th Edition), (pp. 793–828). Chichester: John Wiley and Sons.

Brown H (2018) Reciprocal roles in an unequal world. Chapter 2 pp 20 – 37 in Cognitive Analytic Therapy & The Politics of Mental Health, Lloyd & Pollard (eds)

Brown H (2019) Owning Privilege and Acknowledging Racism. Ch15. in Lloyd P and Pollard R (2019) *Cognitive Analytic Therapy and the Politics of Mental Health*. Routledge

Brown H (2019). Reciprocal Roles in an Unequal World. In J. Lloyd, & R. Pollard, *Cognitive Analytic Therapy and the Politics of Mental Health* (pp. 20-38). New York: Routledge.

Brown R (in press) 'CAT in social context', Chapter in Laura Brummer, Marisol Cavieres, and Ranil Tan (eds), The Oxford Handbook of Cognitive Analytic Therapy (online edn, Oxford Academic, 2022), https://doi.org/10.1093/oxfordhb/9780198866572.013.10, Accessed September 2023.

Burnham J (2012) 'Developments in the Social GGRRAAACCEEESSS: Visible, invisible and voiced-unvoiced' in Krause I (ed) *Culture and Reflexivity in Systemic Psychotherapy*: Routledge

Calder J (2020). Language, gender and sexuality in 2019: interrogating normativities in the field. *Gender and Language*, 429-454.

Robertson, A (2020). *#LetsTalkAboutLoneliness: Games can help keep you connected this Christmas*. Online blog, available at: https://www.askaboutgames.com/stayconnectedatchristmas (accessed September 2023)

CALM (2022). *How Gaming and Streaming can help your head: the lowdown*. Published online by Campaign Against Living Miserably on 2nd Nov 2022. Available at; https://www.thecalmzone.net/streaming-the-lowdown Accessed September 2023

Campling P (2015). Reforming the culture of healthcare: the case for intelligent kindness. BJPsych Bull. 2015 Feb;39(1):1-5. doi:10.1192/pb.bp.114.047449

Carman M, Rosenberg S, Bourne A & Parsons M (2020). *Research Matters: What does LGBTIQ mean?* Victoria: Rainbow Health Victoria.

Carr M, Jones C, Lee W, Smith AB, Marshall K & Duncan J (2010). *Learning in the making: Disposition and design in early education*. Brill.

Carradic A (2004). Applying Cognitive Analytic Therapy to Guide Indirect Working. *Reformulation*, Autumn, pp.18-23.

Cecchin G (1987). "Hypothesizing, circularity, and neutrality revisited: An invitation to curiosity." *Family process* 26, no. 4: 405-413.

Chanen AM (2023). Bringing personality disorder in from the cold: Why personality disorder is a fundamental concern for youth mental health. *Australasian Psychiatry*. 31(3):267-269. doi:10.1177/10398562231159511

Chanen AM, Betts JK, Jackson H, et al. A Comparison of Adolescent versus Young Adult Outpatients with First-Presentation Borderline Personality Disorder: Findings from the MOBY Randomized Controlled Trial. *The Canadian Journal of Psychiatry*. 2022;67(1):26-38. doi:10.1177/0706743721992677

Chanen AM, Betts JK, Jackson H, et al. Effect of 3 Forms of Early Intervention for Young People With Borderline Personality Disorder: The MOBY Randomized Clinical Trial. *JAMA Psychiatry*. 2022;79(2):109–119. doi:10.1001/jamapsychiatry.2021.3637

Chanen AM, McCutcheon L, Kerr IB (2014). HYPE: A Cognitive Analytic Therapy-Based Prevention and Early Intervention Programme for Borderline Personality Disorder. In: Sharp, C., Tackett, J. (eds) *Handbook of Borderline Personality Disorder in Children and Adolescents*. Springer, New York, NY. https://doi.org/10.1007/978-1-4939-0591-1_23

Chanen AM, Sharp C, Nicol K, & Kaess M (2022). Early Intervention for Personality Disorder. *Focus*, 20(4), 402-408. https://focus.psychiatryonline.org/doi/10.1176/appi.focus.20220062

Chapman R & Botha M (2023) Neurodivergence-informed therapy. *Dev Med Child Neurol*. Mar;65(3):310-317.

Chapman R & Botha M (2022). Neurodivergence-informed therapy. *Dev Med Child Neurol*. 2023 Mar;65(3):310-317. doi: 10.1111/dmcn.15384. Epub. PMID: 36082483.

Collins English dictionary (2020) Available at http://www.collinsdictionary.com/english/creative Accessed September 2023.

References

Cooke A (2017) *Understanding Psychosis and Schizophrenia: why some people hear voices, believe things that others find strange, or appear out of touch with reality and what can help.* (Revised edition, originally published 2014) A report by the Division of Clinical Psychology, British Psychological Society. ISBN: 978-1-85433-748-1. Available at; https://www.bps.org.uk/guideline/understanding-psychosis-and-schizophrenia Accessed - September 2023

CQC, Care Quality Commission (2017) *Brief guide : Positive behaviour support for people with behaviours that challenge* (online) Available at: www.cqc.org.uk/sites/default/files/20180705_900824_briefguide-positive_behaviour_support_for_people_with_behaviours_that_challenge_v4.pdf (accessed September 2023)

Cribb J, Waters T, Wernham T & Xu X (2022) Living standards, poverty and inequality in the UK: 2022 [online]. Available at https://ifs.org.uk/publications/living-standards-poverty-and-inequality-uk-2022 (accessed September 2023)

Crutzen P (2002). Geology of mankind. Nature 415, 23. https://doi.org/10.1038/415023a

Cuijpers P, Javed A & Bhui K (2023). The WHO World Mental Health Report: A call for action. *The British Journal of Psychiatry*, 222(6), 227-229. https://doi.org/10.1192/bjp.2023.9

Dansey D, Shbero D & John M (2019). "Keeping secrets: How children in foster care manage stigma." *Adoption & Fostering* 43, no. 1: 35-45.

Darvesh N, Radhakrishnan A, Lachance CC et al (2020) Exploring the prevalence of gaming disorder and Internet gaming disorder: a rapid scoping review. Systematic Reviews 9 (68) https://doi.org/10.1186/s13643-020-01329-2

Degnan A, Shattock L & Edge D (2020) Cultural Variations in Attachment and Psychosis The application of attachment theory to inform therapeutic work with Black Caribbean Families Ch12 in Berry K, Bucci S, Danquah A N (2020) *Attachment Theory and Psychosis Current Perspectives and Future Directives* Routledge.

Diagnostic and Statistical Manual of Mental Disorders (DSM-5) Published (2013)

Dix P (2017). *When the Adults Change, Everything Changes: Seismic shifts in school behaviour.* Independent Thinking Press.

Durcan G, Zlotowitz S & Stubbs J (2017) Meeting Us Where We're At [online]. Available at: www.centreformentalhealth.org.uk/sites/default/files/centreformentalhealth_meeting_us_where_were_at_briefing_.pdf (accessed September 2023)

Emerson E & Hatton C (2007). Mental health of children and adolescents with intellectual disabilities in Britain. *The British Journal of Psychiatry*, 191(6), 493–499.

Erikson EH (1950). *Childhood and society.* New York: W. W. Norton

Erikson EH (1968). *Identity: Youth, and crisis.* New York: W. W. Norton

Esposito L & Perez FM (2014). Neoliberalism and the Commodification of Mental Health. Humanity & Society, 38(4), 414–442. https://doi.org/10.1177/0160597614544958

Felitti V & Anda R (2010). The relationship of adverse childhood experiences to adult medical disease, psychiatric disorders and sexual behavior: Implications for healthcare. In R. Lanius, E. Vermetten, & C. Pain (Eds.), *The Impact of Early Life Trauma on Health and Disease: The Hidden Epidemic* (pp. 77-87). Cambridge: Cambridge University Press. doi:10.1017/CBO9780511777042.010

Ferfolja T & Ullman J (2020). *Gender and Sexuality Diversity in a Culture of Limitation.* Routledge Taylor & Francis Group.

Ferguson H (2012) *Hearing Voices Qualitive Enquiry in Early Psychosis.* Wilfrid Laurier University Press

Fitzgerald (2020). Serious Games, Gamification, and Serious Mental Illness: A Scoping Review. Psychiatric Services 2020; 71:170–183; doi: 10.1176/appi.ps.201800567

Galaxy House (2023) Music and Galaxy House Project. Available at: https://mft.nhs.uk/rmch/camhs-galaxy-house/music-at-galaxy-house-project/ (accessed September 2023)

Gardiner WI (1972). *Behaviour Modification in Mental Retardation.* University of London Press. p174

Gibbs G (1988). *Learning By Doing: A Guide to Teaching and Learning Methods.* London: FEU.

Goldsmith LP, Lewis SW, Dunn G & Bentall RP (2015). Psychological treatments for early psychosis can be beneficial or harmful, depending on the therapeutic alliance: an instrumental variable analysis. *Psychological medicine*, 45(11), 2365–2373. https://doi.org/10.1017/S003329171500032X

Gopal DP, Chetty U, O'Donnell P & Gajria C (2021). Implicit bias in healthcare: Clinical practice, research and decision making. *Future Healthcare Journal*, 8(1), 40-48. https://doi.org/10.7861/fhj.2020-0233

Gorrese A & Ruggieri R (2012). Peer Attachment: A Meta-Analytic Review of Gender and Age Differences and Associations with Parent Attachment. *Journal of Youth and Adolescence*, 41, 650-672.

Gottman JM (2001). *The relationship cure*. New York: Three Rivers Press.

Gray S & Kellas A (2020). The BMJ Opinion, *"Covid-19 has highlighted the inadequate, and unequal, access to high quality green spaces"* 3rd July 2020. Available at https://blogs.bmj.com/bmj/2020/07/03/covid-19-has-highlighted-the-inadequate-and-unequal-access-to-high-quality-green-spaces/ Accessed September 2023

Greenwood J (2016). "Influencing systems." In *Clinical Practice at the Edge of Care: Developments in Working with At-Risk Children and their Families*. First edition, edited by L. Smith. 29-47. London: Palgrave.

Grierson J (2023) We Musn't be too Snowflakey About Raab Bullying Claims, Says Rees-Mogg. The Guardian. Available at: www.theguardian.com/politics/2023/jan/31/snowflakey-dominic-raab-bullying-claims-jacob-rees-mogg (accessed September 2023)

Gururaj G, Varghese M, Benegal V, Rao G, Pathak K, Singh L, Mehta RDR et al (2016) National Mental Health Survey of India. National Institute of Mental Health and Neurosciences, NIMHANS Publication, 130

Hart A, Gagnon E, Eryigit-Madzwamuse S, Cameron J, Aranda K, Rathbone A & Heaver B (2016). Uniting Resilience Research and Practice With an Inequalities Approach. SAGE Open, 6(4). https://doi.org/10.1177/2158244016682477

Hartley S, Baker C, Birtwhistle M, Burgess JL, Chatburn E, Cobbaert L, Howley M, Huggett C, MacKenzie-Nash C, Newton A, Parry S, Smith J, Taylor CDJ, Taylor PJ & Timoclea R (2022) Commentary: Bringing together lived experience, clinical and research expertise – a commentary on the May 2022 debate (should CAMH professionals be diagnosing personality disorder in adolescence?). *Child Adolesc Ment Health*, 27: 246-249. https://doi.org/10.1111/camh.12586

Harvey F (2023) - Banks still investing heavily in fossil fuels despite net zero pledges. Accessed on 1.5.23 at https://www.theguardian.com/environment/2023/jan/17/banks-still-investing-heavily-in-fossil-fuels-despite-net-zero-pledges-study Accessed September 2023

Havighurst SS, Wilson KR, Harley AE, Kehoe C, Efron D & Prior MR (2013) "Tuning into kids": Reducing young children's behavior problems using an emotion coaching parenting program." *Child Psychiatry & Human Development* 44 (2) 247-264

Hayes N, O'Toole L & Halpenny A (2023) Introducing Bronfenbrenner: A guide for practitioners and students in early years education (2nd Edition). London: Routledge

Heads Up Report (2022) Rethinking Mental Health Services for Vulnerable Young People [online]. Available at: https://thecommissiononyounglives.co.uk/wp-content/uploads/2022/07/COYL-Heads-Up-Report-July-2022.pdf (accessed September 2023)

Healthtalk.org (2019) Psychosis (Young People) [online]. Available at: www.healthtalk.org/psychosis-young-people/overview (accessed September 2023)

Hearing the Voice Project (2019) (Durham University) Research and Resource Website. Available at: https://hearingthevoice.org/ (accessed September 2023)

Hepple J (2012). Cognitive-Analytic Therapy in a Group: Reflections on a Dialogic Approach. *British Journal of Psychotherapy*, 28, 474-495

Heriot-Maitland C, McCarthy-Jones S, Longden E & Gilbert P (2019) Compassion Focused Approaches to Working With Distressing Voices. *Frontiers in Psychology* (online publishing)

Hickman C (2021). Climate anxiety in children and young people and their beliefs about government responses to climate change: a global survey. Hickman, C et al, Lancet Planetary Health. Vol 9, Issue 12. Available at https://doi.org/10.1016/S2542-5196(21)00278-3 (Accessed September 2023)

Hickman L (2022). Melting 'snowflakes'? How climate change became a new front in the right's culture war. The Guardian, 23rd July 2022. Available at https://www.theguardian.com/commentisfree/2022/jul/23/snowflakes-climate-change-right-culture-war-daily-mail (Accessed September 2023)

Hill A (2021). Youth Organisations in England face wholesale closure. Guardian, 3rd Jan 2021. Available at https://www.theguardian.com/uk-news/2021/jan/03/youth-organisations-in-england-face-wholesale-closure Accessed: 26.6.23.

Hill A, Bourne A, McNair R, Carman M & Lyons A (2020) Private Lives 3: The health and wellbeing of LGBTIQ people in Australia. Melbourne: Australian Research Centre in Sex, Health & Society La Trobe University.

Hill A et al (2021). *Writing Themselves In 4: The health and wellbeing of LGBTQA + young people in Australia.* Melbourne: Australian Research Centre in Sex, Health & Society La Trobe University.

Hill D (2020). Learning Dispositions in Early Childhood Education: How Interaction Between Children and Teachers Nurture and Support Young Children's Learning Dispositions. *Doctoral dissertation, University of Arizona.*

Holmes S (2018) The role of sociocultural perspectives in eating disorder treatment: A study of health professionals. Health (London). Nov;22(6):541-557. doi: 10.1177/1363459317715778. Epub 2017 Jun 24. PMID: 28649862.

Holquist M (1990). *Dialogism.* Routledge. p. 15.

Holt-White (2023). COSMO Briefing No. 5 - Health Impacts and Behaviours. Available at - https://cosmostudy.uk/publication_pdfs/health-impacts-and-behaviours.pdf (accessed September 2023)

Horton (2022). Criminalising our right to protest': green groups' anger over public order bill. The Guardian, 10 May 2022. Accessed on 1.5.23 and available at https://www.theguardian.com/environment/2022/may/10/criminalising-our-right-to-protest-green-groups-anger-over-public-order-bill-queens-speech https://doi.org/10.15123/uel.885xw.

HSJ Awards (2015). Time 2 Talk project awarded Innovation in Mental Health Award. For information see - https://www.hsj.co.uk/the-hsj-awards/hsj-awards-2015-innovation-in-mental-health/7000296.article (accessed 10.10.23)

Hughes DA & Baylin J (2012) *Brain-Based Parenting. The neuroscience of caregiving and healthy attachment.* W.W. Norton and co. London.

Hutsebaut J, Clarke SL & Chanen AM (2023) The diagnosis that should speak its name: why it is ethically right to diagnose and treat personality disorder during adolescence. *Frontiers in Psychiatry/Frontiers Research Foundation*, 14 1130417. https://www.frontiersin.org/articles/10.3389/fpsyt.2023.1130417

ICATA, 2023. https://www.internationalcat.org/event-details/responding-to-dilemmas-and-feelings-about-the-climate-and-ecological-emergency

Imtiaz A (2021). Grit: The dark side of deciding to tough it out. BBC Workplace, 4th June 2021. Available at - https://www.bbc.com/worklife/article/20210601-grit-the-dark-side-of-deciding-to-tough-it-out (Accessed September 2023)

Infantino G (2022) FIFA President press conference, on the eve of Qatari World Cup, November 2022, from article *Fact check: 11 eye-catching lines from Gianni Infantino's speech in Qatar.* MacInnes, P. The Guardian 19 Nov 2022, Available at; https://www.theguardian.com/football/2022/nov/19/world-cup-gianni-infantino-speech-fact-check-qatar (Accessed September 2023)

IPCC, 2023 - *AR6 Synthesis Report: Climate Change 2023, United Nations' International Governmental Panel on Climate Change.* Report. Available at https://www.ipcc.ch/report/sixth-assessment-report-cycle/ (accessed September 2023)

Institute for Solution Focused Therapy (2020, April) - *What is Solution Focussed Therapy?* Available at: https://solutionfocused.net/what-is-solution-focused-therapy/ (accessed September 2023)

Islam N (2019). Diasporic identity and transnational belonging: reflections from supporting mental health services in the Rohingya camps. *Intervention: Journal of Mental Health and Psychosocial Support in Conflict Affected Areas.* 17 (2), pp. 310-315. https://doi.org/10.4103/INTV.INTV_22_19

Jefferis S, Fantarrow Z & Johnston L (2021), The torchlight model of mapping in cognitive analytic therapy (CAT) reformulation: A qualitative investigation. Psychol Psychother Theory Res Pract, 94: 137-150. https://doi.org/10.1111/papt.12311

Jellema A, Crowley V, Griffiths T, Twist G & Gray S (2003). Developing and Promoting CAT in the NHS - Problems and Possibilities. *Reformulation*, Spring, pp.13-15.

Jenaway A (2007). Using Cognitive Analytic Therapy with parents: some theory and a case report. *Reformulation*, Winter, pp.12-15.

Jenaway A (2018). Parenting – The Middle Way. Blog published, 8th September, 2018. Available at; https://parentingthemiddleway.wordpress.com/2018/09/08/the-story-begins/ (accessed September 2023)

Jenaway A & Rattigan N (2011). Using a template to draw diagrams in Cognitive Analytic Therapy. *Reformulation*, Summer, pp.46-48.

Jennings S & Evans R (2020). "Inter-professional practice in the prevention and management of child and adolescent self-harm: foster carers' and residential carers' negotiation of expertise and professional identity." *Sociology of Health & Illness* 42, (5) 1024-1040.

Johns MM, Lowry R, Andrzejewski J, Barrios LC, Demissie Z, McManus T, Rasberry CN, Robin L & Underwood JM (2019) Transgender Identity and Experiences of Violence Victimization, Substance Use, Suicide Risk, and Sexual Risk Behaviors Among High School Students – 19 States and Large Urban School Districts, 2017. Morbidity and Mortality Weekly Report 68 (3) 67-71.

Johnson S (2016). "NHS staff lay bare a bullying culture", in the Guardian, 26th Oct, 2016. https://www.theguardian.com/society/2016/oct/26/nhs-staff-bullying-culture-guardian-survey . (accessed September 2023)

Johnstone L, Boyle M, Cromby J, Dillon J, Harper D & Kinderman P (2018). The Power Threat Meaning Framework (overview) [online]. The British Psychology Society. Available at: www.bps.org.uk/member-networks/division-clinical-psychology/power-threat-meaning-framework (accessed September 2023)

Kaess M, Edinger A, Fischer-Waldschmidt G et al. (2020). Effectiveness of a brief psychotherapeutic intervention compared with treatment as usual for adolescent nonsuicidal self-injury: a single-centre, randomised controlled trial. *Eur Child Adolesc Psychiatry* 29, 881–891. https://doi.org/10.1007/s00787-019-01399-1

Keegan-Bull R (2022). *Don't Put us away. Memories of a man with intellectual disabilities*. Critical Publishing. St Albans. (P 5)

Kemp N, Bickerdike A & Bingham C (2017) 'Map and Talk' – A cognitive analytic therapy informed approach to reflective practice in a forensic setting. *International Journal of Cognitive Analytic Therapy and Relational Mental Health*, 1(1) pp 147-163.

Kerr IB, Birkett PB & Chanen A (2003). Clinical and service implications of a cognitive analytic therapy model of psychosis. *The Australian and New Zealand journal of psychiatry*, 37(5), 515–523. https://doi.org/10.1046/j.1440-1614.2003.01200.x

Kline R (2023). Paradigm lost? Reflections on the effectiveness of NHS approaches to improving employment relations. *BMJ Leader* Published Online 20th April, 2023. doi:10.1136/leader-2022-000729

Kolb DA (1984). *Experiential Learning: Experience as the Source of Learning and Developing*. Upper Saddle River, NJ: Prentice Hall.

Lammy D (2017) Lammy review: An independent review into the treatment of, and outcomes for Black, Asian and Minority Ethnic individuals in the criminal justice system [online]. Available at: https://assets.publishing.service.gov.uk/government/uploads/system/uploads/attachment_data/file/643001/lammy-review-final-report.pdf (accessed September 2023)

Lange B (2016) Adverse childhood experiences and their relation to parenting stress and parenting practices. *Community Mental Health Journal* 55 (4) 651-662

Laver C (2021) You don't take things too seriously or unseriously: Beyond recovery to liminal and liminoid possibility in a community arts and mental health project. *Community and Applied Social Psychology* 32 (4) 653-664

References

Leiman M (2023) www.researchgate.net/profile/Mikael-Leiman

Lester RJ (2019) Chapter 2 "Rethinking Eating Disorders". *Famished: Eating Disorders and Failed Care in America*, Berkeley: University of California Press, pp. 31-61. https://doi.org/10.1525/9780520972902-005

Liberty (2023) – Holding our own – A Guide to non-policing solutions to serious youth violence. Available at https://www.libertyhumanrights.org.uk/wp-content/uploads/2023/04/HoldingOurOwn_Digital-DoubleSpreads.pdf (accessed September 2023)

Linington M (2002). 'Whose Handicap?' Psychotherapy with people with learning disabilities. *British Journal of Psychotherapy*, 18 (3), 409-414.

Lloyd J & Pollard R (2018). Introduction: cognitive analytic therapy and the politics of mental health. In J. Lloyd, & R. Pollard, *Cognitive Analytic Therapy and the Politics of Mental Health* (pp. 1-20). New York: Routledge.

Longden E (2013) Learning from the Voices in my Head. TED Conferences. Available at https://www.ted.com/speakers/eleanor_longden (accessed September 2023)

Lötter HP (2011). *Poverty, Ethics and Justice*. Cardiff: University of Wales Press

Lucassen MF, Merry SN, Hatcher S & Frampton CM (2015). Rainbow SPARX: A novel approach to addressing depression in sexual minority youth. *Cognitive and Behavioral Practice*, 22(2), pp.203-216.

MAC-UK (2020) Our Approach [online]. Available at: https://mac-uk.org/our-approach/ (accessed September 2023)

MacRuairc G (2009). Dip Dip Sky Blue, Who's It? NOT YOU: Children's Experiences of Standardised Testing, a Socio-cultural Analysis. *Irish Educational Studies* 28(1), 47–66.

Markham S (2019) Catalyst for Harm: Risk-aversion in mental health settings [online]. Available at: https://thepolyphony.org/2019/09/24/catalyst-for-harm-risk-aversion-in-mental-health-settings/ (accessed September 2023)

Marmot (2020) *Build Back Fairer: The COVID-19 Marmot Review* [online]. Available at: www.instituteofhealthequity.org/about-our-work/latest-updates-from-the-institute/build-back-fairer (accessed September 2023)

Marmot M (2020) *The Marmot Review, 10 years On* [online]. Institute of Health Equity. Available at: www.instituteofhealthequity.org/the-marmot-review-10-years-on (accessed September 2023)

Marshall J & Kirkland J (Eds) (2021) *Reflective Practice in Forensic Settings: A Cognitive Analytic Approach to Developing Shared Thinking*. West Sussex: Pavilion Publishing

Martin E, Bryne G, Connon G & Power L (2020) An exploration of group cognitive analytic therapy for anxiety and depression. *Psychology and Psychotherapy: Theory, research and practice* 94 79-95.

Marx K (1844). "On James Mill." Accessed via https://www.marxists.org/archive/marx/works/1844/james-mill/ .

McCormack M, Swarbrick B & Greenhill B (2014). Bringing sexuality into dialogue using a CAT approach to the sexual rights and sexual relationships of people with Intellectual Disabilities. *Reformulation*, 22-28.

McCrorie P, Olsen JR, Caryl FM, Nicholls N & Mitchell R (2021) Neighbourhood natural space and the narrowing of socioeconomic inequality in children's social, emotional, and behavioural wellbeing. Wellbeing, Space and Society, 2, 100051. (doi: 10.1016/j.wss.2021.100051)

McCutcheon LK, Kerr IB & Chanen AM (2019) Chapter 6 - Cognitive Analytic Therapy: A Relational Approach to Young People With Severe Personality Disorder, In U. Kramer (Ed), *Case Formulation for Personality Disorders*, (pp 95-111). Academic Press. https://doi.org/10.1016/B978-0-12-813521-1.00006-0.

McDermott E, Eastham R, Hughes E, Pattinson E, Johnson K, Davis S, Pryjmachuk S, Mateus C & Jenzen O (2021). Explaining effective mental health support for LGBTQ+ youth: A meta-narrative review. *SSM- Mental Health*, 1-9.

McDonagh C, Roche M, Sullivan B & Glenn M (2020) *Enhancing Practice through Classroom Research: A Teacher's Guide to Professional Development*. London: Routledge.

McGarvey D (2022) The Reith Lectures 2022: The Four Freedoms. Available at: https://downloads.bbc.co.uk/radio4/reith2022/Reith_2022_Lecture3.pdf (accessed September 2023)

McGarvey D (2022). The Social Distance Between Us: How Remote Politics Wrecked Britain. Ebury Publishing. ISBN: 9781529104080

McGowan P (2009). The Legacy of Child Abuse. Headway 4 (1), McGill University

McGrath L, Griffin V, Mundy E, Curno T et al (2016). The psychological impact of austerity: A Briefing paper. *Educational Psychology Research and Practice*. 2 (2), 46-57.

McKay C & Macomber G (2021). The Importance of Relationships in Education: Reflections of Current Educators. *Journal of Education*, 0 (0). https://doi.org/10.1177/00220574211057044

McKenzie K & Shah J (2015) Understanding the Social Aetiology of Psychosis. In Kirmayer, L.J. et al (Eds.) *Re-Visioning Psychiatry: Cultural Phenomenology, Critical Neuroscience, and Global Mental Health*. Cambridge University Press

Mellor C et al. (2022). Seeding hope: restoring nature to restore ourselves. Nature restoration as an essential mental health intervention. *International Review of Psychiatry*, 34 5, 541-545, https://doi.org/10.1080/09540261.2022.2092391

Mellow Parenting (2021) About Us [online]. Available at: https://www.mellowparenting.org/ (accessed September 2023)

Merry SN, Stasiak K, Shepherd M, Frampton C, Fleming T & Lucassen MF (2012). The effectiveness of SPARX, a computerised self help intervention for adolescents seeking help for depression: randomised controlled non-inferiority trial. *BMJ*, 344, p.e2598.

Milton DE (2012) on the ontological status of Autism : the 'double empathy problem'. *Disability and) society*. 27, pp883-887.

Minuchin S, Reiter MD & Border C (2014). *The Craft of Family Therapy: Challenging certainties.* New York: Routledge

Mitchel (2021). Autism and the double empathy problem: Implications for development and mental health. *British Journal of Developmental Psychology*. 39, (1)1-18.

Monbiot G (2013). *Feral: Rewilding the land, sea and human life*. Penguin

Moncreiff J (2022) The political economy of the mental health system: a Marxist analysis. *Front. Sociol*. 6 771875. doi: 10.3389/fsoc.2021.771875

Monson K, Herrman H, Moeller-Saxone K, Humphreys C & Harvey C (2021). "How can mental health practitioners collaborate with child welfare practitioners to improve mental health for young people in out of home care?." *Early Intervention in Psychiatry* 15, (6) 1768-1776.

Monson K, Moeller-Saxone K, Humphreys C, Harvey C & Herrman H (2020). "Promoting mental health in out of home care in Australia." *Health promotion international* 35, (5) 1026-1036.

Morley L (2022). "Contemporary practitioner experiences of relational social work: The case of child welfare." *Australian Social Work* 75 (4) 458-470.

Morrison A (2017) A manualised treatment protocol to guide delivery of evidence-based cognitive therapy for people with distressing psychosis: learning from clinical trials. *Psychological Social and integrative Approaches Volume 9* (3)

Mulhall J (2010). Thoughts and Experiences of the Application of Cognitive Analytic Therapy to Clinical Work with Adolescents. *Reformulation*, 34, 34-36.

Mulhall J (2013) Cognitive Analytic Therapy (CAT) and (Open) Groups with Adolescents within an Inpatient Psychiatric Setting: Initial Thoughts and Experiences. *Reformulation*, Winter, p.37,38,39.

Murphy N (2008) CAT used therapeutically and contextually for a client with learning disabilities and Asperger's syndrome. *Reformulation*, Summer (30) 26-30

Naar-King S & Suarez M (Eds.). (2011) *Motivational Interviewing With Adolescents and Young Adults*. New York, NY: Guilford Press

National Institute for Clinical Excellence (NICE) (2016) Implementing the Early Intervention in Psychosis Access and Waiting Time Standard: *Guidance Version number: 1*

National Institute for Health and Care Excellence (NICE) (2017) Eating Disorders: recognition and treatment [online]. Available at: www.nice.org.uk/guidance/ng69 (accessed September 2023)

Newell A (2012) Using Cognitive Analytic Therapy to Understand and Treat People with Eating Disorders. In: JRE Fox and KP Goss (Eds.) *Eating and Its Disorders*. John Wiley & Sons

Newland RP & Crnic KA (2017) developmental risk and goodness of fit in the mother-child relationship: links to parenting stress and children's behaviour problems. *Infant Child Development* Mar-Apr 26 (2)

Ng FYY, Townsend ML, Miller CE, Jewell M & Grenyer BFS (2019) The lived experience of recovery in borderline personality disorder: a qualitative study. *Borderline Personality Disorder and Emotional Dysregulation* 6, 10. https://doi.org/10.1186/s40479-019-0107-2

NICE (2015) Challenging behaviour and intellectual disabilities: prevention and interventions for people with intellectual disabilities whose behaviour challenges. NICE guideline [NG11] Published: 29 May 2015.

Nicholls G, Bailey T, Grindle CF & Hastings RP (2023) Challenging behaviour and its risk factors in children and young people in a special school setting: A four wave longitudinal study. *Journal of Applied Research in Intellectual Disabilities* 36 (2) 366-373

Nicolle L (2023) *BBC uncovers 'worst scandal since Winterbourne View* [online]. Learning Disability Today. Available at: www.learningdisabilitytoday.co.uk/bbc-uncovers-worst-care-scandal-since-winterbourne-view (accessed September 2023)

Ninja Theory, 2017. https://www.hellblade.com/

Nowak-Łojewska A, O'Toole L, Regan C & Ferreira M (2019). 'To learn with' in the view of the holistic, relational and inclusive education. *Kwatalnik Pedagogiczny / Issues in Early Education*, 251 (1), 151-162.

O'Toole L, Regan C & Nowak-Łojewska A (2019) 'To learn with' as an alternative voice for children's education. Introduction to a European project: Teaching for Holistic, Relational and Inclusive Early Childhood Education (THRIECE). *Kwatalnik Pedagogiczny* 64 (1(251)) 175-182

O'Toole L (2020) Participant Action Research in Primary and Early Childhood Education: The example of the THRIECE project. *Kwatalnik Pedagogiczny / Issues in Early Education* 49 (2) 31-44

O'Toole L & Hayes N (2020) *Supporting Positive Behaviour in Early Years Settings and Primary Schools: Relationships, reciprocity and reflective practice*. London: Routledge

O'Toole L, Dowling G & McElheron T (2023) A new publicness for early childhood education and care in Ireland. In: Säfström CA and Biesta G *The New Publicness of Education: Democratic Possibilities after the Critique of Neoliberalism*. London: Routledge

Oppenheim M (2022). Domestic abuse soars by almost 50% after England win World Cup matches, study finds. Independent, 2.12.22 – Available at https://www.independent.co.uk/news/uk/home-news/domestic-abuse-world-cup-england-win-b2237666.html (accessed September 2023)

Partington (2021). UK workforce shrinks after sharp rise in people choosing to leave work. *The Guardian*, 23rd November 2021. Available at - https://www.theguardian.com/business/2021/nov/23/uk-workforce-shrunk-people-leaving-work-resolution (accessed September 2023)

Peebles MJ (2022) *When Psychotherapy Feels Stuck*. Routledge. New York

Penn P (1982) "Circular questioning." *Family process* 21 (3) 267-280.

Perry A (2012) CAT with People who Hear Distressing Voices *Reformulation* 38 16-22

Perry BD & Winfrey O (2021). *What happened to you? Conversations on trauma resilience and healing* (First). Flatiron Books.

Perry B (2022) Introduction to the Neuro sequential model. Slides available at: www.bdperry.com/_files/ugd/5cebf2_06ffbb61c4e84744819eab12fc0e55af.pdf (accessed September 2023)

Pilkington (2022) Covid has had a devastating toll on poor and low income communities. *The Guardian* 4th April 2022. Available at: www.theguardian.com/world/2022/apr/04/us-covid-devastating-toll-poor-low-income-communities (accessed September 2023)

Pollard R & Toye J (2006) Updating the Psycho-Social Checklist. *Reformulation*, Winter, pp19-21

Potter S (2010) Words with Arrows: The Benefits of Mapping Whilst Talking *Reformulation* 34 37-45

Potter S (2018) Reciprocal Roles: The Mother of All Ideas. *Reformulation*, Summer, 50, pp9-11

Potter S (2019) The helpers dance list [online]. Available at: https://www.mapandtalk.com/_files/ugd/524d79_bf6793378f8b4c41b7af50c1dbcc63a0.pdf (accessed September 2023)

Potter S (2020) *Therapy with a Map: A Cognitive Analytic Approach to Helping Relationships.* Pavilion Publishing

Potter S (2021a) Relational mapping – an alternative approach to reflective practice. In: J Marshall & J Kirkland (Eds) *Reflective Practice in Forensic Settings: A Cognitive Analytic Approach to Developing Shared Thinking*. West Sussex: Pavilion Publishing

Potter S (2021b) Steps to reflective mapping. In: J Marshall, & J Kirkland (Eds) *Reflective Practice in Forensic Settings: A Cognitive Analytic Approach to Developing Shared Thinking*. West Sussex: Pavilion Publishing

Potter S (2022) *Talking with a Map: A Cognitive Analytic Approach to Everyday Conversational Awareness*. Luminate

Psaila CL & Crowley V (2006) Cognitive Analytic Therapy in People with Learning Disabilities: an Investigation into the Common Reciprocal Roles Found Within this Client Group. *Reformulation*, Winter, 5-11

Public Health England (2020) Improving access to greenspace: A new review for 2020 [online]. Available at: https://assets.publishing.service.gov.uk/government/uploads/system/uploads/attachment_data/file/904439/Improving_access_to_greenspace_2020_review.pdf (accessed September 2023)

Rafi AT & Suresh Prabalkumari S (2019) Cognitive Analytic Therapy: An Innovative Psychotherapy Framework in the Indian Context. *Indian Journal of Psychological Medicine* 0 (0) https://doi.org/10.1177/02537176221081778

Rathod S, Pinninti N, Irfan M, Gorczynski P, Rathod P, Gega L & Naeem F (2017) Mental Health Service Provision in Low- and Middle-Income Countries. *Health Serv Insights*. doi: 10.1177/1178632917694350.

Raworth K (2017) TED Talk – Doughnut Economics. Available at: https://www.kateraworth.com/doughnut/ (accessed September 2023)

RCGP (2021) *The power of relationships: what is relationship-based care and why is it important?* [online]. Available at: www.rcgp.org.uk/getmedia/ca3e21e7-f742-47d7-9538-77e59bbb1ec7/power-of-relationships-rcgp-2021.pdf (accessed September 2023)

RCPsych (2021) *Record number of children and young people referred to mental health services as pandemic takes its toll* [online]. Royal College of Psychiatrists. Available at: www.rcpsych.ac.uk/news-and-features/latest-news/detail/2021/09/23/record-number-of-children-and-young-people-referred-to-mental-health-services-as-pandemic-takes-its-toll (accessed September 2023)

RCPsych (2023) *Presidential Lead for Compassionate and Relational Care* [online]. Available at: www.rcpsych.ac.uk/members/posts-for-members/detail/presidential-lead-for-compassionate-and-relational-care?searchTerms = relational (accessed September 2023)

Realista MN, Dela Cruz DC & Abadiano MN (2019) Sexuality identity development and the coming out process of self-identified gays: a qualitative study. *International Journal of Social Science and Humanities Research* 583-592

Renbarger R & Morgan G (Eds.) (2018) *The Sage Encyclopedia of Educational Research, Measurement and Evaluation* (Vols. 1-4). London: SAGE Publications, Inc.

Research Square (2021) Long COVID - the physical and mental health of children and non-hospitalised young people 3 months after SARS-CoV-2 infection; a national matched cohort study (The CLoCk) Study [online]. Available at: https://www.researchsquare.com/article/rs-798316/v1 (accessed September 2023)

Roberts E & DeBlassie RR (1983) Test bias and the culturally different early adolescent. *Adolescence* 18 (72) 837

References

Robinson K, Bansel P, Denson N, Ovenden G & Davies C (2014) *Growing Up Queer*. Melbourne: Young and Well Cooperative Centre

Rogerson M (2017) *The Health and Wellbeing Impacts of Volunteering with The Wildlife Trust* [online]. University of Essex. Available at: www.wildlifetrusts.org/sites/default/files/2018-05/r3_the_health_and_wellbeing_impacts_of_volunteering_with_the_wildlife_trusts_-_university_of_essex_report_3_0.pdf (accessed September 2023)

Romme M and Escher S (2000) *Making Sense of Voices: A Guide for mental health professionals working with voice hearers*. Mind Publications

Ruberg B & Ruelos S (2020) Data for queer lives: How LGBTQ gender and sexuality identities challenge norms of demographics. *Big Data & Society* 1-12.

Rumping S, Boendermaker L & de Ruyter DJ (2019) Stimulating interdisciplinary collaboration among youth social workers: A scoping review. *Health & Social Care in the Community* 27 (2) 293-305

Ryle A & Kerr I (2002). *Introducing Cognitive Analytic Therapy: Principles and Practice*. John Wiley & Sons Ltd, West Sussex

Ryle A & Kerr I (2020) *Introducing Cognitive Analytic Therapy: principles and practice of a relational approach to mental health* (P5,198). John Wiley and Sons Ltd.

Ryle A (1985) Cognitive theory, object relations and the self. *British Journal of Medical Psychology* 58 1-7

Ryle A (1991) *Cognitive–Analytic Therapy: Active Participation in Change: A New Integration in Brief Psychotherapy* (Wiley series on psychotherapy & counselling) John Wiley & Sons; New edition

Ryle A (1998) The whirligig of time. *Psychiatric Bulletin* 22 (4) 263-267 doi:10.1192/pb.22.4.263

Ryle A (2001) CAT's Dialogic Perspective on the Self. *Reformulation*, ACAT News.

Ryle A & McCutcheon L (2006). Cognitive Analytic Therapy. In G. Stricker & J. Gold (Eds.), *A casebook of psychotherapy integration* (pp. 121–136). American Psychological Association. https://doi.org/10.1037/11436-010

Ryle A (2010) The political sources of reciprocal role procedures. *Reformulation*, Summer (34) 6-7

Ryle A, Kellett S, Hepple J et al (2014) Cognitive analytic therapy at 30. *Advances in Psychiatric Treatment* 20 (4) pp258-268.

Ryle A (2017) Cited at foreword to *International Journal of Cognitive Analytic Therapy and Relational Mental Health, Volume 1*. Available at: https://www.internationalcat.org/volume-1 (accessed September 2023)

Salisbury H (2023) Wellbeing shouldn't be weaponised. *BMJ* 2023; 381 p771 doi: https://doi.org/10.1136/bmj.p771

Salman S (2020). Made Possible: Stories of success by people with learning disabilities- in their own words. Unbound press. London.

Sainsburys Centre for Mental Health (2002). Breaking the Circles of Fear. A review of the relationship between mental health services and African and Caribbean communities. ISBN: 1 870480 55 4. Available at https://www.centreformentalhealth.org.uk/sites/default/files/publication/download/breaking_the_circles_of_fear.pdf Accessed September 2023

Saunders G (2022). A Swim in the Pond in the Rain. Thoughts on "Gooseberries", page 335 - 336. Bloomsbury Publishing, London (3rd Edition).

Schandrin A, Francey S, Nguyen L, Whitty D, McGorry P, Chanen AM & O'Donoghue B (2023). Co-occurring first-episode psychosis and borderline personality pathology in an early intervention for psychosis cohort. *Early Intervention in Psychiatry*, 17(6), 588–596. https://doi.org/10.1111/eip.13352

Schwartz S et al (2022) Climate change anxiety and mental health: Environmental activism as buffer. *Curr Psychol* 42 16708–16721 https://doi.org/10.1007/s12144-022-02735-6

Sefi A (2018) *A Thousand ways to Therapy – Xenzone report* [online]. Available at: www.thethoughtreport.com/a-thousand-ways-to-therapy/ (accessed September 2023)

Series L (2022) *Deprivation of Liberty in the Shadows of the Institution*. Bristol University Press

Shannon K, Butler S, Ellis C, McLaine J & Riley J (2016) Use of Cognitive Analytic Concepts; A relational framework for Organisational service delivery and working with clients with Multiple Complex Needs (MCN) at the Liverpool YMCA. *Reformulation*, Winter, pp12-20

Shannon K, Butler S, Ellis C, McLaine J & Riley J (2017) 'Seeing the unseen': supporting organizational and team working at YMCA Liverpool with multiple complex needs clients. The use of cognitive analytic concepts to enhance service delivery. *Reformulation*, Summer, pp5-15

Sharp C (2022). Personality Disorders. *The New England Journal of Medicine*, 387(10), 916-923. https://www.nejm.org/doi/10.1056/NEJMra2120164

Shechtman Z (2007) *Group Counseling and Psychotherapy With Children and Adolescents: Theory, Research and Practice* (1st Edition). Routledge, New York

Sinason V (1992) *Mental handicap and the human condition. New approaches from the Tavistock*. Free Association Books: London

Skull A (2017) *Madness in Civilization – A Cultural History of Insanity, from the Bible to Freud, from the Madhouse to Modern Medicine*. Princeton University Press, Illustrated edition.

Soja E (2013) Seeking Spatial Justice. London: University of Minnesota Press

Solmi F, Downs JL & Nicholls DE (2021) COVID-19 and eating disorders in young people. *Lancet Child Adolesc Health* 5 (5) 316-318. doi: 10.1016/S2352-4642(21)00094-8

Sontag S (1996) *A letter to Borges* [online]. Available at: www.faena.com/aleph/susan-sontags-admirable-letter-to-jl-borges (accessed September 2023)

Springall G, Cheung M, Sawyer SM and Yeo M (2022) Impact of the coronavirus pandemic on anorexia nervosa and atypical anorexia nervosa presentations to an Australian tertiary paediatric hospital. *Journal of Paediatric Child Health* 58 (3) 491-496. doi: 10.1111/jpc.15755

Stapley E, Town R, Yoon Y, Lereya ST, Farr J, Turner J, Barnes N & Deighton J (2022) A mixed methods evaluation of a peer mentoring intervention in a UK school setting: Perspectives from mentees and mentors. *Children and Youth Services Review* 132 106327, https://doi.org/10.1016/j.childyouth.2021.106327

Steele M (2013) 'So how truly collaborative are we?' *Reformulation* 40 33-35

Steensma TD, Kreukels BPC, de Vries ALC & Cohen-Kettenis PT (2013) Gender identity development in adolescence. *Hormones and Behaviour* 288-297

Stephens J, Bailey A & Parker A (2013) *Evidence Summary: Working with same sex attracted young people*. Melbourne: headspace National Youth Mental Health Foundation Ltd.

Stephenson T (2023) Long COVID - the physical and mental health of children and non-hospitalised young people 3 months after SARS-CoV-2 infection; a national matched cohort study (The CLoCk) Study [online]. Available at: https://www.researchsquare.com/article/rs-798316/v1 (accessed September 2023)

Stiles W (1999) Signs and Voices in psychotherapy (P2-3). *Psychotherapy Research*

Strauss P, Winter S, Waters Z, Wright Toussaint D & Watson V (2022) Perspectives of trans and gender diverse young people accessing primary care and gender-affirming medical services: Findings from Trans Pathways. *International Journal of Transgender Health* 23 (3) 295-307, DOI: 10.1080/26895269.2021.1884925

Stubbs J (2017) *An independent evaluation of Project Future Report, Centre for Mental Health* [online]. Available at: www.centreformentalhealth.org.uk/sites/default/files/2018-09/CentreforMentalHealth_Unlocking_a_different_future.pdf (accessed September 2023)

Tanner C & Connan F (2003) Cognitive Analytic Therapy. In: Treasure J, Schmidt U, van Furth E (Eds) *Handbook of Eating Disorders*. John Wiley & Sons

Tatlow-Golden M & McElvaney R (2015) "A bit more understanding: Young adults' views of mental health services in care in Ireland." *Children and Youth Services Review* 51 1-9

Taylor P, Jones S, Huntley C & Seddon C (2017) What are the key elements of cognitive analytic therapy for psychosis? A Delphi Study. *Psychology and Psychotherapy* 90 (4) 511-529

Taylor P, Perry A, Hutton P, Ranil T, Fisher N, Focone C, Griffiths D & Seddon C (2018) Cognitive Analytic Therapy for Psychosis: A Case Series (P367) *Psychology and Psychotherapy* 92 (3) 359-378

Thara R, Padmavati R & Srinivasan TN (2001) Focus of Psychiatry in India. *The British Journal of Psychiatry* 184 (4) 366-373. https://doi.org/10.1192/bjp.184.4.366

Thatcher M (1987) Quote from interview for "Women's Own". 23rd Sept, 1987.

The Difference (2022) *Impact Report*. 2021-22 [online]. Available at: www.the-difference.com/our-impact-report-2021-22 (accessed September 2023)

The Equality Trust (2023) *How has inequality changed?* [online]. Available at: https://equalitytrust.org.uk/how-has-inequality-changed (accessed September 2023)

The ICARS report England (2023) *Restraint and seclusion in England's schools* [online]. Available at: https://againstrestraint.com/wp-content/uploads/2023/04/icars_report_23.pdf (accessed September 2023)

The Office of the Children's Commissioner (2012) *Nobody made the connection: The prevalence of neurodisability in young people who offend* [online]. Available at: https://assets.childrenscommissioner.gov.uk/wpuploads/2017/07/Nobody-made-the-connection.pdf (accessed September 2023)

The Royal College of Psychiatrists (2016) Challenging Behaviour: A unified approach [online]. Available at: www.rcpsych.ac.uk/docs/default-source/improving-care/better-mh-policy/college-reports/college-report-cr144.pdf?sfvrsn=73e437e8_2 (accessed September 2023)

Thoreaux HD (1865) Journal entry. See www.walden.org/wp-content/uploads/2016/02/Journal-9-Chapter-1.pdf (accessed September 2023)

Treasure J, Todd G, Brolly M, Tiller J, Nehmed A, Denman F,(1995) A pilot study of a randomised trial of cognitive analytical therapy vs educational behavioral therapy for adult anorexia nervosa, *Behaviour Research and Therapy*, 33 (4) 363-367

Treasure J & Ward A (1997) Practitioner report: Cognitive analytical therapy in the treatment of anorexia nervosa. *Clinical Psychology and Psychotherapy* 4 (1) 62–71

Treasure J, Willmott D, Ambwani S, Cardi V, Clark Bryan D, Rowlands K & Schmidt U (2020) Cognitive Interpersonal Model for Anorexia Nervosa Revisited: The Perpetuating Factors that Contribute to the Development of the Severe and Enduring Illness. *Journal of Clinical Medicine* 9 (3) 630

Trevarthen C (2017) The Affectionate, Intersubjective Intelligence of the Infant and Its Innate Motives for Relational Mental Health. *International Journal of Cognitive Analytic Therapy and Relational Mental Health, Volume 1*. pp11-53. Available at: www.internationalcat.org/_files/ugd/ff32b4_ca345666618b48deb998a126447d2480.pdf (accessed September 2023)

Trotton N (2021) *Wild Therapy – Rewilding Our Inner and Outer Worlds, 2nd Edition*. PCCS Books.

Turner D (2021) *Intersections of Privilege and Otherness in Counselling and Psychotherapy*. Mockingbird

Ullman, J (2021). *Free to Be... Yet?: The second national study of Australian high school students who identify as gender and sexuality diverse*. Penrith: Centre for Educational Research, School of Education, Western Sydney University.

UNDP (2023) *How Just Transition can help deliver the Paris Agreement* [online]. Available at: https://climatepromise.undp.org/research-and-reports/how-just-transition-can-help-deliver-paris-agreement (accessed September 2023)

Ungar M (2011) The social ecology of resilience: addressing contextual and cultural ambiguity of a nascent construct. *Am J Orthopsychiatry* 81 (1) 1-17

United Nations, Department of Economic and Social Affairs (2020) *World Social Report 2020 Inequality in a rapidly changing world* [online]. Available at: www.un.org/development/desa/dspd/wp-content/uploads/sites/22/2020/01/World-Social-Report-2020-FullReport.pdf (accessed September 2023)

Van der Kolk BA (2014) *The Body Keeps the Score: Brain, mind, and body in the healing of trauma*. Viking

Varela J (2014) Cognitive analytic therapy and behaviour that challenges. In: J Lloyd, & P Clayton (Eds) *Cognitive Analytic Therapy for People with Intellectual Disabilities and Their Carers* (136-52) Philadelphia, PA: Jessica Kingsley Publishers

Varela J (2016) "Playing" with CAT - Using a CAT Informed Approach with Young Children and their Families. *Reformulation*, Summer, pp.6-10

Varela,J and Franks L (2018) Responding not reacting to challenging behaviour: a reformulation approach. In: J Lloyd & R Pollard (Eds.) *Cognitive Analytic Therapy and the Politics of Mental Health* (1st ed.). Routledge

Varese F et al (2012) Childhood adversities increase the risk of psychosis: A meta-analysis of patient-control, prospective- and cross-sectional cohort studies. *Schizophrenia Bulletin* 38 (4) 661–671 doi.org/10.1093/schbul/sbs050

Victoria (2015). Talking myself into and out of Asperger's Syndrome: Using Cognitive Analytic Therapy (CAT) to rethink normal. *Reformulation*, Summer,18-22.

Vince G (2022) The century of climate migration: why we need to plan for the great upheaval. *The Guardian* 18th August 2022. Available at: www.theguardian.com/news/2022/aug/18/century-climate-crisis-migration-why-we-need-plan-great-upheaval (accessed September 2023)

Vygotsky LS (1978) *Mind in Society: Development of higher psychological processes*. Cambridge, Mass: Harvard university press

Wallace W (2015) Is Transsexualism an Iatrogenic Construction? *Reformulation* 24-29.

Wallace W (2019) Immorality, Illegality and Pathology. In: J Lloyd & R Pollard (Eds) *Cognitive Analytic Therapy and the politics of Mental Health* (pp175-186). New York: Routledge

Ward B (2018) *President Trump's fake news about climate change* [online]. London School of Economics and Political Science. Available at: www.lse.ac.uk/granthaminstitute/news/president-trump-fake-news-climate-change/ (accessed September 2023)

Welch L (2020) Naming the Reciprocal Roles of Britain's Black and Minority Ethnic Communities. *Reformulation*, Summer, pp40-43

Whitburn J (2020) Meta-analysis of human connection to nature and pro environment behavior. *Conservation Biology* 34 (1) 180–193. https://doi.org/10.1111/cobi.13781

White M (2007) *Maps of Narrative Practice*. New York: W.W. Norton and Company

Whitefield C & Midgley N (2015) 'And when you were a child?': How therapists working with parents alongside individual child psychotherapy bring the past into their work. *Journal of Child Psychotherapy* 41 (3) 272–292. doi.org/10.1080/0075417X.2015.1092678

Wicksteed A (2016) Cognitive Analytic Therapy (CAT) for Eating Disorders. In: T Wade (Ed) *Encyclopedia of Feeding and Eating Disorders*. Springer, Singapore. doi.org/10.1007/978-981-287-087-2_166-1

Wicksteed A (2012) Using a Cognitive Analytic Therapy approach in working with eating disorders: Reflections on practice. *Reformulation*, Summer, pp26-31.

Wilberforce D (2014) The problems of caring and being cared for (or how to get your showlaces tied for you). In: J Lloyd & P Clayton (Eds.) *Cognitve Analytic Therapy for People with Intellectual Disabilities and Their Carers* (109–21). Philadelphia, PA: Jessica Kingsley Publishers

Wilkinson R and Pickett K (2010*) The Spirit Level: Why equality is better for everyone*. London: Penguin

Winnicott DW (1965) *The Maturational Processes and the Facilitating Environment*. Maresfield Library, Karnac Books

Winnicott D (1973) *The Child, the Family, and the Outside World*. Penguin

Wise R (2019) *Relationships: From the bottom up to the top down* [online]. Available at: www.scie.org.uk/news/opinions/relationships-matter-in-childrens-care (accessed September 2023)

Wolff J (2021) Musical Performance as a Route to Relational Autonomy and Social Equality. In: N Stoljar and K Voigt (Eds) *Autonomy and Equality*. Routledge

Woods A, Alderson-Day B and Fernyhough C (2022) *Voices in Psychosis Interdisciplinary Perspectives.* Oxford University Press

World Bank database (2019) Gini index. World Bank, Poverty and Inequality platform. Available at: https://data.worldbank.org/indicator/SI.POV.GINI (accessed September 2023)

World Health Organisation database (2023) Out-of-pocket expenditure (% current health expenditure). World Health Organisation Global Health Expenditure database. Available at: https://data.worldbank.org/indicator/SH.XPD.OOPC.CH.ZS (accessed September 2023)

World Health Organisation (2021) *Health Equity in India* [online]. Available at: https://cdn.who.int/media/docs/default-source/wrindia/document/health-equity-in-india7cee19b6-1324-4de4-a9c7-13f24cee0976.pdf?sfvrsn=816d1189_4 (accessed September 2023)

World Health Organisation (2022) *WHO highlights urgent need to transform mental health and mental health care* [online]. Available at: www.who.int/news/item/17-06-2022-who-highlights-urgent-need-to-transform-mental-health-and-mental-health-care (accessed September 2023)

Wufong E, Rhodes P and Conti J (2019) "We don't really know what else we can do": Parent experiences when adolescent distress persists after the Maudsley and family-based therapies for anorexia nervosa. *Journal of Eating Disorders*. Feb 12;7:5. doi: 10.1186/s40337-019-0235-5

Yalom ID & Leszcz M (2005) *The theory and practice of group psychotherapy* (5th ed.) Basic Books/Hachette Book Group

Young Minds, 2020. Blog, "How Gaming Helped My Mental Health", by Wes. 17/02/2020. Available at https://www.youngminds.org.uk/young-person/blog/how-gaming-helped-my-mental-health/ (accessed September 2023)

Yuksel D (2009) A Bakhtinian understanding of social constructivism in language teaching. Journal of Language and Linguistic Studies 5 (1)

Glossary

Cognitive Analytic Therapy or CAT – a model of psychological therapy initially developed in the United Kingdom by Dr Anthony Ryle. This time-limited therapy was developed with the aim of providing effective and affordable psychological treatment and considers relationships as core to understanding distress. It is based on a model of a relational self, developed through how we have been related to, how we relate to ourselves and others, and how we expect to be related to. As the name implies, Ryle took from psychodynamic theory that we are greatly affected by our early caregiver relationship experiences, as well as from cognitive theory that we can become fixed in our way of thinking, and this affects our mood and behaviour and consequences. CAT was further developed by the introduction of Bakhtin's dialogism and Vygotsky's social formation of mind theory through Professor Mikael Leiman from Finland. CAT is a collaborative therapy where the therapeutic relationship is often spoken about and used transparently to reflect on relationship patterns. CAT is very much focused on the therapist and client having a shared formulation that guides a person into recognising their relational patterns that are keeping them stuck and helps them move to revise things.

Contextual reformulation – a formulation or understanding of a setting, often a workplace, where the relationships people in that setting feel drawn to enact, often unhelpfully, are reflected upon using an SDR or map. This understanding considers the wider influences of the socio-cultural and political atmosphere and its relational effects on the work.

Psychotherapy file – the psychotherapy file is a questionnaire used in cognitive analytic therapy to assist in identifying and understanding a person's relational patterns that are causing problems for them. It provides a quick way of getting a lot of information about a person's experiences in relationships with others, and with themselves. Common patterns of relating are defined as traps, dilemmas and snags and exploration of these can aid the reformulation process. The full questionnaire can be found on the ACAT website– see below.

Reciprocal Role (RR) – a core concept of CAT that is used to illustrate how someone relates to themselves and others and how they expect to be related to through internalised relationships. RRs are two parts of a relationship usually drawn out as a dyad with a double-headed arrow showing how both roles or states reciprocally influence one another to make a relationship. The usual convention of how an RR is drawn is with the top pole being the active, or "doing to", one, and is attached above the bottom pole of the impact, or "done to" state. For example:

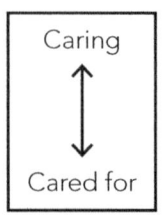

```
┌──────────┐
│  Caring  │
│    ↑     │
│    ↓     │
│ Cared for│
└──────────┘
```

Reciprocal role procedure (RRP) – an aim-directed activity connected to reciprocal roles with the intention to move out or towards a relationship pole or RR. For example, a child may have a procedure of crying to get a caring response from someone and thus move from feeling uncared for to being cared for. In CAT, we would draw this out or map this like so:

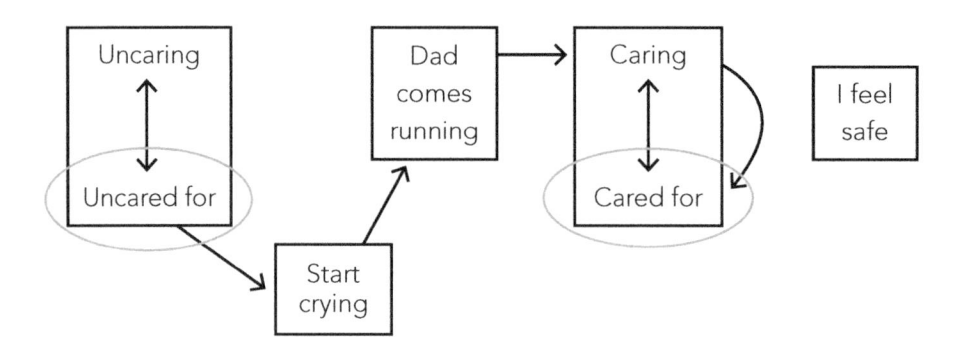

```
┌──────────┐     ┌──────────┐     ┌──────────┐     ┌──────────┐
│ Uncaring │     │   Dad    │ →   │  Caring  │     │  I feel  │
│    ↑     │     │  comes   │     │    ↑     │     │   safe   │
│    ↓     │     │ running  │     │    ↓     │     │          │
│Uncared for│    └──────────┘     │ Cared for│     └──────────┘
└──────────┘           ↑          └──────────┘
       ↘         ┌──────────┐
                 │  Start   │
                 │  crying  │
                 └──────────┘
```

Reformulation – a shared compassionate formulation or narrative of what relationship patterns are making life difficult, how they came about from our early care relationships and how they may be repeated, often expected in present relationships, with self and others. The reformulation is co-created by the therapist and client through the use of the CAT theory and CAT tools of the reformulation letter and map or SDR (see below for definition).

SDR (Sequential diagrammatic diagram), or map – often referred to as 'the map' when using CAT. The SDR is the mapping tool that seeks to simplify the complex relationship patterns one may be stuck in. This map is used to notice compassionately how the patterns play out now in the present, helping the client and therapist plan for ways out of these patterns, often called exits.

Zone of proximal development or ZPD – the learning space that needs to be scaffolded between teacher and learner so that the learner can develop new or more complex skills. This concept was explored initially by Lev Vygotsky, a Russian philosopher and psychologist.

To learn more about these definitions and others related to CAT and relational thinking, the following websites may be helpful:

Association for Cognitive Analytic Therapy (ACAT)
www.acat.me.uk

ACATs public engagement website
www.engage.acat.org.uk/

Catalyse at
https://catalyse.uk.com/

ICATA International Cognitive Analytic Therapy Association
www.internationalcat.org/